PEARSON'S

Anatomy and Physiology for Medical Assisting

VOLUME II

Nina Beaman, MS, RNC, CMA
Bryant and Stratton College
Richmond, VA

Lorraine Fleming-McPhillips, MS, MT, CMA
Medical Assisting Program Coordinator (retired)
Quinebaug Valley Community College
Danielson, Connecticut

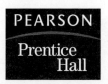

PEARSON
Prentice
Hall

Upper Saddle River, New Jersey 07458

Library of Congress Cataloging-in-Publication Data

Pearson's administrative medical assisting.
  p. ; cm.
  Includes index.
  ISBN 0-13-220904-7 (v. 1)—ISBN 0-13-199042-X (v. 2)—
ISBN 0-13-174206-X (v. 3)—ISBN 0-13-171577-1 (v. 4)
  1. Medical assistants. 2. Medical secretaries. 3. Medical
offices—Management.
  [DNLM: 1. Physician Assistants. 2. Medical Secretaries.
3. Practice Management, Medical. W 21.5 P362 2006]
  I. Title: Administrative medical assisting. II. Pearson/
Prentice Hall.
  R728.8.P43 2006
  610.73'7—dc22
                                                2005036391

Brief Contents

Contents

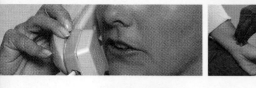

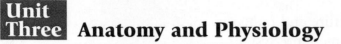

Unit Three **Anatomy and Physiology** 339

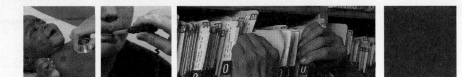

Preface

Pearson's Anatomy and Physiology for Medical Assisting

Pearson's Anatomy and Physiology for Medical Assisting is a brand new approach to learning the profession of Medical Assisting. It is all about Successful Skill Building so that you will be successful in the classroom and in the physician's office. To help ensure that success, Professionalism and Cultural Considerations are also explored. These are skills that will help you, the Medical Assistant, relate to your whole workplace: your responsibilities, your patients, and your physicians. It's about making the connection between your skills and your whole profession.

Medical Assisting is, after all, a "people helping people" profession. What could be more important than the connections that make the Medical Assistant the vital link between people and their personal health and well-being? This textbook helps the student learn the right skills for becoming the very best and most effective Medical Assistant through a step-by-step, competency based approach that covers virtually all the facets of the medical assisting profession. Through up to the minute content and careful planning, *Pearson's Anatomy and Physiology for Medical Assisting* prepares students to make successful connections in class, in their externships, and in their professional placements.

How does *Pearson's Anatomy and Physiology for Medical Assisting* accomplish these goals? A thorough table of contents that covers all the material necessary for student success, a curriculum that follows the AAMA and AMT competencies, a fully developed instructional package that contains everything an instructor needs to successfully connect with the student and challenge their skills, and the latest in interactive technology that will engage students and instructors alike. The entire package is comprehensive, easily implemented, simple to follow, and completely up to date.

Each chapter in *Pearson's Anatomy and Physiology for Medical Assisting* begins with a Role Delineation Chart highlighted with the concepts covered in that chapter. Both students and their instructors easily see which AAMA or AMT competencies will be covered in the chapter. Learning Objectives underscore the chart, listing the skills the student will be able to demonstrate after completing the chapter. Terms to Learn are also included so that the student can immediately see the new vocabulary that she will experience. A case study vignette introduces the reader to central concepts and is followed up on later in the chapter with critical thinking questions. Other learning aids

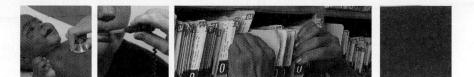

in the book include color photos and photo sequences; full color, detailed drawings; easy to understand charts and tables; and clear, informative guidelines.

A helpful chapter review allows the student to check her knowledge in several ways:
- Chapter review questions test the student's understanding of key chapter concepts.
- Critical Thinking questions relate back to the case study vignette that opens each chapter.
- "On the Job" presents the student with a new scenario with more critical thinking opportunities.
- Certification Exam-style questions help prepare the student for the CMA and RMA exams and review the chapter material.
- An Internet Activity and a MediaLink is also included in each chapter review.

Developed by Pearson Education and Legacy Interactive, Inc., the Medical Assisting Interactive CD-ROM found in the back of the book provides a fascinating journey through the responsibilities, the technical skills, and the "people skills" of the Medical Assistant. The CD-ROM opens to the waiting room of a typical Doctor's office. The player can move from room to room in the medical office or, for the more sequentially-minded student, from chapter to chapter. There are medical assisting terminology memory games to play, interactive animations and simulations, tips from professionals, decision-making and critical thinking scenarios, an audio glossary, a resource library, and many other wonderful things to do.

Special features throughout the book include segments on *Patient Education;* important *Legal and Ethical* concerns: and *Lifespan Considerations* which focus on the pediatric patient and the geriatric patient. *Preparing for Externship* deals with topics and issues relating to students' participation in an externship program as a capstone to their training. It addresses pertinent issues including student responsibilities, caring attitudes, enthusiasm, grooming/dress, interpersonal skills with patients and colleagues, language skills, poise under pressure and other issues.

Cultural Considerations addresses the Medical Assistant's encounters with people of different cultural backgrounds, a brief tip, advice, or general guideline on how to deal with a specific cultural or communication issue. Many different cultural issues arise in any physician's office. There may be taboos against certain procedures, removal of clothing, discussion of birth control, showing emotions or feelings, eating certain foods, or taking certain kinds of medication. In our multi-cultural world today, every Medical Assistant will deal with all kinds of people from many different backgrounds. This feature will help the Medical Assistant react with grace, graciousness, and a professional manner.

In the medical office today, the Medical Assistant must go a step further than mastering a myriad of challenging, detailed, and precise skills. The Medical Assistant must show complete *Professionalism*. This element of each chapter provides a focus on grooming and dress, interpersonal skills, ethical standards, language skills, punctuality, dependability, and a caring attitude. These highly important qualities help the Medical Assistant maintain a completely professional demeanor at all times. Coupled with mastery of technical skills, these "soft" skills will guarantee the professional status of the new Medical Assistant.

Use this book in any of a variety of learning environments and situations including the traditional classroom; the self-paced or individualized course; as a review for those seeking certification and preparing for a certification examination; or in an on-the-job training program in a doctor's office.

All care has been taken to insure that *Pearson's Anatomy and Physiology for Medical Assisting* covers all the current content and competencies of both the American Association of Medical Assistants (AAMA) and the American Medical Technologists (AMT). This text is aimed at preparing you for either the AAMA or the AMT certification examinations.

The Learning Package:

The Student Package:
- Textbook
- Interactive CD-ROM with exercises, learning games, skills review, medical office simulation for real-life application, skills videos, simulations, animations, resources, audio glossary.
- Student Workbook that contains chapter-specific assignments; review questions; terminology review; skill exercise; vocabulary exercises; forms; other activities designed to reinforce the content of the text. This workbook has perforated pages so that assignments can be submitted for grading.
- Vango Notes are chapter highlights and in-depth summaries that are downloaded to an MP3

The Instructional Package:
- Instructor's Resource Guide with detailed CAAHEP Competency Correlation guide

- CD-ROM with Test Gen and over 1000 test questions and Classroom Management software.
- Lesson Plans
- Hundreds of PowerPoint slides for daily lessons
- Syllabus, teaching tips, notes, additional exercises, instructional strategies, answers to all text questions and workbook questions.
- Administrative and Clinical Medical Assisting videos in VHS or DVD format
- Pearson Solutions Medical Assisting Curriculum and Pearson Training Master Instructional Training
- "Klickerz" Classroom Response System for interactive classroom PowerPoint presentations; chapter review and test preparation; and classroom games.
- Transition Guides to help make text implementation easy

Reviewers

The invaluable editorial advice and direction provided by the following educators and health care professionals is deeply appreciated:

James Baird, MBA, CAHI
Medical Program Director
Computer Career Center
El Paso, TX

Suzanne Bitters, RMA, NCPT, NCICS
Former Instructor
CHI Institute
Southampton, PA

Lou Brown, MT (ASCP), CMA
Medical Assisting Program Director
Wayne Community College
Goldsboro, NC

Denise Carsillo, MS, BS, AS, RMA, BXMO
Director of Academic Services
New England Tech
West Palm Beach, FL

Anita Denson, CMA
Director of Health Care Education
National College of Business & Technology
Danville, KY

George Fakhoury, MD, DORCP, CMA
Academic Program Manager Healthcare
Head College's Central Administrative Office
San Francisco, CA

Suzanne Feathers, CMA, EMT
Medical Program Coordinator
Computer Learning Network
Altoona, PA

Robyn Gohsman, RMA, CMAS
Medical Assisting Department Head
Medical Careers Institute
Newport News, VA

Wendy Hall-Campbell, ADN
Medical Assisting Program Director
Concorde Career Institute
Portland, OR

Elizabeth Henisse, BAS, MA
Allied Health Program Director
Florida Metropolitan University
Orlando, FL

Demetria Jackson
Former Program Director
Virginia College
Birmingham, AL

Holly A. Lincoln, BA
Academic Coordinator
St. Louis College of Health Careers
Fenton, MO

Marta Lopez, LM, CPM
Medical Assisting Program Coordinator
Miami Dade College
Miami, FL

Mary M. Marks, MSN, RN-BC, Pbt (ASCP)
Program Coordinator
Mitchell Community College
Mooresville, NC

Tanya Mercer, BS, RN, RMA
Curriculum Specialist
KAPLAN Higher Education
Roswell, GA

Everlee O'Nan, RMA
Director of Health Care Education
National College of Business & Technology
Florence, KY

Karen Patrick, NCMA, CPI
Director
CAPPS College
Dothan, AL

Diane Peavy, RN, ASN, AHI
Director of Educational Services
Capps College
Foley, AL

Christina Rauberts-Conklin, AA, RMA
Medical Department Chair
Florida Metropolitan University
Tampa, FL

Gary Shandrew, MSIA
Campus Director
Certified Careers Institute
Clearfield, UT

Maria L. Simard, LVN
Director of Allied Health Programs
Maric College
San Diego, CA

Lynn Slack, CMA
Medical Programs Director
ICM School of Business and Medical Careers
Pittsburgh, PA

Richard Snyder BA, RMA, CPT
Director of Medical Assisting Program
Hagerstown Business College
Hagerstown, MD

Dr, Ruth Torres, MD, MA
Medical Instructor
Indiana Business College
Terre Haute, IN

Roberta C. Weiss, Ed.D.
Allied Health Curriculum Specialist
and Instructional Designer

Nancy Wright, RN, BS, CNOR
Director Surgical Technology
Virginia College
Birmingham, AL

Authors & Contributors

It is with the greatest appreciation and admiration that we acknowledge the following Health Professions Educators for their contributions to the content of this text. Their dedication to the Medical Assisting profession and to the education of successful Medical Assistants has made this text the premier learning tool.

Authors

Nina Beaman, MS, RNC, CMA
Bryant and Stratton College
Richmond, VA

Lorraine Fleming-McPhillips, MS, MT, CMA
Medical Assisting Program
Coordinator (retired)
Quinebaug Valley Community College
Danielson, Connecticut

Contributors

Kendra Allen, LPN
Program Manager Healthcare Office
Technologies
Ohio Institute of Health Careers
Columbus, OH

Michelle Buchman, BSN, RN, BC
Everest College
Springfield, MO

Susie Huyer, MSN, RN
University of Phoenix Online Affiliate
Faculty
Heartland Hospice, Administrator

Demetria Jackson
Former Program Director
Virginia College
Birmingham, AL

Cathy Kelley-Arney, CMA, MLTC, BSHS
Institutional Director of Health Care
Education
National College of Business and
Technology
Bluefield, VA

Christine Malone, BS
Everett Community College
Everett, WA

Shelly Rainer, LPN
Vatterott College
Springfield, MO

Melanie Sheffield, LPN, AHI
Allied Medical Instructor
Remington College
Mobile, AL

Lynn Slack, CMA
Medical Programs Director
ICM School of Business and Medical
Careers
Pittsburgh, PA

Roberta C. Weiss, Ed.D.
Allied Health Curriculum Specialist
and Instructional Designer

Nancy Wright, RN, BS, CNOR
Virginia College
Birmingham, AL

Acknowledgments

Cover Photo Credits
Photodisc (background); Adam Smith/SuperStock (center); Thinkstock/Age Fotostock (bottom left); Arthur Tilley/Taxi/Getty Images (top left)

Interior Photo Credits
Dorling Kindersley Media Library 361, 363, 444, 445, 473, 489; EyeWire Collection/Getty Images/Photodisc 341(BR); Mike Gallitelli/Pearson Education/PH College 350, 405; Michal Heron/Pearson Education/Prentice Hall College 377, 537(BR); Dave King/Dorling Kindersley Media Library 393, 423, Richard Logan/Pearson Education/PH College 351; Dr. P. Marazzi/Photo Researchers, Inc. 453(TL); Pearson Education/PH College 452(CL/BL), 509; Barbara Penoyar/Getty Images, Inc./Photodisc 461(BR); R. Spencer Phippen/Phototake NYC 453(TR); Simon Smith/Dorling Kindersley Media Library 521; SuperStock, Inc. 452(TL); John Woodcock/Dorling Kindersley Media Library 431

Illustration Credits
All illustrations created by Imagineering Inc. for Prentice Hall.

Special Acknowledgments

The Editor wishes to give special acknowledgments to Teri Zak, the Development Editor of Pearson's Comprehensive Medical Assisting. She worked tirelessly to ensure that this text is the very epitome and most current of Medical Assisting textbooks.

The Editor further gives special thanks to Assistant Editor Bronwen Glowacki. Bronwen's many hours analyzing reviews, monitoring ancillary contributors, and responding to every request—small and large—have helped to ensure this project's success.

Successful Connections

Pearson's Anatomy and Physiology for Medical Assisting

Volume Two

This is the first book to connect skills in the classroom and skills on the job, by helping medical assistant students achieve success in school and in their careers.

With *Pearson's Anatomy and Physiology for Assisting*, students learn what to do and how to do it. Strong integration of tips, hints, and guidelines help students avoid common performance problems, including timeliness, presentation, and interpersonal relations.

Skills in the Classroom

- Preparing for the Certification Exam
- Applied learning activities
- Open design makes using the text easy and clear to the student
- Role Delineation Chart shows student and instructor which skills and competencies will be covered in the chapter

Skills on the Job

- Case Study
- Legal and Ethical Issues
- Cultural Considerations
- Lifespan Considerations
- Professionalism
- Patient Education
- Preparing for Externship

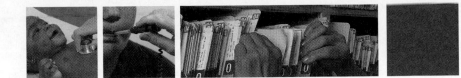

Chapter Opener Features...

Role Delineation Chart

Role Delineation Chart sets the stage and directly links the material that students need to master for passing the Certification Exam.

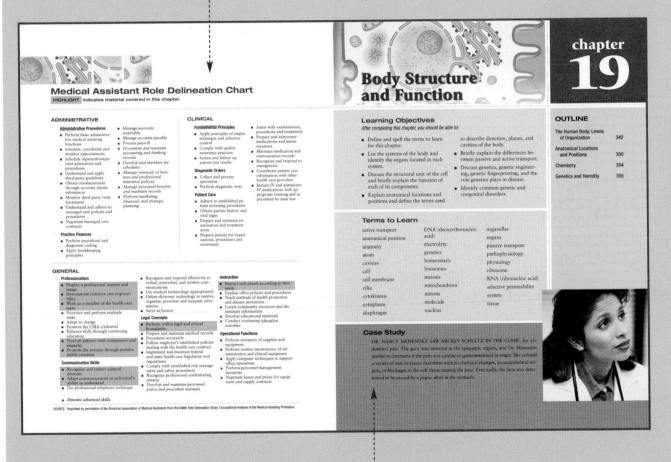

Medical Assistant Role Delineation Chart
HIGHLIGHT indicates material covered in this chapter.

ADMINISTRATIVE

Administrative Procedures
- Perform basic administrative medical assisting functions
- Schedule, coordinate and monitor appointments
- Schedule inpatient/outpatient admissions and procedures
- Understand and apply third-party guidelines
- Obtain reimbursement through accurate claims submission
- Monitor third-party reimbursement
- Understand and adhere to managed care policies and procedures
- *Negotiate managed care contracts*

Practice Finances
- Perform procedural and diagnostic coding
- Apply bookkeeping principles

- Manage accounts receivable
- *Manage accounts payable*
- *Process payroll*
- *Document and maintain accounting and banking records*
- *Develop and maintain fee schedules*
- *Manage renewals of business and professional insurance policies*
- *Manage personnel benefits and maintain records*
- *Perform marketing, financial, and strategic planning*

CLINICAL

Fundamental Principles
- Apply principles of aseptic technique and infection control
- Comply with quality assurance practices
- Screen and follow up patient test results

Diagnostic Orders
- Collect and process specimens
- Perform diagnostic tests

Patient Care
- Adhere to established patient screening procedures
- Obtain patient history and vital signs
- Prepare and maintain examination and treatment areas
- Prepare patient for examinations, procedures and treatments

- Assist with examinations, procedures and treatments
- Prepare and administer medications and immunizations
- Maintain medication and immunization records
- Recognize and respond to emergencies
- Coordinate patient care information with other health care providers
- Initiate IV and administer IV medications with appropriate training and as permitted by state law

GENERAL

Professionalism
- Display a professional manner and image
- Demonstrate initiative and responsibility
- Work as a member of the health care team
- Prioritize and perform multiple tasks
- Adapt to change
- Promote the CMA credential
- Enhance skills through continuing education
- Treat all patients with compassion and empathy
- Promote the practice through positive public relations

Communication Skills
- Recognize and respect cultural diversity
- Adapt communications to individual's ability to understand
- Use professional telephone technique

- Recognize and respond effectively to verbal, nonverbal, and written communications
- Use medical terminology appropriately
- Utilize electronic technology to receive, organize, prioritize and transmit information
- Serve as liaison

Legal Concepts
- Perform within legal and ethical boundaries
- Prepare and maintain medical records
- Document accurately
- Follow employer's established policies dealing with the health care contract
- Implement and maintain federal and state health care legislation and regulations
- Comply with established risk management and safety procedures
- Recognize professional credentialing criteria
- *Develop and maintain personnel, policy and procedure manuals*

Instruction
- Instruct individuals according to their needs
- Explain office policies and procedures
- Teach methods of health promotion and disease prevention
- Locate community resources and disseminate information
- *Develop educational materials*
- *Conduct continuing education activities*

Operational Functions
- Perform inventory of supplies and equipment
- Perform routine maintenance of administrative and clinical equipment
- Apply computer techniques to support office operations
- *Perform personnel management functions*
- *Negotiate leases and prices for equipment and supply contracts*

- *Denotes advanced skills.*

SOURCE: Reprinted by permission of the American Association of Medical Assistants from the AAMA Role Delineation Study: Occupational Analysis of the Medical Assisting Profession.

Body Structure and Function

chapter 19

Learning Objectives
After completing this chapter, you should be able to:

- Define and spell the terms to learn for this chapter.
- List the systems of the body and identify the organs located in each system.
- Discuss the structural unit of the cell and briefly explain the function of each of its components.
- Explain anatomical locations and positions and define the terms used

- to describe direction, planes, and cavities of the body.
- Briefly explain the differences between passive and active transport.
- Discuss genetics, genetic engineering, genetic fingerprinting, and the role genetics plays in disease.
- Identify common genetic and congenital disorders.

OUTLINE

Terms to Learn

active transport	DNA (deoxyribonucleic acid)	organelles
anatomical position		organs
anatomy	electrolyte	passive transport
atom	genetics	pathophysiology
cavities	homeostasis	physiology
cell	lysosomes	ribosome
cell membrane	meiosis	RNA (ribonucleic acid)
cilia	mitochondrion	selective permeability
cytokinesis	mitosis	system
cytoplasm	molecule	tissue
diaphragm	nucleus	

Case Study

DR. NANCY MENENDEZ SAW MICKEY SCHULTZ IN THE CLINIC for abdominal pain. The pain was centered in the epigastric region, and Dr. Menendez needed to determine if the pain was cardiac or gastrointestinal in origin. She ordered a variety of tests to ensure that there were no chemical changes, musculoskeletal origins, or blockages in the soft tissue causing the pain. Eventually, the pain was determined to be caused by a peptic ulcer in the stomach.

Case Study

Case Study provides brief vignettes that help students understand how the chapter information relates to their careers. It increases retention of chapter material because students have a context for the topics.

Additional Features...

Open design is ideal for visual learners. Material is presented in smaller chunks with relevant applications to provide context.

Legal and Ethical Issues

Legal and Ethical Issues

Each state has its own laws regarding individuals with diabetes driving school buses and other forms of public transportation. It is important to understand the regulations in your state. In some states, if there is evidence that the diabetes is controlled, then the individual may be allowed to drive one of these means of transportation. These individuals do typically need regular monitoring with the appropriate documentation sent to the authorities. The medical assistant is often integral in maintaining these records.

Legal and Ethical Issues address the complex topics in a practical and relevant manner, making it easier for students to apply.

Professionalism

Professionalism is one of the most important keys to career success. These featured highlights help students understand the importance of adopting and maintaining a professional demeanor.

Professionalism

The professional medical assistant will occasionally have days on which the physician is seeing patients later than their appointments. This can create discomfort for both the patients and the medical assistant. Explain to patients that the physician is running behind, and give them the option to reschedule their appointment. If they choose to wait, be sure to move them to an exam room as quickly as possible, and plan ahead as much as possible to help the physician be as efficient as possible. Explaining to patients that the physician is providing the same care to other patients that he or she will provide to them will help to alleviate their frustrations with the delays. Always remember that if patients verbalize their frustrations about the delay, their attack is never personal; instead, they are just venting their frustration.

Cultural Considerations

In the current American culture, tobacco smoking has become less acceptable, especially as the medical profession continues to discover more links to chronic, life-threatening diseases. However, not every patient (or medical assistant) is part of a culture that accepts these tenets. Be sure that all information is presented in a nonjudgmental, factual, accepting manner. There are cultures that consider habits such as cigarette smoking as not only acceptable, but expected. These choices are the patient's own, and, although medical professionals will present factual information, they should never force this information on patients.

Cultural Considerations

Cultural Considerations give students the skills to connect with both patients and other health professionals from diverse backgrounds.

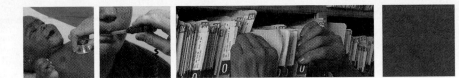

Lifespan
Considerations

THE CHILD
- The development of the circulatory system begins with the development of the fetal heart during the first 2 months of gestation, and the newborn's circulation begins to function just after birth.
- Children have a smaller circulatory system, and their vital signs are typically different than those of adults. Their blood pressure will typically be higher than that of an adult, as will their pulse and respiratory rates.

THE OLDER ADULT
- Cardiac and other circulatory changes once attributed to aging may be minimized with appropriate lifestyle modifications.
- Reduced blood flow, elevated blood lipids, and defective endothelial repair that can be seen in aging may accelerate the course of circulatory disease.

Lifespan Considerations

Lifespan Considerations help students develop the skills to relate to patients of all ages.

Patient Education

Skin care is a very important part of hygiene. Patients should be taught that they should moisturize their skin on a daily basis, or more often as necessary. Sunscreen is one of the easiest ways to avoid skin cancer, and teaching patients about using adequate sun protection may be one duty of the medical assistant. Write down the correct sun protection factor prescribed by the physician so that the patient can easily locate the appropriate lotion in the store. Patients should be taught to avoid sunburn as much as possible. Some medications can increase the risk of sunburn, and education for patients who take these medications is extremely important.

Patient Education

Patient Education provides hints and important tips on how to share information with patients in a professional and complete manner.

Preparing for Externship

Preparing for Externship discusses topics and issues students may encounter during participation in an externship program.

Preparing for
Externship

When preparing for a procedure, *carefully plan the steps you will take. Make sure that you not only do exactly what you have been asked to do or prepare for, but be ready to take the next step. Always think ahead. Ask yourself what the physician might need next, whether it is having paperwork for labs ready to go or a prescription pad or being ready for a follow-up procedure. If the physician will be performing a minor surgical procedure, be sure that all the necessary supplies, including dressings, are ready for use.*

PREPARING FOR THE CERTIFICATION EXAM

1. The medical term for gallstones is:
   A. cholecystectomy
   B. cholecystotomy
   C. choledochal
   D. cholelithiasis
   E. choledochectomy

2. The muscle at the superior portion of the stomach is the
   A. pyloric sphincter
   B. esophageal sphincter
   C. cardiac sphincter
   D. gallbladder
   E. fundus

3. Which substance is not produced by the liver?
   A. heparin
   B. bile
   C. hydrochloric acid
   D. fibrogen and prothrombin
   E. blood proteins

4. Which is not a component of the small intestine?
   A. jejunum
   B. ileum
   C. duodenum
   D. cecum
   E. pyloric sphincter

5. What is the function of the gallbladder?
   A. production of bile
   B. storage of bile
   C. production of pepsin
   D. production of insulin
   E. storage of insulin

6. How many permanent teeth does the body produce?
   A. 20
   B. 24
   C. 28
   D. 32
   E. 36

7. A potentially life-threatening condition that occurs when scarring damages the liver is
   A. pancreatitis
   B. cirrhosis
   C. cholecystitis
   D. colitis
   E. stomatitis

8. An inflammation of the large intestine that may be caused by many different disease processes is
   A. pancreatitis
   B. cirrhosis
   C. cholecystitis
   D. colitis
   E. stomatitis

9. Symptoms of Crohn's disease include all of the following EXCEPT
   A. abdominal pain
   B. diarrhea
   C. weight loss
   D. night sweats
   E. constipation

10. GERD occurs when the muscle of what organ does not close tightly?
    A. stomach
    B. liver
    C. gallbladder
    D. pancreas
    E. large intestine

Certification

Certification Exam Success end-of-the-chapter self-assessment and practice help students build exam confidence.

CRITICAL THINKING

1. Why did the physician include a PSA and digital rectal exam for Mr. Sansone.
2. If Mr. Sansone has BPH, does he have prostate cancer?
3. Why was Mr. Sansone having difficulty starting his stream of urine and having urgency to urinate?

INTERNET ACTIVITY

Do an Internet search of the National Breast Cancer Foundation and other breast cancer awareness organizations. Research the following regarding breast cancer: cancer myths, early detection, and up-and-coming research.

MediaLink More on the reproductive system, including interactive resources, can be found on the Student CD-ROM accompanying this textbook.

applied learning activities

Applied learning activities like "On the Job" scenarios help students increase retention and success by linking concepts to their job functions.

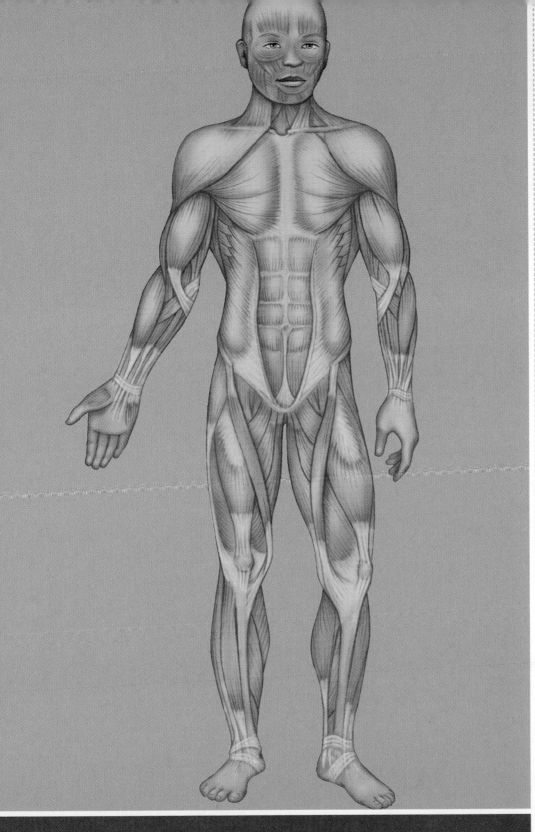

Anatomy
and Physiology

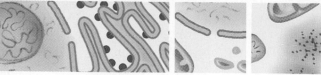

Medical Assistant Role Delineation Chart

HIGHLIGHT indicates material covered in this chapter.

ADMINISTRATIVE

Administrative Procedures

- Perform basic administrative medical assisting functions
- Schedule, coordinate and monitor appointments
- Schedule inpatient/outpatient admissions and procedures
- Understand and apply third-party guidelines
- Obtain reimbursement through accurate claims submission
- Monitor third-party reimbursement
- Understand and adhere to managed care policies and procedures
- *Negotiate managed care contracts*

- Manage accounts receivable
- *Manage accounts payable*
- *Process payroll*
- *Document and maintain accounting and banking records*
- *Develop and maintain fee schedules*
- *Manage renewals of business and professional insurance policies*
- *Manage personnel benefits and maintain records*
- *Perform marketing, financial, and strategic planning*

Practice Finances

- Perform procedural and diagnostic coding
- Apply bookkeeping principles

CLINICAL

Fundamental Principles

- Apply principles of aseptic technique and infection control
- Comply with quality assurance practices
- Screen and follow up patient test results

Diagnostic Orders

- Collect and process specimens
- Perform diagnostic tests

Patient Care

- Adhere to established patient screening procedures
- Obtain patient history and vital signs
- Prepare and maintain examination and treatment areas
- Prepare patient for examinations, procedures and treatments

- Assist with examinations, procedures and treatments
- Prepare and administer medications and immunizations
- Maintain medication and immunization records
- Recognize and respond to emergencies
- Coordinate patient care information with other health care providers
- Initiate IV and administer IV medications with appropriate training and as permitted by state law

GENERAL

Professionalism

- Display a professional manner and image
- Demonstrate initiative and responsibility
- Work as a member of the health care team
- Prioritize and perform multiple tasks
- Adapt to change
- Promote the CMA credential
- Enhance skills through continuing education
- Treat all patients with compassion and empathy
- Promote the practice through positive public relations

Communication Skills

- Recognize and respect cultural diversity
- Adapt communications to individual's ability to understand
- Use professional telephone technique

- Recognize and respond effectively to verbal, nonverbal, and written communications
- Use medical terminology appropriately
- Utilize electronic technology to receive, organize, prioritize and transmit information
- Serve as liaison

Legal Concepts

- Perform within legal and ethical boundaries
- Prepare and maintain medical records
- Document accurately
- Follow employer's established policies dealing with the health care contract
- Implement and maintain federal and state health care legislation and regulations
- Comply with established risk management and safety procedures
- Recognize professional credentialing criteria
- *Develop and maintain personnel, policy and procedure manuals*

Instruction

- Instruct individuals according to their needs
- Explain office policies and procedures
- Teach methods of health promotion and disease prevention
- Locate community resources and disseminate information
- *Develop educational materials*
- *Conduct continuing education activities*

Operational Functions

- Perform inventory of supplies and equipment
- Perform routine maintenance of administrative and clinical equipment
- Apply computer techniques to support office operations
- *Perform personnel management functions*
- *Negotiate leases and prices for equipment and supply contracts*

- *Denotes advanced skills.*

chapter 19

Body Structure and Function

Learning Objectives

After completing this chapter, you should be able to:

- Define and spell the terms to learn for this chapter.
- List the systems of the body and identify the organs located in each system.
- Discuss the structural unit of the cell and briefly explain the function of each of its components.
- Explain anatomical locations and positions and define the terms used

- to describe direction, planes, and cavities of the body.
- Briefly explain the differences between passive and active transport.
- Discuss genetics, genetic engineering, genetic fingerprinting, and the role genetics plays in disease.
- Identify common genetic and congenital disorders.

Terms to Learn

active transport

anatomical position

anatomy

atom

cavities

cell

cell membrane

cilia

cytokinesis

cytoplasm

diaphragm

DNA (deoxyribonucleic acid)

electrolyte

genetics

homeostasis

lysosomes

meiosis

mitochondrion

mitosis

molecule

nucleus

organelles

organs

passive transport

pathophysiology

physiology

ribosome

RNA (ribonucleic acid)

selective permeability

system

tissue

Case Study

DR. NANCY MENENDEZ SAW MICKEY SCHULTZ IN THE CLINIC for abdominal pain. The pain was centered in the epigastric region, and Dr. Menendez needed to determine if the pain was cardiac or gastrointestinal in origin. She ordered a variety of tests to ensure that there were no chemical changes, musculoskeletal origins, or blockages in the soft tissue causing the pain. Eventually, the pain was determined to be caused by a peptic ulcer in the stomach.

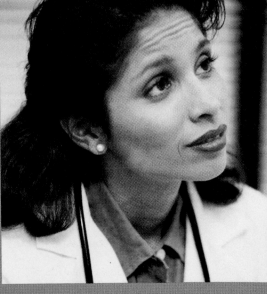

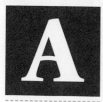**A**natomy can be defined as the study of the structure of an organism. The word *anatomy* is derived from a Greek word meaning "to cut up" (to dissect). **Physiology** can be defined as the study of the function of the organism. Aging or a malfunction of a part of the body can lead to diseases or disorders. The study of these diseases or disorders is called **pathophysiology**.

The human body consists of a series of increasingly complex and larger systems. The basis of the structure of the body is the atom, which makes up molecules. Molecules form organelles, which form cells. A group of cells forms tissues, which create organs. Then organ systems combine to form the completion of the organism (the body). By adjusting for constant changes, all of these systems work together to maintain balance or equilibrium. This is known as **homeostasis**. Homeostasis is one of the fundamental characteristics of living things. It refers to the maintenance of the internal environment within tolerable limits. All sorts of factors affect the suitability of our body fluids to sustain life; these include properties such as temperature, salinity, acidity, and the concentrations of nutrients and wastes. Because these properties affect the chemical reactions that keep us alive, we have built-in physiological mechanisms to maintain them at desirable levels.

When a change occurs in the body, the body can respond in either of two general ways. In negative feedback, the body responds in such a way as to reverse the direction of change. Because this tends to keep things constant, it allows us to maintain homeostasis. On the other hand, positive feedback is also possible. This means that if a change occurs in some variable, the response is to change that variable even more in the same direction. This has a destabilizing effect, so it does not result in homeostasis. Positive feedback is used in certain situations where rapid change is desirable. The nervous system and the endocrine system have the main responsibility for maintaining homeostasis.

The body responds to changes from stimuli, either internal or external. Usually the change is accomplished by a negative feedback mechanism. This means the body's response reverses the stimulus to assist in maintaining homeostasis. For example, if your body temperature rises on a hot day, sweating occurs. This helps to decrease the body's temperature. But, with continued, excessive sweating, dehydration could result. To prevent dehydration, thirst occurs. As the thirst is quenched (through fluid intake), the body's temperature again rises. Thus, sweating and thirst assist in maintaining homeostasis.

In positive feedback, the response to the stimulus does not cause the reversal of the stimulus, but instead actually causes it to continue. One example is childbirth. As oxytocin is secreted, the uterus contracts. As the uterus contracts and the cervix begins to stretch, more oxytocin is secreted. The cycle continues. When delivery of baby and placenta is completed, the sequence is interrupted.

The Human Body: Levels of Organization

The human body is organized in different levels (see Figure 19-1). These include atoms (the smallest unit), molecules, cells, tissues, organs, systems, and finally the body. As you study the body, you will find that organ systems often depend on each other, or at least assist each other, in completing the required functions for a healthy life.

Atoms

The first level of organization of the human body consists of atoms. The **atom** is the smallest chemical unit of matter. Chemical elements are made up of atoms, and the number of protons, neutrons, and electrons that are contained within creates each element. An element cannot be separated into substances that differ from itself by use of ordinary chemical means. A compound is composed of two or more parts that combine in definite proportions by weight.

Atoms are composed of three types of particles: protons, neutrons, and electrons. Protons and neutrons are responsible for most of the atomic mass. The mass of an electron is very small. Both the protons and neutrons reside in the nucleus. Protons have a positive (+) charge, neutrons have no charge—they are neutral. Electrons reside in orbitals around the nucleus. They have a negative charge (−). The number of protons determines the atomic number. The number of protons in an element is constant, but neutron number may vary, so mass number may also vary.

Molecules

A **molecule** is the smallest part of a substance called a compound that can still be considered that substance. For example, a molecule of water is the smallest bit of water that is still water. A molecule of a substance cannot be seen by the naked eye—a drop of water is made up of many, many molecules of water. Molecules are composed of atoms joined together chemically. Molecules do not have an electrical charge.

Scientists believe that molecules are always moving. They can be solids, liquids, or gases, and those that move the most are the farthest apart when they are gases. Molecules are closest together and move the most slowly when they are solids. Molecules whose movement is between those of gases and those of solids are liquids. A formula tells what elements make up a molecule. For example, a molecule of water is made up of two hydrogen atoms and one oxygen atom. The formula for a molecule

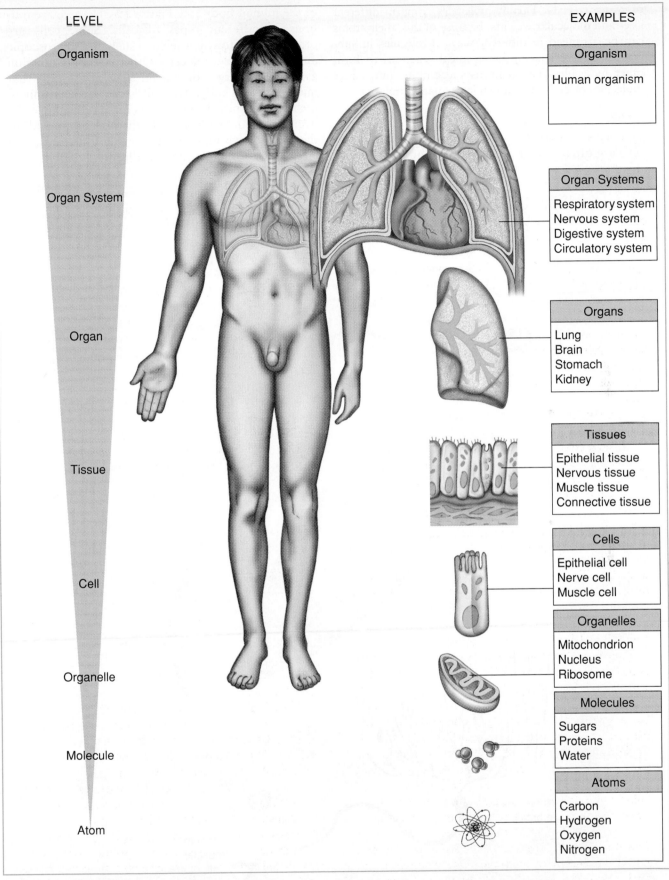

LEVEL

Organism

Organ System

Organ

Tissue

Cell

Organelle

Molecule

Atom

EXAMPLES

Organism
Human organism

Organ Systems
Respiratory system
Nervous system
Digestive system
Circulatory system

Organs
Lung
Brain
Stomach
Kidney

Tissues
Epithelial tissue
Nervous tissue
Muscle tissue
Connective tissue

Cells
Epithelial cell
Nerve cell
Muscle cell

Organelles
Mitochondrion
Nucleus
Ribosome

Molecules
Sugars
Proteins
Water

Atoms
Carbon
Hydrogen
Oxygen
Nitrogen

FIGURE 19-1 Organization of the human body.

of water is H_2O. Finally, molecules come in different sizes and molecular weights. Because of this, their atoms can be arranged in different ways. Molecules in substances can be split up in chemical reactions to form other molecules. They can also recombine into larger molecules or be broken down into smaller molecules.

Cells

The cell is one of the most basic units of life, and cells are often described as the basic building blocks of the human body (see Figure 19-2). There are millions of different types of cells. Some cells are organisms unto themselves, such as microscopic amoebas and bacteria cells. Other cells only function as part of a larger organism, such as the cells that make up your body. The cell is the smallest unit of life in our bodies. The body has brain cells, skin cells, liver cells, stomach cells, and the list goes on. All of these cells have unique functions and features, and all have some recognizable similarities.

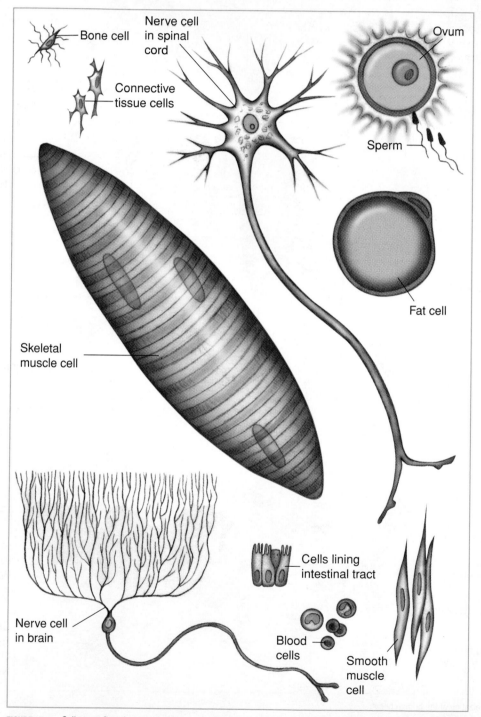

FIGURE 19-2 Cells are often described as the basic building blocks of the human body. There are millions of different cells.

All cells have a "skin," called the cell membrane, that protects them from the outside environment. The cell membrane regulates the movement of water, nutrients, and wastes into and out of the cell. Inside of the cell membrane are the working parts of the cell. At the center of the cell is the cell **nucleus**. The cell nucleus contains the cell's **DNA (deoxyribonucleic acid)**, the genetic code that coordinates protein synthesis. In addition to the nucleus, there are many **organelles** inside of the cell—small structures that help carry out the day-to-day operations of the cell. One important cellular organelle is the **ribosome**. Ribosomes participate in protein synthesis. The transcription phase of protein synthesis takes places in the cell nucleus. After this step is complete, the **RNA (ribonucleic acid)** leaves the nucleus and travels to the cell's ribosomes, where translation occurs. Another important cellular organelle is the **mitochondrion**. Mitochondria (many mitochondrion) are often referred to as the power plants of the cell because many of the reactions that produce energy take place in mitochondria. Also important in the life of a cell are the **lysosomes**. Lysosomes are organelles that contain enzymes that aid in the digestion of nutrient molecules and other materials. Figure 19-3 shows the major parts of the cell and the structures located within each individual cell.

Cell Membrane

The cell membrane is a lipid bilayer that allows for **selective permeability**, meaning it allows certain substances to enter the cell and prevents others from entering. It is responsible for controlling transport in and out of the cell and for helping to maintain the cell's shape.

Cytoplasm

Cytoplasm is basically the substance that fills the cell. It is a jelly-like material that is 80 percent water and usually clear in color. It is more like a viscous (thick) gel than a watery substance, but it liquefies when shaken or stirred. Cytoplasm, which can also be referred to as cytosol, means "cell substance." This name is very fitting because cytoplasm is the substance of life that serves as a molecular soup in which all of the cell's organelles are suspended and held together by a fatty membrane. The cytoplasm is found inside the cell membrane, surrounding the nuclear envelope and the cytoplasmic organelles. Cytoplasm is also the home of the cytoskeleton, a network of cytoplasmic filaments that are responsible for the movement of the cell and give the cell its shape. The cytoplasm contains dissolved nutrients and helps dissolve waste products. The cytoplasm helps materials move around the cell by moving and churning through

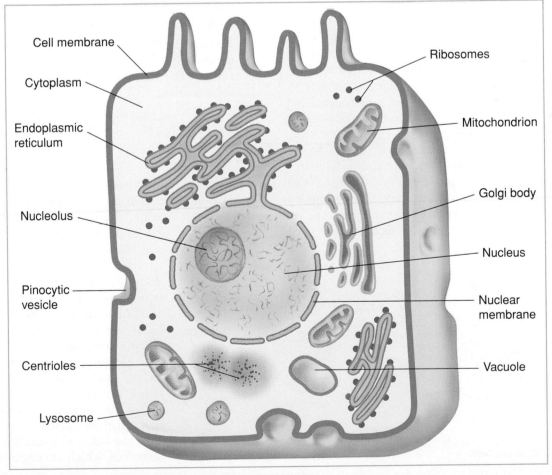

FIGURE 19-3 Major parts of the cell and the structures located inside the cell.

a process called *cytoplasmic streaming*. The nucleus often flows with the cytoplasm changing the shape as it moves. The cytoplasm contains many salts and is an excellent conductor of electricity, which therefore creates a medium for the vesicles, or mechanics of the cell. The function of the cytoplasm and the organelles within it are critical to the cell's survival.

Nucleus

The nucleus, which is known as the control center of the cell, is a remarkable organelle because it forms the package for our genes and their controlling factors. Its functions include the storage of genes on chromosomes, organization of genes into chromosomes to allow cell division, transport of genetic products via nuclear pores, production of messages through RNA, production of ribosomes, and organizing the uncoiling of DNA to replicate key genes.

The nucleus is necessary for growth, metabolism reproduction, and transmission of cell characteristics. Within the nucleus is a sphere that is made up of fibers and granules. This is known as the *nucleolus* and it is necessary for protein synthesis. Surrounding the nucleus is the nuclear membrane, which contains chromosomes. These thread-like structures are made up of DNA that can be described as a double helix. This means that it is formed from two long chains of nucleic acid that twist around each other. Nucleic acid, present in chromosomes of cells, is the chemical basis of heredity. The DNA provides the cell's genetic makeup, or "blueprint." DNA is absolutely necessary for cell reproduction. RNA is a single chain of chemical bases. RNA molecules direct the formation of proteins. The two types of RNA are mRNA and tRNA. Each of these is important for protein synthesis.

The portions of the cell that provide for work and storage include the following:

- Endoplasmic reticulum—This is a network of tubules through the nucleus and cytoplasm.

- Mitochondria—Mitochondria supply most of the ATP (energy) so they are referred to as the "power house" of the cell.

- Golgi apparatus—The Golgi apparatus is a series of flat, membranous sacs. It secretes substances such as mucus.

- Lysosomes—Lysosomes contain digestive enzymes. They phagocytize bacteria. (*Phag/o* means "to ingest or engulf" or "to eat.")

- Centrioles—The function of centrioles is to organize the spindle fibers during cell division. Centrioles are necessary for mitosis.

- Ribosomes—Ribosomes are the site of protein synthesis. Some are located on the surface of the rough endoplasmic reticulum. Some float freely within the cytoplasm.

Small hair-like projections, called **cilia,** increase the surface area of the cell. Cilia propel substances along a cell's surface and increase the cell's ability to absorb water and nutrients.

Mitosis and Cell Division

Mitosis is nuclear division plus **cytokinesis,** or the actual cellular division, that produces two identical daughter cells during prophase, metaphase, anaphase, and telophase (see Figure 19-4). Interphase is often included in discussions of mitosis, but interphase is technically not part of the process of mitosis. During interphase, the cell is engaged in metabolic activity and preparing for mitosis (the next four phases that lead up to and include nuclear division). Chromosomes are not clearly distinguishable in the nucleus, although a dark spot called the nucleolus may be visible. The cell may contain a pair of centrioles, which are organizational

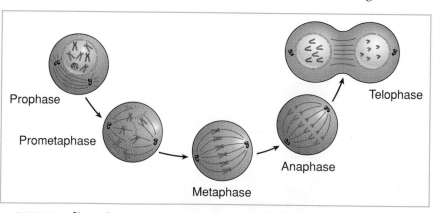

FIGURE 19-4 Stages of mitosis.

sites for microtubules. Chromatin in the nucleus begins to condense and becomes visible in the light microscope as chromosomes. The nucleolus disappears. Centrioles begin moving to opposite ends of the cell and fibers extend from the centromeres. Some fibers cross the cell to form the mitotic spindle. During the prophase, the nuclear membrane disperses. Proteins attach to the centromeres, creating the kinetochores. Microtubules attach at the kinetochores and the chromosomes begin moving.

During the metaphase, spindle fibers align the chromosomes along the middle of the cell nucleus. This line is referred to as the metaphase plate. This organization helps to ensure that in the next phase, when the chromosomes are separated, each new nucleus will receive one copy of each chromosome.

Anaphase occurs when the paired chromosomes separate at the kinetochores and move to opposite sides of the cell. Motion results from a combination of kinetochore movement along the spindle. This is followed by the telophase. During this process, the chromatids arrive at opposite poles of the cell, and new membranes form around the daughter nuclei. The chromosomes then disperse and are no longer visible under the light microscope. The spindle fibers also disperse, and cytokinesis, or the partitioning of the cell, may also begin during this stage.

Meiosis

Meiosis is a two-part cell division process in organisms that sexually reproduce which results in gametes with one-half the number of chromosomes of the parent cell. Meiosis I encompasses four stages: prophase I, metaphase I, anaphase I, and telophase I. The largest differences between mitosis and meiosis occur in prophase I. Prophase I is usually longer in duration when compared to prophase in mitosis and it is usually much more complex. It can take days for prophase I to complete. It is estimated that prophase I accounts for some 85 to 95 percent of the total time for meiosis. Metaphase I is of much shorter duration and complexity when compared to prophase I. Anaphase I is also very similar to anaphase in mitosis. Likewise, telophase I is similar to telophase in mitosis. Meiosis II is the second part of the meiotic process. Much of the process is similar to mitosis and meiosis I. In prophase II, if needed, the nuclear membrane and nuclei break up while the spindle "network" appears and the chromosomes begin migrating to the metaphase II plate (at the cell's equator). During metaphase II, the chromosomes line up at the metaphase II plate at the cell's center. The kinetochores of the sister chromatids point toward opposite poles. In anaphase II, the sister chromatids separate and move toward the opposite cell poles. And in telophase II, distinct nuclei form at the

opposite poles and cytokinesis occurs. Finally, at the end of meiosis II, there are four daughter cells each with one-half the number of chromosomes of the original parent cell.

Tissues

A grouping of cells creates a **tissue**. Each tissue performs a specialized function, depending on the types of cells that create it. There are four types of tissues in the body: epithelial, connective, muscle, and nerve (see Figure 19-5).

Epithelial Tissue

Epithelial tissue is a flat arrangement of cells that forms the skin, lines and covers the organs, lines the walls of cavities, and forms tubes, ducts, and some glands. Epithelial cells have four functions: protection, absorption, secretion, and excretion.

Connective Tissue

Connective tissue is the most abundant tissue in the body. All parts of the body have connective tissue either assisting in the construction of or holding different organs in place. Bones are dense connective tissue. Tendons (the structures that hold muscle to bone) and muscle sheaths are other examples of connective tissue. Blood is also a type of connective tissue. Blood is the only liquid tissue in the body.

Muscle Tissue

Muscle is used for movement. The primary function of muscle tissue is to contract or shorten. The three types of muscle tissue are skeletal, smooth, and cardiac. Skeletal muscle tissue is part of the skeleton and assists with voluntary movement of the body. The tissue is striated, meaning that it appears to have stripes.

Smooth muscle tissue is found in the viscera (internal organs). It is nonstriated and is involuntary muscle. It is not controlled through active participation of movement. An example of this is peristalsis (wave-like contractions) such as occurs during the movement of food through the intestinal tract.

Cardiac muscle tissue is found only in the heart. The cardiac muscle is called the *myocardium* and has the function of pumping blood.

Nerve Tissue

Nerve tissue is the functional part of the nervous system. Neurons, or nerve cells, have the properties of excitability, which means they are active, and conductivity, which means that they transmit impulses.

Body Organs and Systems

The human body is made up of **organs**, which are groups of tissues that serve a common purpose or function. When a group of organs works together to perform a specific function, it is called a **system** (see Figure 19-6).

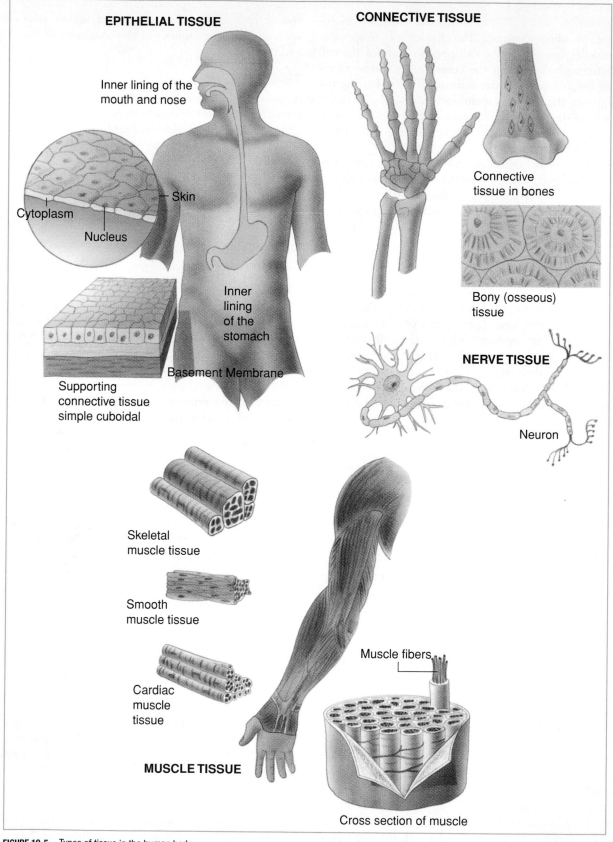

EPITHELIAL TISSUE

Inner lining of the mouth and nose

Cytoplasm

Nucleus

Skin

Inner lining of the stomach

Basement Membrane

Supporting connective tissue simple cuboidal

CONNECTIVE TISSUE

Connective tissue in bones

Bony (osseous) tissue

NERVE TISSUE

Neuron

Skeletal muscle tissue

Smooth muscle tissue

Cardiac muscle tissue

Muscle fibers

MUSCLE TISSUE

Cross section of muscle

FIGURE 19-5 Types of tissue in the human body.

Organ System	Major Functions

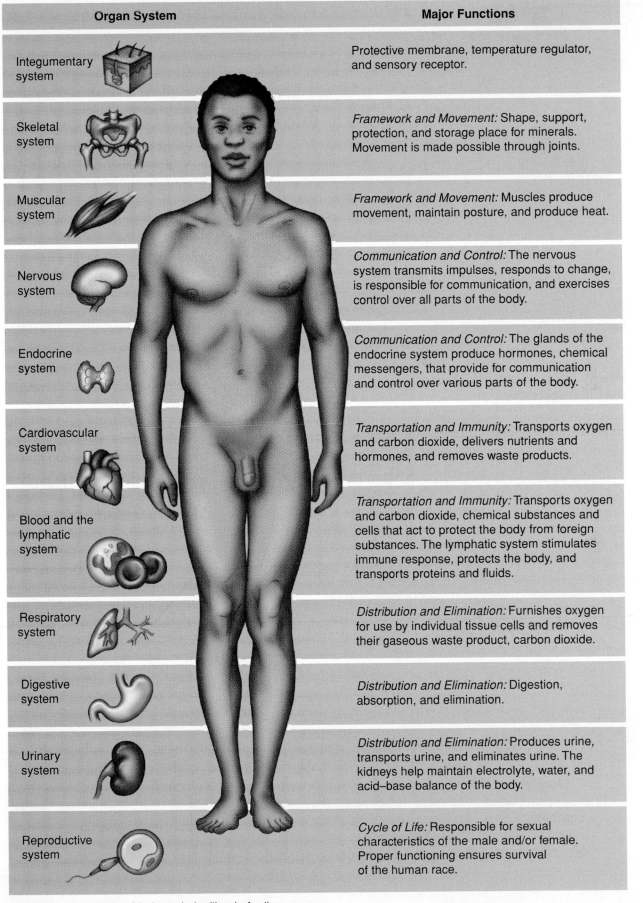

Integumentary system
Protective membrane, temperature regulator, and sensory receptor.

Skeletal system
Framework and Movement: Shape, support, protection, and storage place for minerals. Movement is made possible through joints.

Muscular system
Framework and Movement: Muscles produce movement, maintain posture, and produce heat.

Nervous system
Communication and Control: The nervous system transmits impulses, responds to change, is responsible for communication, and exercises control over all parts of the body.

Endocrine system
Communication and Control: The glands of the endocrine system produce hormones, chemical messengers, that provide for communication and control over various parts of the body.

Cardiovascular system
Transportation and Immunity: Transports oxygen and carbon dioxide, delivers nutrients and hormones, and removes waste products.

Blood and the lymphatic system
Transportation and Immunity: Transports oxygen and carbon dioxide, chemical substances and cells that act to protect the body from foreign substances. The lymphatic system stimulates immune response, protects the body, and transports proteins and fluids.

Respiratory system
Distribution and Elimination: Furnishes oxygen for use by individual tissue cells and removes their gaseous waste product, carbon dioxide.

Digestive system
Distribution and Elimination: Digestion, absorption, and elimination.

Urinary system
Distribution and Elimination: Produces urine, transports urine, and eliminates urine. The kidneys help maintain electrolyte, water, and acid–base balance of the body.

Reproductive system
Cycle of Life: Responsible for sexual characteristics of the male and/or female. Proper functioning ensures survival of the human race.

FIGURE 19-6 Organ systems of the human body with major functions.

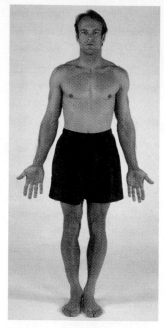

FIGURE 19-7   Anatomical position.

Anatomical Locations and Positions

In discussing the anatomy and physiology of the body, specific terms are used to determine relationships of the parts of the body. For example, in the **anatomical position** (see Figure 19-7), the body is assumed to be standing, with the feet together, the arms to the side, and the head, eyes, and palms of the hands facing forward. To ensure consistency of description, it is important to keep the anatomical position constantly in mind. This last point is an important one, because in the normal relaxed position of the body, the thumb points anteriorly. In anatomical parlance, the thumb is a lateral structure, not an anterior one. (Note, however, as discussed in Patient Education, that your patients may not understand this terminology.)

Directions of the Body

Directional terms describe the positions of structures relative to other structures or locations in the body.

The directional anatomical terms are shown in Figure 19-8 and include the following:

- **Superior or cranial:** toward the head end of the body; upper (example: the hand is part of the superior extremity)
- **Inferior or caudal:** away from the head; lower (example: the foot is part of the inferior extremity)
- **Anterior or ventral:** front (example: the kneecap is located on the anterior side of the leg)
- **Posterior or dorsal:** back (example: the shoulder blades are located on the posterior side of the body)
- **Medial:** toward the midline of the body (example: the middle toe is located at the medial side of the foot)
- **Lateral:** away from the midline of the body (example: the little toe is located at the lateral side of the foot)
- **Proximal:** toward or nearest the trunk or the point of origin of a part (example: the proximal end of the femur joins with the pelvic bone)
- **Distal:** away from or farthest from the trunk or the point or origin of a part (example: the hand is located at the distal end of the forearm)

Planes of the Body

Medical professionals often refer to sections of the body in terms of anatomical planes (flat surfaces). These planes are imaginary lines—vertical or horizontal—drawn through an upright body. The following terms are used to describe a specific body part (see Figure 19-9):

- **Coronal plane (frontal plane):** A vertical plane running from side to side; divides the body or any of its parts into anterior and posterior portions.
- **Sagittal plane (median plane):** A vertical plane running from front to back; divides the body or any of its parts into right and left sides.
- **Axial plane (transverse plane):** A horizontal plane; divides the body or any of its parts into upper and lower parts.

Patient Education

As a medical assistant, you will become accustomed to using medical language. Remember that the patient may not understand medical terminology and will thus require explanations. You may be asked to explain prescription instructions or procedure preparations to patients. Always use terms that the patient understands, yet without making the patient feel you are talking down to him or her. Ask the patient for confirmation of his or her understanding of the information. An informed patient will be more compliant. Document patient education on the chart.

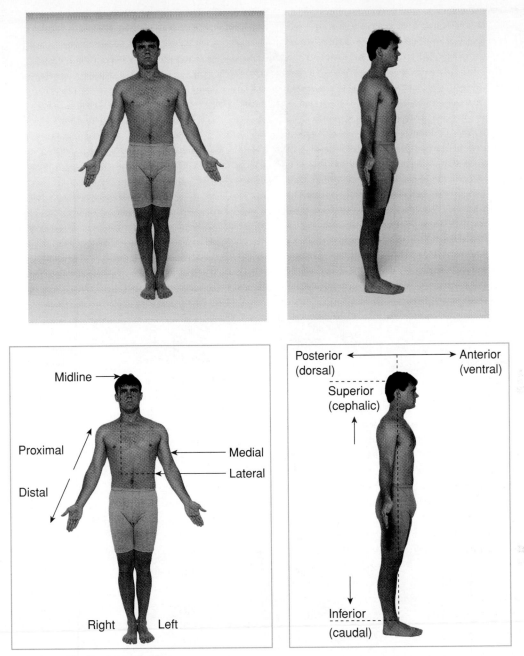

FIGURE 19-8 Directional anatomical terms.

Body Cavities and Abdominal Regions

The **cavities**, or spaces, of the body contain the internal organs, or viscera (see Figure 19-10). The two main cavities are called the *ventral* and *dorsal cavities*. The ventral is the larger cavity and is subdivided into two parts (thoracic and abdominopelvic cavities) by the **diaphragm**, a dome-shaped respiratory muscle. The thoracic cavity consists of the upper ventral, or chest, cavity and contains the heart, lungs, trachea, esophagus, large blood vessels, and nerves. The thoracic cavity is bound laterally by the ribs (covered by costal pleura) and the diaphragm caudally (covered by diaphragmatic pleura).

The abdominopelvic cavity is the lower part of the ventral cavity. It can be further divided into two portions: the abdominal portion and the pelvic portion. The abdominal cavity contains most of the gastrointestinal tract as well as the kidneys and adrenal glands. The abdominal cavity is bound cranially by the diaphragm, laterally by the body wall, and caudally by the pelvic cavity. The pelvic cavity contains most of the urogenital system as well as the rectum. The pelvic cavity is bounded cranially by the abdominal cavity, dorsally by the sacrum, and laterally by the pelvis. The dorsal cavity is the smaller of the two main cavities. As its name implies, it contains organs lying more posterior in the body. The dorsal cavity,

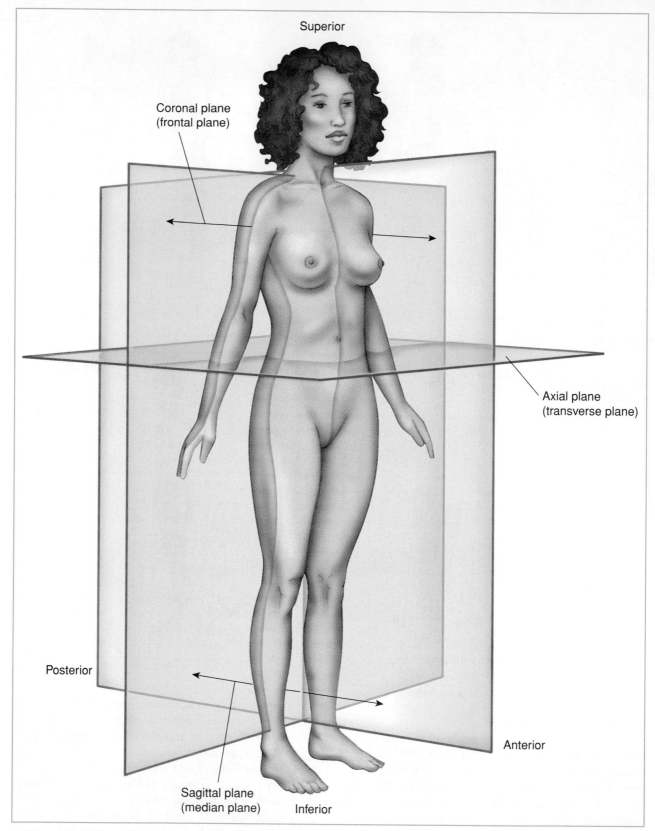

FIGURE 19-9 Anatomical planes.

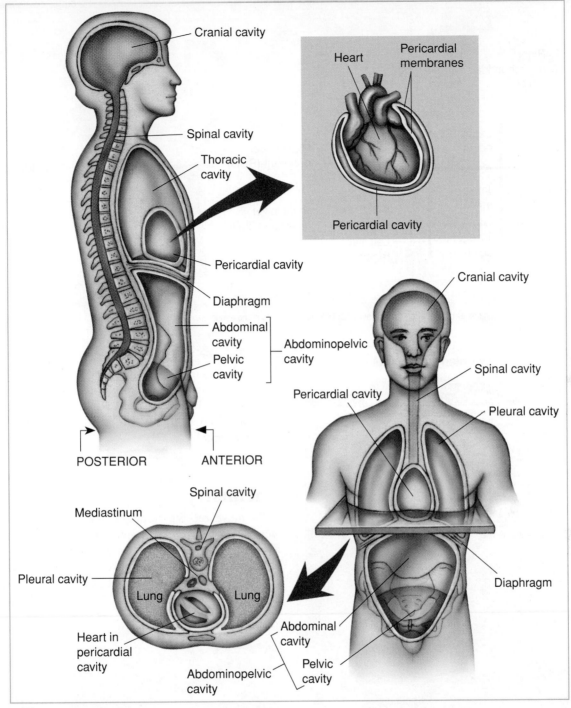

FIGURE 19-10 Body cavities.

again, can be divided into two portions. The upper portion, or the cranial cavity, houses the brain, and the lower portion, or vertebral canal houses the spinal cord.

Abdominal Regions and Quadrants

The abdominopelvic cavity, which can be seen in Figure 19-11, is frequently divided into nine regions, including:

- Right and left hypochondriac
- Right and left lumbar
- Right and left iliac

- Epigastric
- Umbilical
- Hypogastric

The abdomen is also divided into four quadrants. These are:

- Right upper quadrant (RUQ)
- Left upper quadrant (LUQ)
- Right lower quadrant (RLQ)
- Left lower quadrant (LLQ)

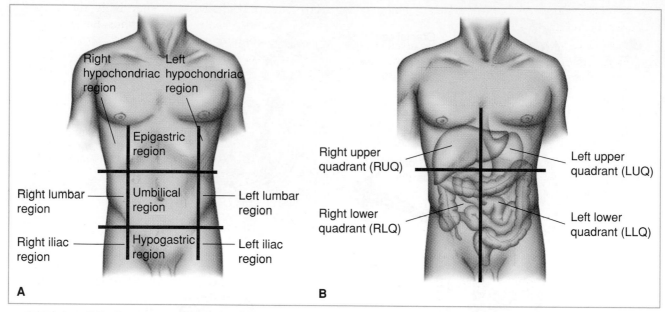

FIGURE 19-11   (A) The nine regions of the abdominopelvic cavity. (B) The four quadrants of the abdomen.

Landmarks

The body has many landmarks. Table 19-1 provides a listing of the most frequently noted landmarks. Landmark terms should be used when charting information or when relaying information to other health care personnel.

Chemistry

Cells must receive nourishment and also eliminate wastes. For this to occur, materials must be transported to and from the cell, or even within the cell. There are two mechanisms in which this occurs. The first, which does not require energy from the cell, is through **passive**

TABLE 19-1 Frequently Noted Landmarks

Landmark/Term	Refers to
Antecubital	Bend of the elbow
Axillary	Armpit
Buccal	Cheek
Cervical	Neck
Deltoid	Shoulder
Femoral	Thigh
Gluteal	Buttocks
Hepatic	Liver
Lumbar	Lower back
Occipital	Back of the head
Patellar	Kneecap
Popliteal	Behind the knee
Pulmonary	Lungs
Renal	Kidney
Sural	Calf of the leg
Thoracic	Chest
Volar (palmer)	Palm of the hand

Cultural Considerations

An interpreter might be needed for patients who speak a language other than English, or who perhaps have English as a second language. Dictionaries can assist the staff with commonly used words and may be purchased from local bookstores. Anything that can be done to make the patient more at ease in your office setting will be beneficial.

transport Passive transport may involve any number of processes, including the following:

- Diffusion: This is movement of dissolved particles from an area of greater concentration to an area of lesser concentration. This action requires no cell energy.

- Osmosis: This is a type of diffusion in which water is pulled through a semipermeable membrane. Molecules are again transported from an area of greater concentration to an area of lesser concentration. This also requires no cell energy.

- Filtration: In filtration, dissolved particles are diffused through membranes but only mechanical pressure is required. Whether or not filtration occurs depends on the size of the cell's pores. Only liquids are allowed through the barrier.

The second method by which cells may become nourished and their wastes eliminated is through **active transport**. Active transport requires energy to carry material from areas of lesser concentration to an area of greater concentration. In this method, the cell is able to obtain what it requires from the tissue fluid. These mechanisms include:

- Phagocytosis: In this method, the cell engulfs a solid particle, such as bacteria.

- Pinocytosis: In this method, the cell "drinks" the fluid required.

Electrolytes

Electrolyte is a "medical/scientific" term for salts, specifically ions. The term *electrolyte* means that this ion is electrically charged and moves to either a negative (cathode) or positive (anode) electrode. Ions that move to the cathode are positively charged and are called *cations*. Ions that move to the anode and are negatively charged are called *anions*. Body fluids, such as blood, plasma, and interstitial fluid (the fluid between cells), are like seawater and have a high concentration of sodium chloride. The electrolytes in sodium chloride include sodium ion (Na^+), the cation, and chloride ion (Cl), the anion. The major electrolytes in the human body include sodium (Na^+), potassium (K^+), chloride (Cl), calcium (Ca), magnesium (Mg), bicarbonate (HCO_3), phosphate (PO_4), and sulfate (SO_4).

Electrolytes are important because they are what your cells (especially nerve, heart, muscle) use to maintain voltages across their cell membranes and to carry electrical impulses (nerve impulses, muscle contractions) across themselves and to other cells. Your kidneys work to keep the electrolyte concentrations in your blood constant despite changes in your body. For example, when you exercise heavily, you lose electrolytes in your sweat, particularly sodium and potassium. These electrolytes must be replaced to keep the electrolyte concentrations of your body fluids constant. Therefore, many sports drinks have sodium chloride or potassium chloride added to them. They also have sugar and flavorings to provide your body with extra energy and to make the drink taste better.

Genetics and Heredity

Genetics is the study of the makeup of animals or plants. DNA carries all the information needed for protein synthesis and replication of cells. In living organisms DNA is organized in chromosomes and is located in the nucleus of each cell.

Genetic Engineering

Genetic engineering is defined as making or changing an organism's DNA. There are many forms of genetic engineering, some occurring naturally whereas others are human-made. Genetic engineering in the current state is a relatively new science, the effects of which are not yet known. This causes controversy as to whether or not genetic engineering is safe or ethical.

Genetic engineering has been going on for years in the form of natural selection and artificial breeding. Natural selection, or "survival of the fittest" as it is sometimes known, occurs when the environment chooses the traits that are best suited to the current environment and allows animals with those traits to reproductively mature and reproduce. This changing of the genes within a species is nature's way of ensuring survival. Artificial breeding is human intervention in the process of natural selection. Humans choose traits for an animal that they think are beneficial and then breed those traits into the animal's offspring. An example of this is domestic dogs, all of which are descended from the wolf family through artificial breeding.

Genetic Fingerprinting

The chemical structure of everyone's DNA is the same. The only difference between people (or any animal) is the order of the base pairs. There are so many millions of base pairs in each person's DNA that although—it is possible to have the exact same DNA sequences—it is very unlikely. This means that every person has a different sequence from which he or she can be identified. DNA fingerprinting is carried out by obtaining a small amount of the person's DNA, usually from hair, sexual fluid, blood, or saliva, but any part of a human can be used. This piece of DNA is put through various tests to extract and isolate part of the strand of DNA. This is done by using chemicals such as enzymes and by using electricity to separate the different parts of DNA. This process results in a profile of the person that matches one person and one person only; the only exception to this is for identical twins. The sample is analyzed by a picture showing the DNA patterns in the form of an x-ray photo. If the two patterns

*In preparing for a medical assistant externship,
make sure that your writing is very clear. Practice your penmanship to ensure that others can
read your entries in the medical record (chart).
Entries on a chart should always be written
neatly, in black ink. All entries should be made
with permanent ink only. If a mistake is made, it
should have one line drawn through the mistake,
and then be initialed and dated per clinic protocol. Never use white-out liquids or tapes to cover
mistakes. Always follow the facility's protocol regarding corrections to the medical record.*

from the two DNA samples match, they are very likely to have come from the same person. In the case of proving parentage, DNA from the child is matched to that of the people requesting the test. The tests show the relationship of the people to the particular child by matching both the maternal (mother's) and paternal (father's) DNA finger-prints to the child's. If the DNA fingerprint shows significant similarities, then the people having the test are the parents.

Genetics, Heredity, and Disease

Heredity is the genetic transmission from parent to child. The genes for certain traits are passed down in families from parents to children, and hereditary traits are determined by specific genes.

Individuals carry two genes for each trait, one from the mother's egg and one from the father's sperm. When an individual reproduces, the two genes split up (segregate) and end up in separate gametes.

Genetic Disorders

Genetic disorders are medical conditions caused by mu-tations in a gene or a set of genes. Mutations are changes in the DNA sequence of a gene. They can happen at any time, from when we are a single cell to when we are 90— or even older! Some people say that there are disorder genes. It is not a gene or genes, however, that cause the illness, but a mutation that causes the normal genes to operate improperly. It is better to say that mutated genes cause genetic disorders. A genetic disorder that is present at birth is frequently referred to as a *congenital disorder*. They may also be called *birth defects*. Listed here are some of the more common congenital disorders:

- Albinism is a congenital, but nonpathological disorder. A recessive gene mutation causes hered-itary lack of pigment in the skin, hair, and eyes.

The patient may complain of photophobia and is prone to sunburn because protective melanin is not present.

- Attention deficit hyperactivity disorder (ADHD) is a disease that can affect both children and adults. It is characterized by the person having difficulty organizing and completing a task. The cause may be due to genetic factors, and it is 10 times more prevalent in boys than in girls. There is no known cure, but treatment often includes medications or counseling. Abstinence from certain foods or food additives may be recommended if these are deter-mined to be a part of the cause of hyperactivity. However, symptoms may subside or even disap-pear with time.

- Cleft palate is a congenital defect in the roof of the mouth that occurs when the palatine bones of the skull do not close properly. The cleft causes a passageway between the mouth and nasal cavi-ties. It may also be associated with a cleft upper lip, and it affects females more often than males. Initially, the infant has special needs for feeding. Surgical repairs are usually performed within the first year of life and are generally successful in re-pairing the defect.

- Color deficiency is a disorder that was previ-ously called color blindness. It often entails diffi-culty in distinguishing between reds and greens. It is an inherited, sex-linked disorder, usually passed from mother to son. In total color defi-ciency, the person is unable to perceive any color at all due to a defect in or absence of cones in the retina.

- Cystic fibrosis (CF) is a chronic and progressive disease usually diagnosed in childhood that causes mucus to become thick, dry, and sticky. The mu-cus builds up and clogs passages in many of the body's organs, but primarily the lungs and the pancreas. In the lungs, the mucus can lead to seri-ous breathing problems and lung disease. In the pancreas, the mucus can lead to malnutrition and problems with growth and development. People with CF have an average life expectancy of about 32 years, although new treatments offer hope for longer and healthier lives.

- Down syndrome (trisomy 21) is a disorder caused by the person having an extra chromosome, usu-ally number 21 (hence, the name). A few of the ma-jor features seen include marked sloping of the forehead, a short broad hand with a single palmer crease (known as a simian crease), and a flat nose. A mother who gives birth after the age of 40 has a higher risk at delivering an infant with Down syn-drome. Amniocentesis is generally used as a tool for diagnosing this disorder.

- Fragile X syndrome, also known as Martin-Bell syndrome, Marker X syndrome, and FRAXA syndrome, is the most common form of inherited mental retardation. Individuals with this condition have developmental delays, variable levels of mental retardation, and behavioral and emotional difficulties. They may also have characteristic physical traits. Generally, males are affected with moderate mental retardation and females with mild mental retardation. Fragile X is caused by a mutation in the FMR-1 gene, located on the X chromosome. The role of this gene is unclear, but it is probably important in early development.

- Hemochromatosis is an inherited disorder of excessive body accumulation of iron. It is common among the white population, affecting approximately 1 in 400 individuals of European ancestry. Hemochromatosis patients are believed to absorb excessive amounts of iron from the diet. Since the human body has limited ways of eliminating the absorbed iron, the iron accumulates over time in the liver, bone marrow, pancreas, skin, and testicles. This accumulation of iron in these organs causes them to function poorly. Patients with early hemochromatosis have no symptoms and are unaware of their condition. The disease may be discovered when elevated iron blood levels are noted as a result of routine blood testing. In males, symptoms may not appear until 40 to 50 years of age. Iron deposits in the skin cause darkening of the skin. Because females lose iron through menstrual blood loss, they develop organ damage from iron accumulation 15 to 20 years later than men on average.

- Hemophilia is a hereditary, sex-linked disorder in which the blood coagulation time is greatly increased. It is due to a recessive gene mutation in the X chromosome. Females carry the recessive gene and transmit the disorder to their male offspring.

- Klinefelter's syndrome is a congenital endocrine disorder. Primary testicular failure occurs that usually is not evident until puberty. The testes are small and firm and gynecomastia may be present. The boy has abnormally long legs. This disorder also can lead to subnormal intelligence.

- Muscular dystrophy is a genetic disease characterized by a gradual atrophy and weakening of the muscle. It is more frequent in males. The most common type is Duchenne's Muscular dystrophy, which accounts for 50% of all cases. The onset is at an early age, and the patient is usually confined to a wheelchair by the age of 12. Death often occurs within 10 to 15 years of onset of symptoms. Unfortunately, there is no successful

Professionalism

A large part of the medical assistant's job is taking messages for the physician. This means that the medical assistant may speak to a patient, gather data for the physician, and then transcribe the information. When doing this, it is essential to first confirm the spelling of the patient's name and the birth date. Many offices use the birth date as a double check to ensure that the correct medical record is accessed. The patient's chief complaint or question is listed first, along with pertinent information about his or her complaint, the medications being taken, and any questions. Be sure that all of the writing is legible and that the message is timed, dated, and signed. Many offices have specific protocols regarding taking messages, the form on which the message is written, and the method of delivering the messages to the physician. These messages are part of the medical record, and should never be scratched out or scribbled on, and should always look professional. Never write messages on scraps of paper. Use the appropriate forms provided by your work facility.

treatment, although physical therapy and exercise are recommended to prevent more atrophy of muscles.

- PKU (phenylketonuria) is due to a recessive gene mutation. A defective enzyme causes the body to be unable to oxidize an amino acid, known as phenylalanine, to tyrosine. If the condition is not treated early, mental retardation occurs due to brain damage. Many states require testing at birth to detect PKU.

- Sickle cell anemia is a hereditary, chronic form of anemia that is due to a recessive gene mutation. It affects millions of people throughout the world and it is particularly common among people whose ancestors came from sub-Saharan Africa; Spanish-speaking regions (South America, Cuba, Central America); Saudi Arabia; India; and Mediterranean countries, such as Turkey, Greece, and Italy. In the United States, sickle cell disease occurs in about 1 in every 500 African-American births and 1 in every 1,000 to 1,400 Hispanic-American births. Erythrocytes, which are usually round, "sickle out," meaning that they take on a half-moon shape. The abnormally shaped cells block blood vessels and can cause a sickle cell "crisis" during times of stress or illness. Sickle cell crisis is characterized by joint pain, thrombosis, and fever.

- Spina bifida is a congenital neural tube defect. The posterior vertebral arch has a developmental anomaly. In some cases, the spinal cord and its membranes may protrude. Most often the abnormality occurs in the lumbar region.

- Talipes (clubfoot) is a congenital deformity of the foot. Treatment may include casting of the foot or special orthopedic shoes to assist with walking.

- Tay-Sachs disease (TSD) is an inherited disorder that tends to affect people of central and northern European Jewish (Ashkenazi) or French-Canadian ancestry. The faulty gene targets the nervous system. Symptoms first appear at around 6 months of age in a previously healthy baby. Over a short period of time, the baby stops moving and smiling, becomes paralyzed, and eventually dies. Most children with TSD die before their fifth birthday. There is no cure.

- Turner's syndrome is a congenital disorder caused by failure of the ovaries to respond to the stimulation of pituitary hormones. Intelligence may be impaired, amenorrhea may be present, and the patient is usually short in stature.

SUMMARY

In this chapter, you have learned of the organizational components of the body. A group of cells with similar functions forms tissues, and tissues with similar functions form organs. These organs then form systems that make up the human body. As each of these systems performs its function, the body can remain in homeostasis. Although disease processes may occur, the body is remarkable in its ability to fight off infections, or in some cases, as in cellular development, even regenerate.

Chapter Review

COMPETENCY REVIEW

1. Define and spell the terms to learn for this chapter.
2. What does the term anatomy mean?
3. What is the substance within the cell called?
4. What are the three types of muscle tissue?
5. What are the four functions of epithelial tissue?
6. What are the two properties of nerve tissue?
7. Which part of the cell is known as the control center?
8. Name the three distinct cavities of the ventral cavity.
9. What is the plane that vertically divides the body into right and left sides?
10. Where is cardiac muscle located?

PREPARING FOR THE CERTIFICATION EXAM

1. What is the basic structural unit of the body?
   A. tissue
   B. organ system
   C. cell
   D. molecule
   E. electrolyte

2. Which plane divides the body into superior and inferior parts?
   A. frontal
   B. midsagittal
   C. sagittal
   D. transverse

3. The cavity containing the heart and lungs is the
   A. abdominopelvic cavity
   B. dorsal cavity
   C. buccal cavity
   D. thoracic cavity

4. Which type of tissue is the most widespread and abundant tissue in the body?
   A. muscle tissue
   B. connective tissue
   C. nervous tissue
   D. epithelial tissue

continued on next page

5. Which plane divides the body into anterior and posterior parts?
   A. sagittal
   B. coronal
   C. transverse
   D. midsagittal

6. Which term means nearer the point of attachment?
   A. proximal
   B. distal
   C. ventral
   D. dorsal
   E. lateral

7. Which of the following would NOT describe smooth muscle?
   A. found in the heart
   B. involuntary
   C. nonstriated
   D. found in visceral organs

8. Which cell organelle phagocytizes bacteria?
   A. endoplasmic reticulum
   B. lysosomes
   C. mitochondria
   D. ribosomes

9. The cell membrane allows diffusion of dissolved particles through membranes while requiring mechanical pressure. This is known as
   A. filtration
   B. facilitated diffusion
   C. osmosis
   D. phagocytosis

10. Homeostasis means
    A. blood stoppage
    B. spreading
    C. maintaining inner balance
    D. study of the function of an organism

CRITICAL THINKING

1. Where is the epigastric region?

2. If Dr. Menendez ordered a test that required the patient to be supine, how would you position the patient?

3. Visualize the imaginary lines dividing the abdomen into quadrants. In which quadrant would Mr. Schultz's pain be localized?

ON THE JOB

Ben is a medical assistant who is taking a medical history on Tyler Jackson. Tyler has a lot of bruises on his left calf on the outside as a result of falling down the stairs. He also has a fracture on his right arm closer to the wrist as a result of the same fall.

1. How would Ben chart these injuries on the medical record using correct directional terms?

INTERNET ACTIVITY

Use the Internet to look up different anatomical direction descriptions (such as lateral wrist).

MediaLink   More on body structure and function, including interactive resources, can be found on the Student CD-ROM accompanying this textbook.

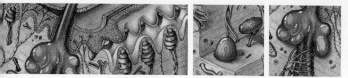

Medical Assistant Role Delineation Chart

HIGHLIGHT indicates material covered in this chapter.

ADMINISTRATIVE

Administrative Procedures

- Perform basic administrative medical assisting functions
- Schedule, coordinate and monitor appointments
- Schedule inpatient/outpatient admissions and procedures
- Understand and apply third-party guidelines
- Obtain reimbursement through accurate claims submission
- Monitor third-party reimbursement
- Understand and adhere to managed care policies and procedures
- *Negotiate managed care contracts*

Practice Finances

- Perform procedural and diagnostic coding
- Apply bookkeeping principles

- Manage accounts receivable
- *Manage accounts payable*
- *Process payroll*
- *Document and maintain accounting and banking records*
- *Develop and maintain fee schedules*
- *Manage renewals of business and professional insurance policies*
- *Manage personnel benefits and maintain records*
- *Perform marketing, financial, and strategic planning*

CLINICAL

Fundamental Principles

- Apply principles of aseptic technique and infection control
- Comply with quality assurance practices
- Screen and follow up patient test results

Diagnostic Orders

- Collect and process specimens
- Perform diagnostic tests

Patient Care

- Adhere to established patient screening procedures
- Obtain patient history and vital signs
- Prepare and maintain examination and treatment areas
- Prepare patient for examinations, procedures and treatments

- Assist with examinations, procedures and treatments
- Prepare and administer medications and immunizations
- Maintain medication and immunization records
- Recognize and respond to emergencies
- Coordinate patient care information with other health care providers
- Initiate IV and administer IV medications with appropriate training and as permitted by state law

GENERAL

Professionalism

- Display a professional manner and image
- Demonstrate initiative and responsibility
- Work as a member of the health care team
- Prioritize and perform multiple tasks
- Adapt to change
- Promote the CMA credential
- Enhance skills through continuing education
- Treat all patients with compassion and empathy
- Promote the practice through positive public relations

Communication Skills

- Recognize and respect cultural diversity
- Adapt communications to individual's ability to understand
- Use professional telephone technique

- Recognize and respond effectively to verbal, nonverbal, and written communications
- Use medical terminology appropriately
- Utilize electronic technology to receive, organize, prioritize and transmit information
- Serve as liaison

Legal Concepts

- Perform within legal and ethical boundaries
- Prepare and maintain medical records
- Document accurately
- Follow employer's established policies dealing with the health care contract
- Implement and maintain federal and state health care legislation and regulations
- Comply with established risk management and safety procedures
- Recognize professional credentialing criteria
- *Develop and maintain personnel, policy and procedure manuals*

Instruction

- Instruct individuals according to their needs
- Explain office policies and procedures
- Teach methods of health promotion and disease prevention
- Locate community resources and disseminate information
- *Develop educational materials*
- *Conduct continuing education activities*

Operational Functions

- Perform inventory of supplies and equipment
- Perform routine maintenance of administrative and clinical equipment
- Apply computer techniques to support office operations
- *Perform personnel management functions*
- *Negotiate leases and prices for equipment and supply contracts*

- *Denotes advanced skills.*

SOURCE: Reprinted by permission of the American Association of Medical Assistants from the AAMA Role Delineation Study: Occupational Analysis of the Medical Assisting Profession.

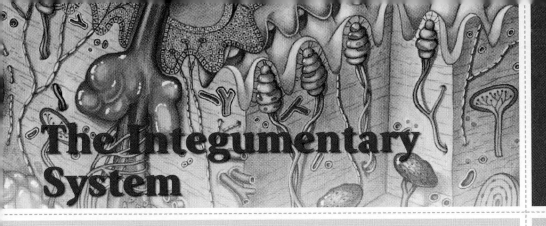

The Integumentary System

chapter
20

Learning Objectives

After completing this chapter, you should be able to:

- Define and spell the terms to learn for this chapter.
- Describe the integumentary system and identify its accessory structures.
- List the functions of the skin.
- Explain skin differences of the child and the older adult.
- Identify and explain common disorders associated with the integumentary system.

OUTLINE

Terms to Learn

acne vulgaris

alopecia

cellulitis

contact dermatitis

decubitus ulcer

dermis

eczema

epidermis

folliculitis

herpes simplex

herpes zoster

impetigo

malignant melanoma

pediculosis

psoriasis

rosacea

scabies

sebaceous glands

squamous cell carcinoma

sudoriferous glands

sweat glands

wart

Case Study

CELINE JACKSON IS A 42-YEAR-OLD FEMALE seen by Dr. Black for moderate itching of her fist, with small vesicles on her forearms and redness and swelling on bilateral hands and arms. When questioned, she states that she was working in her backyard, which opens into a wooded area. Although she was not specifically looking, she knows that there is poison ivy growing in the wooded area. There is no redness or itching anywhere else, and she has no history of other allergies and does not take any medications.

Dr. Black diagnoses her with contact dermatitis poison ivy and treats her with antiallergy medicines and corticosteroid therapy. Temovate cream to be applied to the irritated areas twice a day and a Medrol dose pack (low-dose oral steroids) to take as directed.

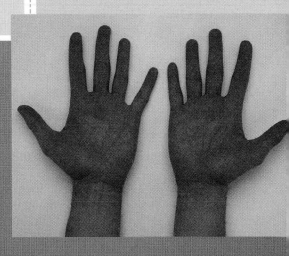

Overview of the Integumentary System

The integumentary system consists of the skin, which is the largest organ in the body. The skin contains 12 to 15 percent of the body's weight, and has a surface area of 1 to 2 meters. Skin is continuous with, but structurally distinct from, mucous membranes that line the mouth, anus, urethra, and vagina. Two distinct layers occur in the skin: the dermis and epidermis. The basic cell type of the epidermis is the keratinocyte, which contains keratin, a fibrous protein. Basal cells are the innermost layer of the epidermis. Melanocytes produce the pigment melanin, and are also located in the inner layer of the epidermis. The dermis, which consists of connective tissue, is located under the epidermis, and contains nerve endings, sensory receptors, capillaries, and elastic fibers. The skin is innervated from the nervous system, and is well supplied by blood vessels from the circulatory system. The accessory structures in the integumentary system include the hair, nails, sebaceous (oil) glands, and sweat glands.

Functions of the Integumentary System

The integumentary system has multiple roles in homeostasis, including protection, temperature regulation, sensory reception, and secretion. All body systems work in an interconnected manner in order to maintain the internal conditions essential to the function of the body.

Protection

The skin serves as a protective membrane, providing a barrier over the internal compartments of the body that serves to hold potential harmful agents (such as bacteria, viruses, pollution) outside of the body. The thicker coverings of the skin protect the more delicate structures below from harm. By producing melanin (pigment) the external skin coverings protect the underlying structures from ultraviolet light's harmful rays while producing vitamin D, which works in conjunction with calcium for multiple body processes. The skin also protects the body from excess fluid and electrolyte loss while providing a reservoir for emergency supplies of nutrients and fluids.

Regulation

The skin also serves as a temperature regulator. When the body is too warm, the skin notifies the rest of the body, so sweating begins for cooling and the vascular system dilates and sends blood to the surface to cool the interior. When the body is too cool, the skin notifies the body so that the circulatory system constricts the blood vessels for heat conservation, and the muscles begin shivering to produce extra warmth.

Sensory Reception

Millions of sensory receptors (nerves) are located in the skin for the sensations of pain, touch, heat, cold, and pressure. The nerve endings in the skin are specialized to react to specific sensory stimulation (temperature, pressure, etc.) and send that information to the cerebral cortex of the brain. When the message reaches the brain, the necessary response is triggered. For example, if the hand touches a hot plate, the message goes to the brain that the hand is on the hot plate, then the brain sends the message back to the hand to move off the plate.

Secretion

The skin contains millions of sweat glands, which secrete perspiration or sweat, and sebaceous glands, which secrete oil for lubrication. Perspiration is mostly water with a small amount of salt and other chemical compounds. If the secretions are allowed to accumulate, especially among body hair in the axillary region, then bacteria grow, creating body odor. Sebaceous glands produce sebum, which acts to protect the body from dehydration and the possible absorption of harmful substances.

Layers of the Skin

The skin is composed of two layers: the **epidermis** and the **dermis** (see Figure 20-1).

The Epidermis

The epidermis is divided into four layers or strata: the stratum corneum, stratums lucidum, stratum granulosum, and stratum germinativum.

Stratum Corneum

The stratum corneum is the outermost layer of skin consisting of dead cells filled with a protein called keratin. It forms a protective covering for the body, and the thickness of the layer depends on the part of the body. Because of the ongoing pressure on their surfaces, the soles of the feet and the palms of the hands have thicker layers than do the eyelids or forehead.

Stratum Lucidum

The stratum lucidum is a translucent layer lying directly beneath the stratum corneum. In thinner skin, it is often absent. Cells in this layer are either dead or dying.

Stratum Granulosum

The stratum granulosum consists of several layers of living cells that are becoming part of the stratum lucidum and stratum corneum. These cells are actively becoming keratinized or hardened, after they lose their nuclei.

Stratum Germinativum

The stratum germinativum is made of several layers of living cells, still capable of mitosis, or cell division. This layer, occasionally referred to as the mucosum, is most responsible for the regeneration of the epidermis. If damage, such as a severe burn, occurs to this layer, the skin is unable to regenerate itself, and skin grafting must be done. This layer also contains the melanocytes, the cells that produce melanin, the pigment that gives the skin its color.

The Dermis

The dermis is also known as the "true skin." It is composed of connective tissue containing nerves and nerve endings, blood vessels, sebaceous and sweat glands, hair follicles, and lymph vessels. The dermis is divided into two layers, the papillary, or upper, layer and the reticular, or lower, layer. The papillary layer is arranged in parallel layers of microscopic papillae. These papillae are what form the ridges that are fingerprints. The reticular layer is composed of white fibrous tissues, which support blood vessels. Underneath, the dermis is attached to the subcutaneous tissue, which supports, nourishes, insulates, and cushions the skin.

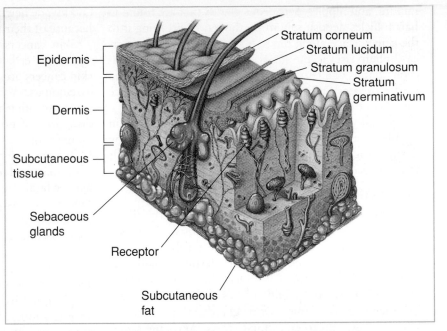

FIGURE 20-1 The integument: the epidermis, dermis, subcutaneous tissue, and its appendages.

Accessory Structures of the Skin

The accessory structures of the skin include the hair follicles, nails, sebaceous glands, and sweat glands. Hair follicles are tube-like depressions located in the dermis of the skin (see Figure 20-1). The shaft is the visible portion of the hair. The root is embedded within the follicle. At the base of each follicle is the hair papilla, which is a loop of capillaries enclosed in the connective tissue. The pilomotor muscle is attached to the side of each follicle. Contraction of the pilomotor muscle causes "goose pimples" or the sensation of the hair "standing on end." This is both a result of an emotional reaction and the skin's attempt at self-warming. The entire body has a very thin layer of hair, except for the palms of the hands and the soles of the feet. Hair is thicker on the scalp than on other portions of the body. The hair around the eyes, ears, and nose serves to filter out foreign particles and prevent their entrance into the sensory organs. Hair color is a result of genetics, and is determined by the amount of pigmentation within the hair shaft. Gray hair has little or no pigmentation. Hair grows about one-half inch a

month, and cutting the hair does not affect its growth rate.

Nails

Fingers and toenails are horny cell structures of the epidermis and are composed of hard keratin. The nail consists of the body, the root, and the matrix, or nail bed (see Figure 20-2). The lunula is the crescent-shaped white area at the base of the nail. Average nail growth is about 1 mm per week. A lost fingernail may take 3½ to 5½ months to regrow, while a lost toenail may take as long as 6 to 8 months to regrow. Nail growth is affected by disease and hormonal insufficiencies.

Sebaceous Glands

The **sebaceous glands** are located in the dermis. They secrete an oily substance called sebum that is made of fat (lipids) and the debris of dead fat-producing cells. Sebum acts to protect and waterproof hair and skin. Sebaceous glands can usually be found in hair-covered areas where they are contained in hair follicles, but can also be found in the hairless areas of the lips, eyelids, penis, labia

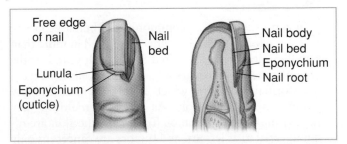

FIGURE 20-2 The fingernail, an appendage of the integument.

minora, and nipples. Sebaceous glands that are found in hair follicles deposit sebum on the hairs and bring it to the skin surface along the hair shaft. At the hairless areas, sebum rises to the surface through ducts. The sebaceous glands of a fetus *in utero* secrete a substance called *vernix caseosa*, a "waxy" or "cheesy" white substance found coating the skin of the newborn baby.

Typically, sebaceous glands can be involved in skin problems such as acne, which is studied and treated by dermatologists. A blocked sebaceous gland can result in a sebaceous cyst.

Sudoriferous (Sweat) Glands

Sudoriferous, or **sweat glands,** occur in nearly all regions of the skin, but are most numerous in the palms and soles. Each gland consists of a tiny tube that originates as a ball-shaped coil in the dermis or subcutaneous layer of the skin. The coiled portion of the gland is closed at its deep end and is lined with sweat-producing cells. Some sweat glands, the "apocrine glands," respond to emotional stress. Apocrine secretions typically have odors, and the glands are considered to be scent glands. They begin to function at puberty and are responsible for some skin regions becoming moist when a person is emotionally upset, frightened, or experiencing pain. They are also active when a person is sexually stimulated. In adults, the apocrine glands are most numerous in the armpits, groin, and the regions around the nipples. They are usually associated with hair follicles. Other sweat glands, the "eccrine glands," are not connected to hair follicles. They function throughout life by responding to elevated body temperature due to environmental heat or physical exercise. These glands are common on the forehead, neck, and back, where they produce profuse sweating on hot days and when a person is physically active. They also are responsible for the moisture that may appear on the palms and soles when a person is emotionally stressed.

Common Disorders Associated with the Integumentary System

Skin is vulnerable to many disorders because it is the most exposed of all the body systems.

Skin Cancer

Skin cancer is the most common of all human cancers, and some form of skin cancer is diagnosed in more than 1 million people in the United States each year. It is the type of cancer that occurs when normal cells undergo a transformation during which they grow and multiply without normal controls. As the cells multiply, they form a mass called a tumor. Tumors of the skin are often referred to as lesions, and tumors are cancerous only if they are malignant. This means that they encroach on and invade neighboring tissues, especially lymph nodes, because of their uncontrolled growth.

Skin cancers are of three major types: basal cell, squamous cell, and melanoma. The vast majority of skin cancers are basal cell carcinomas or squamous cell carcinomas. While malignant, these are unlikely to spread to other parts of the body. They may be locally disfiguring if not treated early. A small but significant number of skin cancers are malignant melanomas. Malignant melanoma is a highly aggressive cancer that tends to spread to other parts of the body. These cancers may be fatal if not treated early. Like many cancers, skin cancers start as precancerous lesions. These precancerous lesions are changes in skin that are not cancer, but could become cancer over time. Health care professionals often refer to these changes as dysplasia. One example of this is a dysplastic neve, or an abnormal mole. These can develop into melanoma over time. Moles are simply growths on the skin. They are very common. Very few moles become cancerous. Dysplastic nevi are not cancer, but they can become cancer. People with dysplastic nevi often have a lot of them, perhaps as many as 100 or more. They are usually irregular in shape, with notched or fading borders, and may be flat or raised, and the surface may be smooth or rough ("pebbly").

Signs and Symptoms

Nonmelanoma skin cancer may appear as a change in the skin, such as a growth, an irritation or sore that does not heal, or a change in a wart or mole. Basal cell carcinoma usually affects the head, neck, back, chest, or shoulders. The nose is the most common site. Signs of basal cell carcinoma can vary and may include skin changes such as a:

- Firm, pearly bump with tiny blood vessels in a spiderlike appearance (telangiectasias)
- Red, tender, flat spot that bleeds easily
- Small, fleshy bump with a smooth, pearly appearance, often with a depressed center
- Smooth, shiny bump that may look like a mole or cyst
- Scar-like patch of skin, especially on the face, that is firm to the touch
- Bump that itches, bleeds, crusts over, and then repeats the cycle and has not healed in 3 weeks
- Change in the size, shape, or color of a wart or mole

Treatment

The goals of treatment for nonmelanoma skin cancer are to remove the entire skin cancer and a margin of skin tissue around the cancer to reduce the chance of recurrence, to preserve nearby skin tissue that is free of cancer, and to minimize scarring after surgery. Treatment for nonmelanoma skin cancer depends on the size

THE CHILD

- *In children, skin conditions can be acute or chronic, local or systemic, and some can be congenital. Age-related skin conditions, include milia (the white pimples occurring in newborns) and acne.*
- *Skin infections in children present as systemic infections with symptoms such as fever and malaise. Because the sebaceous glands do not produce sebum until the child is about 8 to 10 years old, a child's skin is drier and chaps more easily. For that reason, it is important to teach children good hygiene habits at an early age.*

THE OLDER ADULT

- *As a person ages, the papilla grow less dense and the skin becomes looser. There is less collagen and fewer elastic fibers in the upper dermis, and the skin loses its elastic tone, causing wrinkles to occur more easily. The occurrence of premalignant and malignant skin lesions may also increase with aging, especially on the nose, eyelids, and cheeks. Eighty percent of skin cancers found in older adults are basal cell carcinomas.*
- *By age 50, approximately half of adults have some gray hair. The scalp hair continues to thin in men and women as aging progresses, and the hair becomes dry and brittle. The nails may flatten and become more discolored, dry, and brittle.*

and location of the cancer, whether it is basal cell or squamous cell, and the age and overall health of the patient. Because skin cancer usually grows slowly, it often can be detected and successfully treated early in its development. The most common treatment is surgery to destroy or remove the entire skin growth, including a margin of cancer-free tissue around the growth. Most surgical treatments are very effective, with cure rates higher than 90 percent.

Squamous Cell Carcinoma

Squamous cell carcinoma is a malignant tumor that affects the middle layer of the skin. Any change in an existing wart, mole, or other skin lesion, or the development of a new growth that ulcerates and does not heal well, could indicate skin cancer. This type of cancer has a high cure rate if it is treated early, but neglect can allow the cancer to spread, causing great disability or even death. It is important to note that more than 90 percent of skin cancers occur on areas of the skin that are regularly exposed to sunlight or other ultraviolet radiation. This is considered the primary cause of all squamous cell carcinomas. Other risks include genetic predisposition (skin cancers are more common in those who have light-colored skin, blue or green eyes, and blond or red hair), chemical pollution, and overexposure to x-rays or other forms of radiation. Exposure to arsenic, which may be present in some herbicides, presents another risk for development of skin cancers.

Squamous cell cancer is more aggressive than basal cell cancer, but still may be relatively slow growing. It is more likely than basal cell cancer to spread (metastasize) to other locations, including internal organs. Squamous cell cancer is usually painless initially, but may become painful with the development of ulcers that do not heal. This cancer may begin in normal skin; in the skin of a burn, injury, or scar; or at a site of

Patient Education

Skin care is a very important part of hygiene. Patients should be taught that they should moisturize their skin on a daily basis, or more often as necessary. Sunscreen is one of the easiest ways to avoid skin cancer, and teaching patients about using adequate sun protection may be one duty of the medical assistant. Write down the correct sun protection factor prescribed by the physician so that the patient can easily locate the appropriate lotion in the store. Patients should be taught to avoid sunburn as much as possible. Some medications can increase the risk of sunburn, and education for patients who take these medications is extremely important.

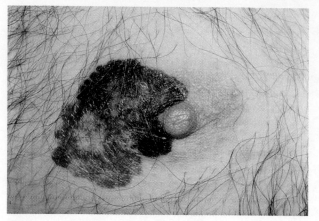

FIGURE 20-3 Melanoma.

chronic inflammation (which may occur with many skin disorders). It most often originates from sun-damaged skin areas, such as actinic keratosis. It usually begins after age 50.

Symptoms include any skin lesion, growth, or bump that is small, firm, reddened, nodular, coned, or flat in shape. Also, if the surface is scaly or crusted and the lesion or growth is located on the face, ears, neck, hands, or arms, there is a good possibility it is a squamous cell carcinoma. Occasionally the growth may occur on the lip, mouth, tongue, or genitals.

The treatment varies with the tumor's size, depth, location, and how much it has spread or metastasized. Surgical removal of the tumor, which may include removal of the skin around the tumor (wide excision), is

often recommended. Microscopic shaving (Mohs' surgery) may remove small tumors. Skin grafting may be needed if wide areas of skin are removed. The tumor may also be reduced in size by radiation treatments. Chemotherapy can be used if surgery and radiation fail, but it is usually minimally effective.

Melanoma

Malignant melanoma is a type of cancer arising from the melanocyte cells of the skin (see Figure 20-3). Melanocytes are cells in the skin that produce a pigment called *melanin*. Malignant melanoma develops when the melanocytes no longer respond to the normal control mechanisms of cellular growth. They may then invade nearby structures or spread to other organs in the body (metastasis), where again they invade and compromise the function of that organ. The primary tumor begins in the skin, often from the melanocytes of a preexisting mole. Once it becomes invasive, it may progress beyond the site of origin to the regional lymph nodes or travel to other organ systems in the body and become systemic in nature. Cancer, as it invades in its place of origin, may also work its way into blood vessels. If this occurs, it provides yet another route for the cancer to spread to other organs of the body. When the cancer spreads elsewhere in the body, it has become systemic in extent and the tumor appearing elsewhere is known as a *metastasis*.

Untreated malignant melanoma follows a classic progression. It begins and grows locally, penetrating vertically. It may be carried via the lymph to the regional nodes, known as regional metastasis. It may go from the lymph to the bloodstream or penetrate blood vessels, allowing it a direct route to go elsewhere in the body. When systemic disease or distant metastases occur, melanoma commonly involves the lung, brain, liver, or occasionally bone. The malignancy causes death when its uncontrolled growth compromises vital organ function.

The predisposing causes to the development of malignant melanoma are environmental and genetic. A small percentage of melanomas arise within burn scar tissue. As of 2003, researchers did not fully understand the relationship between deep burns and an increased risk of skin cancer. Malignant melanomas are usually diagnosed by using the ABCDE rule (see Table 20-1), which is an excellent way of identifying changes of significance in a mole. This includes checking the mole for the following: asymmetry, border irregularity, color variegation, diameter greater than 6 mm (0.24 in.), and elevation above surrounding tissue.

Another summary of important changes in a mole is the Glasgow seven-point scale. The symptoms and signs, which are listed below, can occur anywhere on the skin, including the palms of the hands, soles of the feet, and also the nail beds. In this scheme, change is

TABLE 20-1   The ABCDEs of Melanoma Changes in a Mole

A—Asymmetry	The mole does not have two halves that match each other.
B—Border	The border is ragged, notched, or blurred together.
C—Color	Color is uneven; shades of black, brown, or tan are present; there may be areas of white, red, or blue present.
D—Diameter	There may be a change in size, and the mole is typically greater than 6 mm in diameter.
E—Elevation	The mole sits above the surrounding tissue.

emphasized along with size. Bleeding and sensory changes are relatively late symptoms.

- Change in size
- Change in shape
- Change in color
- Inflammation
- Crusting and bleeding
- Sensory change
- Diameter greater than 7 mm (0.28 in.)

The key to successful treatment of melanoma is early diagnosis. Patients identified with localized, thin, small lesions nearly always survive. For those with advanced lesions, the outcome is poor in spite of progress in systemic therapy.

Acne Vulgaris

Acne vulgaris (acne) is a common skin condition that occurs when oil and dead skin cells clog the skin's pores (see Figure 20-4). These clogs cause blemishes in the skin that are often red and swollen, and it most often affects teens, with more than 85 percent of them developing at least a mild form of this condition. Severe acne can mean hundreds of pimples or sores that can cover the face, neck, chest, and back. While mild acne is merely annoying, severe acne can lead to emotional and physical scars. Most people outgrow acne by the time they are in their 40s and 50s.

Acne develops most often on the face, neck, chest, shoulders, or back and can range from mild to severe. It can last for a few months, many years, or come and go your entire life. In a mild case of acne, only whiteheads and blackheads may be present. At times, these may develop into an infection in the skin pore (pimple). Severe acne can produce hundreds of pimples that cover large areas of skin. Cystic lesions are pimples that are large and deep. These lesions are often painful and can leave scars on your skin. Acne can also lead to low self-esteem and sometimes depression. These conditions need treatment along with the acne.

Treatment for acne depends greatly on whether the person has a mild, moderate, or severe form. Sometimes the health care provider will combine treatments to get the best results and to avoid developing drug resistant bacteria. Treatment could include lotions or gels applied to blemishes or sometimes entire areas of skin, such as the chest or back (topical medications) and oral antibiotics.

Alopecia

Alopecia (see Figure 20-5) is baldness or loss of hair. The most common form is male-pattern baldness (also known as androgenic alopecia), but both women and men can experience hair loss. Alopecia areata is another type of hair loss, involving patches of baldness

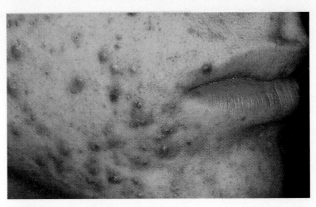

FIGURE 20-4   Acne vulgaris.

that may come and go. It affects about 1 in 100 people, mostly teenagers and young adults. In some cases, hair loss is a side effect of having cancer treatment drugs, but in many cases the hair grows back. Male-pattern baldness is hereditary, which means it runs in families. It usually starts to happen around the late 20s and 30s although this can vary. By the age of 60, most men have some degree of hair loss. It is called male-pattern baldness because it tends to follow a set pattern. The first stage is usually a receding hairline, followed by thinning of the hair on the crown and temples. When these two areas meet in the middle, there is a horseshoe shape of hair around the back and sides of the head. Eventually the person may be completely bald. Women's hair gradually thins with age but they only tend to lose hair from the top of the head. This usually becomes more noticeable after menopause. It is called androgenetic alopecia, or female-pattern hair loss, and also tends to run in families.

Alopecia areata causes patches of baldness that are about the size of a large coin. They usually appear on the scalp but can occur anywhere on the body, including the beard, eyebrows, and eyelashes. There are usually no other symptoms.

If the hair loss is caused by an infection, or other condition such as anemia, it can be treated to prevent

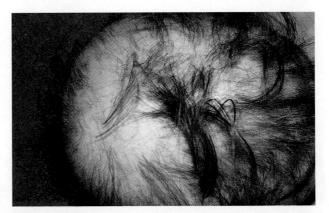

FIGURE 20-5   Alopecia.

further hair loss. In some cases, including after cancer treatment, hair may start to grow again. Drugs are available to treat male-pattern and female-pattern baldness but they do not work for everyone and the effects are not long lasting. There are also lotions that can be rubbed on the scalp, although these do not work for everyone nor do they have long-lasting effects. Shampoos and formulas are available for improving circulation to the scalp, and some people try herbal treatments. Unfortunately, hair loss can lead to problems with confidence and self-esteem.

Cellulitis

Cellulitis is an acute spreading bacterial infection below the surface of the skin characterized by redness (erythema), warmth, swelling, and pain. It can also cause fever, chills, and enlarged lymph nodes (see Figure 20-6). Cellulitis commonly appears in areas where there is a break in the skin from an abrasion, a

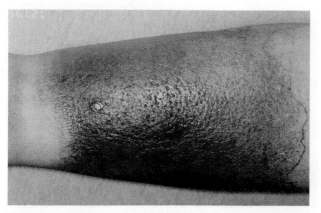

FIGURE 20-6 Cellulitis.

cut, or a skin ulcer. It can also be due to local trauma, such as an animal bite. Only rarely is cellulitis due to the bacteremic spread of infection, that is, bacteria arriving from a distant source via the bloodstream.

Risk factors for cellulitis include diabetes and impairment of the immune system (from, for example, HIV/AIDS or immunosuppressant drugs). Cellulitis is not contagious because it is an infection of the skin's deeper layers, the dermis and subcutaneous tissue, and the skin's top layer (the epidermis) provides a cover over the infection.

The main bacterium that causes cellulitis is staph (*Staphylococcus aureus*), and strep (Group A Streptococcus) is the next most common cause. It can be caused by many other types of bacteria. In children under six, H. flu (*Haemophilus influenzae*) can cause cellulitis, especially on the face, arms, and upper torso. Cellulitis from a dog or cat bite or scratch may be caused by the *Pasteurella multocida* bacteria. Cellulitis after an injury from a saltwater fish or shellfish can be due to *Erysipelothrix rhusiopathiae*. These same bacteria can also cause cellulitis after a skin injury on the farm, especially while working with pigs or poultry.

Antibiotics such as derivatives of penicillin that are most effective against the staph germ are used to treat cellulitis. If other bacteria, as determined by culture tests, turn out to be the cause, or if patients are allergic to penicillin, other appropriate antibiotics are substituted.

Contact Dermatitis

Contact dermatitis is an allergic reaction of the skin caused by irritating substances coming in contact with it. Most frequently, the obvious response is red, irritated skin, but vesicles (small blisters) and rash may also result. Oftentimes, the skin itches, and pain may also be present. Serious allergic reactions may result in urticaria, or hives.

Causes of contact dermatitis often include exposures to poison ivy, poison oak, nickel (especially on jewelry or jean snaps), lotions, detergents, or other chemicals. Most of these allergic reactions are treated with antihistamines (antiallergy medicines) and topical corticosteroid creams to reduce the inflammation. Widespread or excessively uncomfortable reactions may also be treated with systemic corticosteroids (oral medications) that help to further decrease the inflammation caused by the allergic reaction.

Decubitus Ulcer

Decubitus ulcers, also called pressure sores or bedsores, refer to an area of skin and tissue that breaks down. These typically happen when constant pressure is maintained on a specific area of the skin, such as on the coccyx in a patient lying in bed for too long a period of time without being repositioned. The constant pressure on the area decreases the blood supply, causing death to the affected tissue. The most common location for a decubitus ulcer to occur is over bony prominences, such as the coccyx, hips, heels, ankles, shoulders, back, and the back of the head.

According to the National Pressure Ulcer Advisory Panel, the four stages of decubitus ulcers include:

- Stage I: A reddened area on the skin that does not blanch (turn white) when pressed. This is an early stage, and if the pressure is kept off of the area, healing may occur.

- Stage II: The skin has a blister or an open sore. The area around the site may be red and irritated.

- Stage III: The skin breakdown looks like a crater with damage to the tissue below the skin.

- Stage IV: The wound becomes so deep that there is damage to the tissues beneath the initial ulcer, including damage to bone and muscle.

Treatment of decubitus ulcers starts with relieving the pressure. Special pillows, cushions, and sheepskin are frequently used to ensure that there is no pressure on the area. Regular repositioning must be routine. Decubitus ulcers are typically debrided, that is, cleaned of all the toxins and then medicated and covered with special gauze dressings to help in healing. Protecting the wound from any further injury is essential in order to protect the patient from infections and other serious complications and systemic sepsis.

Eczema

Eczema, called atopic dermatitis, is a chronic skin condition caused by an allergic-type reaction on the skin. It is characterized by scaling, itching, and rashes. Typically, there is a family history of allergies and eczema, and the patient may also suffer from other allergic conditions. Eczema is most common in infants, and about half of the cases disappear by age 3. Adults may also suffer from chronic episodes of eczema.

Treatment of eczema often depends on the stage, or appearance, of the lesions that have formed on the skin. These lesions range from dry and scaly, to "weeping." Weeping lesions are treated with mild soaps and dressings, whereas severe cases and dry scaly lesions may be treated with mild, anti-itch lotions or low-potency topical corticosteroids. Chronically thickened areas may be treated with ointments or creams that contain tar compounds, medium- to high-potency corticosteroids, and lubricating ingredients. Very severe cases may require systemic corticosteroids and topical immunomodulators (TIMs).

Folliculitis

Folliculitis is an inflammation or infection of hair follicles. While folliculitis can occur anywhere there is body hair, it most often appears in areas that become irritated by shaving, the rubbing of clothes, or where

Cultural Considerations

In many cultures, modesty is very important, and being sure that a patient is properly draped is a major consideration. The medical assistant can always ask the patient if there is anything that the medical team needs to know regarding special draping and who needs to be present during the exam. Always be very respectful of the patient's rights and need for modesty.

Some cultures may use special tattoos or marks as part of their heritage, and it is important to be respectful of these marks, because they may have special meaning to the patient. Being judgmental about such adornments is never acceptable. If a patient has body piercings, they may require special attention due to the potential for infection. Always remember to note any swelling or redness around a piercing site, and report it to the physician in a professional manner without doing or saying anything to embarrass the patient.

follicles and pores are blocked by oils and dirt. Common sites of folliculitis include the face, the scalp, under the arms, and on the legs.

The appearance of folliculitis may vary from person to person, but generally the symptoms include a reddened rash; raised, red, often pus-filled lesions around hair follicles (pimples); pimples that eventually crust over and occur in areas of a high concentration of hair follicles such as the face (especially in the area of men's beards and moustaches), under the arms, on the scalp, and in the groin; and itching at the site of the rash and pimples.

Diagnosis of folliculitis is generally made by examining the appearance of the skin. On occasion, a skin biopsy will be done, not to diagnosis the folliculitis but to rule out other types of skin lesions. A culture of the lesion may show which bacteria or fungus has caused the infection.

Treatment for folliculitis generally involves taking steps to minimize damage to hair follicles by avoiding clothing that will rub against the skin, damaging hair follicles, shaving with an electric razor as opposed to a blade razor, and keeping the skin clean using soap and water and skin cleansers. When folliculitis is present, treatment usually includes the application of antibiotic ointments.

Herpes Simplex

Herpes simplex is an infection that primarily affects the mouth or genital area. There are two different strains of herpes simplex viruses:

- Herpes simplex virus type 1 (HSV-1) is usually associated with infections of the lips, mouth, and face. It is the most common herpes simplex virus and is usually acquired in childhood. HSV-1 often causes lesions inside the mouth such as cold sores (fever blisters) and is transmitted by contact with infected saliva. By adulthood, up to 90 percent of individuals will have antibodies to HSV-1.

- Herpes simplex virus type 2 (HSV-2) is sexually transmitted. Symptoms include genital ulcers or sores. In addition to oral and genital lesions, the virus can also lead to complications such as meningoencephalitis (infection of the lining of the brain and the brain itself) or cause an infection of the eye, in particular the conjunctiva and cornea. However, some people have HSV-2 but do not display symptoms. Up to 30 percent of U.S. adults have antibodies against HSV-2. Cross-infection of type 1 and 2 viruses may occur from oral–genital contact.

A finger infection, called herpetic whitlow, is another form of herpes infection. It usually affects health care providers who are exposed to oral secretions during procedures. Sometimes, young children contract the disease.

A herpes virus can infect the fetus and cause congenital abnormalities. It may also be transmitted to a newborn during vaginal delivery in mothers infected with herpes viruses, particularly if the mother has active infection at the time. It can also be transmitted even in the absence of symptoms or visible lesions. Symptoms of herpes simplex include:

- Mouth sores
- Genital lesions—may be preceded by burning or tingling sensation
- Blisters or ulcers—most frequent on the mouth, lips, and gums or genitalia
- Fever blisters
- Fever—may be present especially during the first episode
- Enlargement of lymph nodes in the neck or groin

Some cases of herpes simplex are relatively mild and may not require treatment. In severe or prolonged cases, however, or in individuals who are immunosuppressed or who have frequent recurrences, antiviral medications such as acyclovir may be used. In individuals with more than six recurrences of genital herpes per year, chronic antiviral medications may be offered to reduce recurrences.

Herpes Zoster

Herpes zoster, which is also known as *shingles*, is a viral infection that causes a painful rash. It is caused by the varicella-zoster virus, the same virus that causes chickenpox. After you've had chickenpox, the virus lies dormant in your nerves. Years later, the virus may reactivate as shingles. Although painful, typically this condition isn't a serious one. Sometimes, however, the rash can lead to a debilitating complication called postherpetic neuralgia. This condition causes the skin to remain painful and sensitive to touch for months or even years after the rash clears up. Early treatment can help shorten a shingles infection and reduce the risk of complications.

The signs and symptoms of herpes zoster may include pain, burning, tingling, itching, numbness or extreme sensitivity in a certain part of the body, a red rash with fluid-filled blisters that begins a few days after the pain, fever, headache, chills, and an upset stomach. Typically, the rash occurs on only one side of the body. It often appears as a band of blisters that wraps from the middle of your back around one side of your chest to your breastbone, following the path of the nerve where the virus had been dormant.

Although the herpes zoster rash may resemble chickenpox, the virus typically causes more pain and less itching the second time around. And while an episode of herpes zoster usually heals on its own within a few weeks, prompt treatment can ease pain, speed healing, and reduce the risk of complications. Complications are more likely for people who have weak immune systems and people older than age 65.

Doctors typically prescribe oral antiviral medications, preferably beginning within 48 to 72 hours of the first sign of the rash. Sometimes, antiviral medications are combined with corticosteroids to reduce swelling and pain. If the pain is severe—particularly if the patient develops postherpetic neuralgia—the health care provider may prescribe oral analgesics or a skin patch that contains a pain-relieving medication.

Impetigo

Impetigo is a skin infection caused by bacteria. It is most common in children and is contagious. Impetigo forms round, crusted (see Figure 20-7), oozing spots that grow larger day by day. It may affect the skin anywhere on the body but commonly occurs in the area around the nose and mouth. Impetigo is characterized by blisters that may burst, ooze fluid, and develop a honey-colored crust. Impetigo may itch, and it can be spread by scratching. The infection usually spreads along the edges of an affected area, but may also spread to other areas of the body. While the bacteria causing impetigo may have been caught from someone else with impetigo or boils, impetigo usually begins out of the blue without any apparent source of infection.

Antibiotics taken by mouth usually clear up impetigo in 4 or 5 days.

Pediculosis

Pediculosis is an infestation of the hairy parts of the body or clothing with the eggs, larvae or adults of lice (see Figure 20-8). The crawling stages of this insect feed on human blood, which can result in severe itching. Head lice are usually located on the scalp, crab lice in the pubic area, and body lice along seams of clothing. Body lice travel to the skin to feed and return back to the clothing. Anyone may become louse infested under suitable conditions of exposure. Pediculosis is easily transmitted from person to person during direct contact. Head lice infestations are frequently found in school settings or institutions. Crab lice infestations can be found among sexually active individuals. Body lice infestation can be found in people living in crowded, unsanitary conditions where clothing is infrequently changed or laundered.

For both head lice and body lice, transmission can occur during direct contact with an infested individual. Sharing of clothing and combs or brushes may also result in transmission of these insects. Although other means are possible, crab lice are most often transmitted through sexual contact. Usually, the first indication of an infestation is itching or scratching in the area of the body where the lice feed. Scratching at the back of the head or around the ears should lead to an examination for head louse eggs (nits) on the hair. Itching around the genital area should lead to an examination for crab lice or their eggs. (See Legal and Ethical Issues for a discussion of a patient's right to privacy during an examination.) Scratching can be sufficiently intense to result in secondary bacterial infection in these areas.

Medicated shampoos or cream rinses containing pyrethrins are preferred for treating people with head lice. Lindane-based shampoos are also available but not recommended for infants, young children, and pregnant or lactating women. Products containing pyrethrins are available over the counter, but those containing lindane are available only through a physician's prescription. Retreatment after 7 to 10 days is recommended to ensure that no eggs have survived. Nit combs are available to help remove nits from hair. Dose and duration of shampoo treatment should be followed carefully according to label instructions.

Psoriasis

Psoriasis is characterized by frequent episodes of redness, itching, and thick, dry scales on the skin. It is a common condition that affects approximately 3 millions Americans, beginning most commonly between the ages of 1 and 35. It is believed to be genetic, but

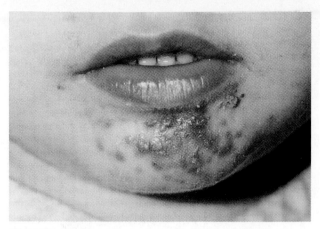

FIGURE 20-7 Impetigo.

also has characteristics related to autoimmune disorders. Typically, the movement of new skins from the lower layers of the skin to the top takes about a month. In psoriasis, however, the cells move in a few days, causing a buildup of dead skin cells and the formation of thick scales. The condition is most commonly seen on the trunk, elbows, knees, scalp, skin folds, and fingernails, but can appear on any area of the skin.

The onset of psoriasis can be gradual or abrupt. Typically, it appears for a time, then goes away for a while. Medications, viral or bacterial infections, excessive alcohol consumption, obesity, lack of sunlight, sunburn, stress, general poor health, cold climate, and frequent skin friction are associated causes of flares. Psoriasis is not contagious.

The treatment of psoriasis depends on the extent and severity of the disorder. Lesions can be serious and extensive enough to require hospitalization. When the case is severe and widespread, large quantities of fluid can be lost, causing dehydration and severe secondary infections that can be serious. Treatment involves analgesics, sedation, intravenous fluids, retinoids (such as Retin-A) and antibiotics. Mild cases are treated at

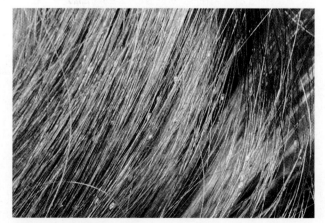

FIGURE 20-8 Pediculosis capitis.

home with topical medications such as prescription or nonprescription dandruff shampoos, cortisone or other corticosteroids, and antifungal medications.

Rosacea

Rosacea is a chronic and potentially life-disruptive disorder primarily of the facial skin, often characterized by flare-ups and remissions. It typically begins after age 30 as a redness on the cheeks, nose, chin, or fore-

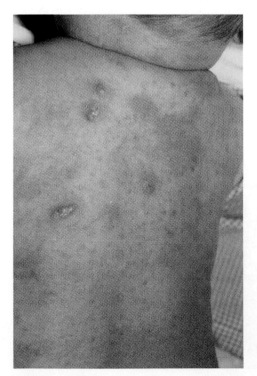

FIGURE 20-9   Scabies.

head that may come and go. In some cases, rosacea may also occur on the neck, chest, scalp, or ears. Symptoms of rosacea can include redness on the cheeks, nose, chin, or forehead, small visible blood vessels on the face, bumps or pimples on the face, and watery or irritated eyes. Over time, the redness becomes ruddier and more persistent. Left untreated, bumps and pimples often develop, and in severe cases the nose may grow swollen and bumpy from excess tissue. This condition affects an estimated 14 million Americans— and most of them don't know they have it.

Although rosacea can affect all segments of the population, individuals with fair skin who tend to flush or blush easily are believed to be at greatest risk. The disease is more frequently diagnosed in women, but more severe symptoms tend to be seen in men— perhaps because they often delay seeking medical help until the disorder reaches advanced stages.

Although there is no cure for rosacea and the cause is unknown, medical therapy is available to control or reverse its signs and symptoms. Individuals who suspect they may have rosacea are urged to see a dermatologist or other knowledgeable physician for diagnosis and appropriate treatment.

Scabies

Scabies is a contagious disorder of the skin (see Figure 20-9) caused by very small, wingless insects or mites called the human itch mite or scabies itch mite *Sarcoptes scabiei* var. *hominis* (Hering). The female insect burrows into the skin where she lays one to three eggs daily. A very small, hard-to-see, zigzag blister usually marks the trail of the insect as she lays her eggs. Other more obvious symptoms are an intense itching (especially at night) and a red rash that can occur at the area that has been scratched. The most common locations for scabies are on the sides of fingers, between the fingers, on the backs of the hands, on the wrists, heels, elbows, armpits, and inner thighs, and around the waist (belt line). If untreated, the female will continue to lay eggs for about 5 weeks. The eggs hatch and the new mites begin the cycle all over again. The mites themselves are too small to be seen without magnification. One of the biggest problems with scabies always has been misdiagnosis. Scabies is spread by personal contact, such as by shaking hands or sleeping together or by close contact with infected articles such as clothing, bedding, or towels. It is usually found where people are crowded together or have frequent contact, and is most common among schoolchildren, families, roommates, and sexual partners. Scabies can be spread by the insect itself or by the egg. Prompt action is required to rid a person of the insects and eggs. Sulfur has been used (6 to 10 percent in lotion or cream) since Roman times as a scabicide; however, some patients may be allergic to sulfur.

Warts

Warts are a type of infection caused by viruses in the human papillomavirus (HPV) family. There are at least 60 types of HPV viruses. Warts can grow on all parts of the body, including the skin, the inside of the mouth, the genitals, and the rectal area. Warts located on the skin can be passed from one person to another when that person touches the warts. It is also possible to get warts from using towels or other objects that were used by a person who has warts. Often warts disappear on their own, although it may take many months, or even years, for the warts to go away; sometimes they never disappear.

Burns

Burns occur when heat, chemicals, or electricity destroys a portion of the skin. Burns are classified as either partial thickness or full thickness. Partial-thickness burns, previously known as first- and second-degree burns, destroy only a portion of the skin. These burns can be painful, may blister, and have a chance of recovery, depending on the amount of skin burned and the depth of the burn. Examples of partial-thickness burns include sunburn, scalds, and chemical burns. Full-thickness burns, previously called third-degree burns, destroy the entirety of the skin in a specified location. These burns are usually not initially painful, because the nerve endings in the skin have also been destroyed. Full-thickness burns are typically caused by direct exposure to fire. Recovery from full-thickness burns is possible, but the chances tend to decrease significantly if the burn covers a large area. The usual cause of death from burns is by infections that set in as the skin can no longer perform its protective function.

The extent of the body surface areas affected and the severity of a burn are often the most important factors in predicting the risk of death resulting from burn injuries. Several factors are used to determine the severity of this injury, including the patient's age, size and depth of the burn, and the location of the burn.

Professionalism

While in a professional environment, courtesy and manners are very essential to the medical assistant's practice. Unless instructed to do otherwise, always call adult patients (especially the elderly) by Mr., Mrs., or Ms. Using the phrases "please" and "thank you" also helps to establish you as a courteous, caring professional. Never address any patient by the endearments of "honey" or "sweetie." Although some individuals may find this cute, many others will find the phraseology demeaning. Convey an attitude of being caring, professional, and sincere. Speak in full sentences, using complete words and avoiding slang, and your patients will know that you truly are a professional.

SUMMARY

The skin provides many protective functions for the body, including preventing infection and preserving the internal environment. Skin also helps to promote optimum temperature levels. Disorders of the skin can be uncomfortable, but most can be treated without too much discomfort.

Chapter Review

COMPETENCY REVIEW

1. Define and spell the terms to learn for this chapter.
2. What is the primary organ of the integumentary system?
3. Name the four accessory structures of the integumentary system.
4. Name the four functions of the skin.
5. Name the two layers of the skin.
6. What is the protein substance in the dead cells of the epidermis that serves as a protective mechanism?
7. Name the four layers of the epidermis.

8. What is the name of the cresecent-shaped area of the nail?
9. What is the name of the cell that gives color to the skin?
10. What are the ABCDEs of skin cancer?

PREPARING FOR THE CERTIFICATION EXAM

1. The black pigment that gives skin its color is
   A. basal layer
   B. keratin
   C. melanin
   D. cyano
   E. chloro

2. The dermis layer of the skin contains
   A. keratin
   B. melanin
   C. stratified squamous epithelium
   D. blood vessels
   E. basal layer

3. The medical term for a dangerous form of skin cancer caused by an overgrowth of melanin-producing cells is
   A. Kaposi's sarcoma
   B. malignant melanoma
   C. basal cell carcinoma
   D. squamous cell carcinoma
   E. lupus erythematosus

4. Urticaria is the medical term for
   A. ringworm
   B. hives
   C. verruca
   D. furuncle
   E. scabies

5. A chronic inflammatory condition consisting of crusty, silvery papules forming patches with pink, circular borders is called
   A. eczema
   B. psoriasis
   C. cellulitis
   D. scleroderma
   E. neoplasm

6. Which is not a function of the skin?
   A. protection
   B. sensation
   C. regulation
   D. germination
   E. secretion

7. What type of decubitus is a red place over a bony prominence that does not blanch?
   A. stage I
   B. stage II
   C. stage III
   D. stage IV
   E. This is not a decubitus.

8. What kind of burn destroys all the layers of skin?
   A. chemical
   B. second degree
   C. partial thickness
   D. full thickness
   E. electrical

9. What is the name of a common skin condition that occurs when oil and dead skin cells clog the skin pores?
   A. acne vulgaris
   B. contact dermatitis
   C. eczema
   D. psoriasis
   E. pediculosis

10. What is another medical term for shingles?
    A. impetigo
    B. pediculosis
    C. herpes zoster
    D. herpes simplex
    E. psoriasis

CRITICAL THINKING

1. If the patient had been aware of poison ivy in her environment, what are three precautions that she could have followed to either decrease or prevent her exposure to the poison ivy?

2. Why was the patient given topical steroids for her poison ivy rash?

INTERNET ACTIVITY

Several organizations have been established to help in the prevention and treatment of diseases affecting the integumentary system. Perform an Internet search to learn more about these organizations and what each provides to people afflicted with specific skin disorders.

MediaLink   More on the integumentary system, including interactive resources, can be found on the Student CD-ROM accompanying this textbook.

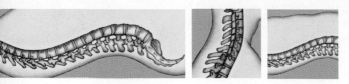

Medical Assistant Role Delineation Chart

HIGHLIGHT indicates material covered in this chapter.

ADMINISTRATIVE

Administrative Procedures

- Perform basic administrative medical assisting functions
- Schedule, coordinate and monitor appointments
- Schedule inpatient/outpatient admissions and procedures
- Understand and apply third-party guidelines
- Obtain reimbursement through accurate claims submission
- Monitor third-party reimbursement
- Understand and adhere to managed care policies and procedures
- *Negotiate managed care contracts*

- Manage accounts receivable
- *Manage accounts payable*
- *Process payroll*
- *Document and maintain accounting and banking records*
- *Develop and maintain fee schedules*
- *Manage renewals of business and professional insurance policies*
- *Manage personnel benefits and maintain records*
- *Perform marketing, financial, and strategic planning*

Practice Finances

- Perform procedural and diagnostic coding
- Apply bookkeeping principles

CLINICAL

Fundamental Principles

- Apply principles of aseptic technique and infection control
- Comply with quality assurance practices
- Screen and follow up patient test results

Diagnostic Orders

- Collect and process specimens
- Perform diagnostic tests

Patient Care

- Adhere to established patient screening procedures
- Obtain patient history and vital signs
- Prepare and maintain examination and treatment areas
- Prepare patient for examinations, procedures and treatments

- <mark>Assist with examinations, procedures and treatments</mark>
- Prepare and administer medications and immunizations
- Maintain medication and immunization records
- Recognize and respond to emergencies
- Coordinate patient care information with other health care providers
- Initiate IV and administer IV medications with appropriate training and as permitted by state law

GENERAL

Professionalism

- <mark>Display a professional manner and image</mark>
- Demonstrate initiative and responsibility
- Work as a member of the health care team
- Prioritize and perform multiple tasks
- Adapt to change
- Promote the CMA credential
- Enhance skills through continuing education
- <mark>Treat all patients with compassion and empathy</mark>
- Promote the practice through positive public relations

Communication Skills

- <mark>Recognize and respect cultural diversity</mark>
- <mark>Adapt communications to individual's ability to understand</mark>
- Use professional telephone technique

- Recognize and respond effectively to verbal, nonverbal, and written communications
- Use medical terminology appropriately
- Utilize electronic technology to receive, organize, prioritize and transmit information
- Serve as liaison

Legal Concepts

- <mark>Perform within legal and ethical boundaries</mark>
- Prepare and maintain medical records
- Document accurately
- Follow employer's established policies dealing with the health care contract
- Implement and maintain federal and state health care legislation and regulations
- Comply with established risk management and safety procedures
- Recognize professional credentialing criteria
- *Develop and maintain personnel, policy and procedure manuals*

Instruction

- <mark>Instruct individuals according to their needs</mark>
- Explain office policies and procedures
- <mark>Teach methods of health promotion and disease prevention</mark>
- Locate community resources and disseminate information
- *Develop educational materials*
- *Conduct continuing education activities*

Operational Functions

- Perform inventory of supplies and equipment
- Perform routine maintenance of administrative and clinical equipment
- Apply computer techniques to support office operations
- *Perform personnel management functions*
- *Negotiate leases and prices for equipment and supply contracts*

- *Denotes advanced skills.*

SOURCE: Reprinted by permission of the American Association of Medical Assistants from the AAMA Role Delineation Study: Occupational Analysis of the Medical Assisting Profession.

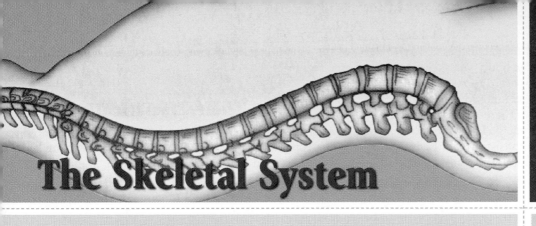

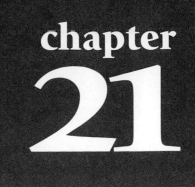

chapter 21

The Skeletal System

Learning Objectives

After completing this chapter, you should be able to:

- Define and spell the terms to learn for this chapter.
- Describe the skeletal system of the body.
- Explain various types of body movement.
- Discuss the vertebral column and explain its function.
- Identify abnormal curvatures of the spine.
- Discuss the male and female pelvis and explain the differences between them.
- List and explain common disorders of the skeletal system.
- Identify various types of fractures.

Terms to Learn

abduction	diaphysis	medullary canal
adduction	diarthrotic joint	osteoarthritis
amphiarthrotic joint	dislocation	osteoporosis
appendicular skeleton	dorsiflexion	periosteum
arthritis	endosteum	pronation
articulation	epiphysis	protraction
axial skeleton	eversion	retraction
bursitis	extension	rheumatoid arthritis
cancellous (spongy) bone	flexion	rotation
	gout	supination
circumduction	inversion	synarthrotic joint
compact bone		

Case Study

JOSEPHINE IS A 62-YEAR-OLD FEMALE seen by Dr. Penningworth for a chief complaint of constant back pain, the development of a humpback, and loss of height. She is postmenopausal, has been a two-pack-a-day smoker for 45 years and drinks three beers a day. She also has a history of asthma and has regularly taken steroids in the past. She has broken her hip once and her wrist once. Dr. Penningworth diagnosed Josephine as having osteoporosis and kyphosis. He prescribed increased calcium, vitamin D, and Fosamax. He also prescribed physical therapy to develop a home exercise program focusing on weight-bearing exercises.

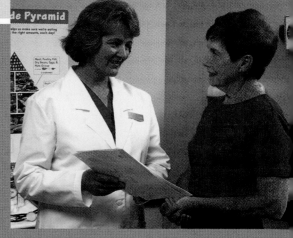

he skeletal system makes up the framework of the body. The skeletal system has 206 bones. The rest of the skeletal system is composed of cartilage and ligaments. There are two different divisions of the skeletal system: the **axial skeleton**, consisting of 80 bones from the axis of the body, including the skull and vertebral system, and the **appendicular skeleton**, which consists of the remaining 126 bones, including the extremities (see Figure 21-1).

Bones and Their Classification

The primary organs of the skeletal system are the bones, which consist of 50 percent water and 50 percent solid matter. The solid matter, or osseous tissue, is made of calcified, rigid tissue. Bones are classified according

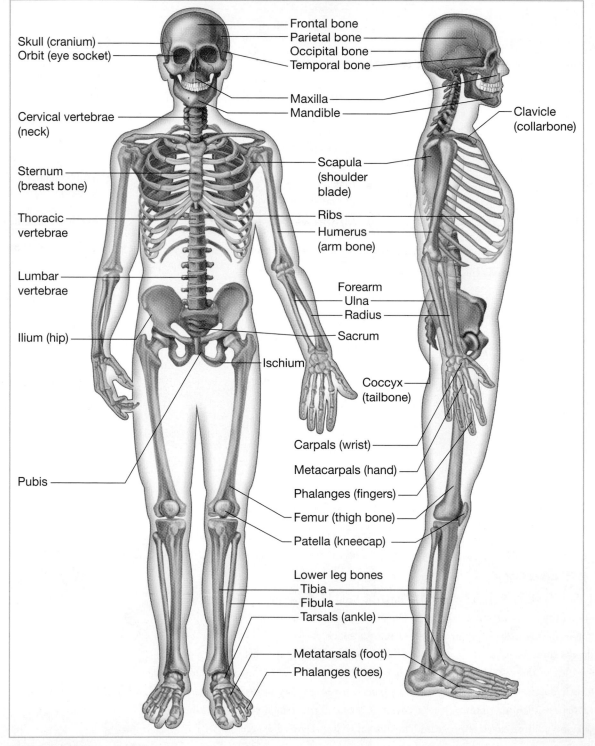

FIGURE 21-1   The human skeleton.

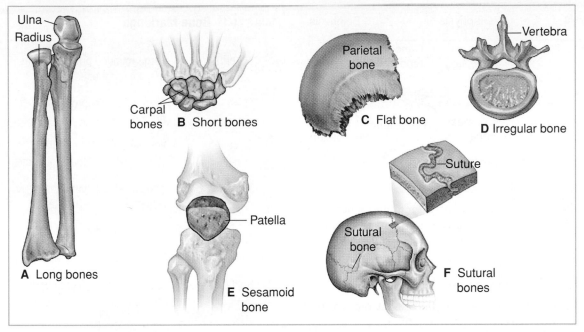

FIGURE 21-2 Classification of bones by shape.

to shape (see Figure 21-2). The six common shapes of bones are long, short, flat, irregular, sesamoid, and sutural (wormian) bones.

Functions of Bones

The bones of the skeleton have six main functions:

- Providing shape, support, and the framework of the body
- Providing protection for the body's internal organs
- Serving as a storage place for mineral salts, calcium, and phosphorus
- Playing an important role in the formation of blood cells as hemopoiesis takes place in the bone marrow
- Providing an area for the attachment of skeletal muscle
- Helping to make movement possible through articulation

Lifespan

Considerations

THE CHILD

- Bones develop from cartilage. Babies are born with a large amount of cartilage and more bones than adults. These bones eventually fuse together to form the normal number of adult bones. Bone tissue begins to develop at the center of the cartilage, and blood vessels carry nutrients to the developing bone. As more bone tissue is formed, the bones grow longer. Eventually, the center of the bone is fully formed.
- A baby's bones are soft, but they gradually become harder as more minerals are deposited. This hardening process is called ossification.
- As a child grows, new bone tissue is made between the head of the bone and its shaft in special areas called growth plates or growth zones. This is how children grow taller.

THE OLDER ADULT

- Women build bone until about age 35 and then begin to lose about 1 percent of their bone mass annually. Men start losing bone mass approximately 10 to 20 years later. During the aging process, most of the skeletal system changes are a result of changes in connective tissue. Most bone loss is due to the loss of bone mineral content, especially calcium salts later in life. The calcium salts are deposited in the bone matrix and the cartilage becomes hard and brittle.
- As individuals age, they begin to have less joint movement, thus an increase in joint diseases, such as arthritis, begins to occur.
- Because of impaired functioning of the osteoblasts, which are the cells present in the bones, in the older adult, bone healing is slower than in children.

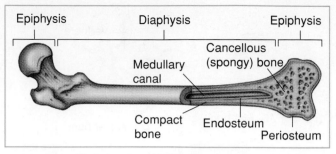

FIGURE 21-3 The features found in a long bone.

Structure of a Long Bone

Long bones, such as the tibia, femur, humerus, or radius, have most of the features found in all bones (see Figure 21-3). These features include the following:

- **Epiphysis**—the ends of a developing bone
- **Diaphysis**—the shaft of the long bone
- **Periosteum**—membrane that forms the covering of bones, except at their articular surfaces
- **Compact bone**—the dense, hard layer of bone tissue
- **Medullary canal**—the narrow space or cavity throughout the length of the diaphysis. The medullary canal contains yellow bone marrow, which is made of fat cells
- **Endosteum**—the tough, connective tissue membrane lining the medullary canal and containing the bone marrow
- **Cancellous or spongy bone**—the reticular tissue that makes up most of the volume of bone. The spongy bone contains red bone marrow, which manufactures most of the red blood cells found in the body and is found in the long bone.

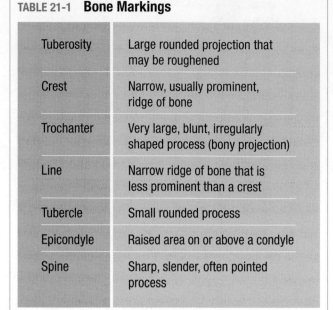

TABLE 21-1	**Bone Markings**
Tuberosity	Large rounded projection that may be roughened
Crest	Narrow, usually prominent, ridge of bone
Trochanter	Very large, blunt, irregularly shaped process (bony projection)
Line	Narrow ridge of bone that is less prominent than a crest
Tubercle	Small rounded process
Epicondyle	Raised area on or above a condyle
Spine	Sharp, slender, often pointed process

See Lifestyle Considerations for information about the skeletal systems of children and older adults.

Bone Markings

The markings of bones are used to indicate the position of different structural features of the bones. These features mark the attachment of tendons and ligaments to muscles, joining of bones, and as passageways for blood vessels and nerves (see Table 21-1).

Joints and Movement

A joint, which is also called an **articulation**, is located at the place where two bones connect (see Figure 21-4). The positioning of the bones at the joint determines the type of movement that the joint performs. Because of this, joints are always classified according to the type of movement they provide. A joint that produces no movement is called a **synarthrotic joint**. While the bones may actually touch, there is no joint cavity. An example of a synarthrosis is the bones in the cranium. **Amphiarthrotic joints** permit very slight movement. An example of this joint is the vertebrae. **Diarthrotic joints** allow for free movement in a variety of directions. Examples of this type of joint are the elbow, wrist, hip, and knee.

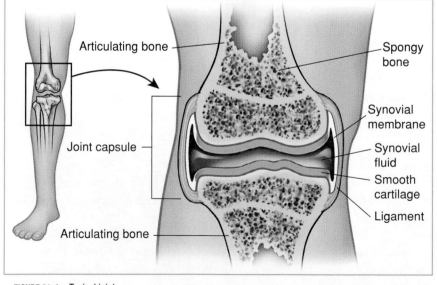

FIGURE 21-4 Typical joint.

Professionalism

The mark of a professional is not being afraid to learn more. Each team member, from the physician on through the entire staff, should continue to ask questions, research answers, and learn from the experiences each day provides. Asking questions is the most important method of learning, along with continuing education programs, reading journals, and attending medical conferences. By learning and keeping current with medical information, the medical assistant can assist the medical office to continue to provide high quality-medical care for all patients.

The diarthrotic joint allows for several types of body movement. These movements, which can be seen in Figure 21-5, include the following:

- **Abduction**—movement of a body part *away* from the midline
- **Adduction**—movement of a body part *toward* the midline
- **Circumduction**—the process of moving a body part in a circular motion
- **Dorsiflexion**—the process of bending a body part backward
- **Eversion**—the process of turning outward
- **Extension**—the process of straightening a flexed limb
- **Flexion**—the process of bending (or curving) the spine
- **Inversion**—the process of turning inward
- **Pronation**—the process of lying prone or face down; the process of turning the hand so that the palm points downward
- **Protraction**—the process of moving a body part forward
- **Retraction**—the process of moving a body part backward
- **Rotation**—the process of moving a body part around a central axis
- **Supination**—the process of lying supine or face upward; also the process of turning the palm or foot upward

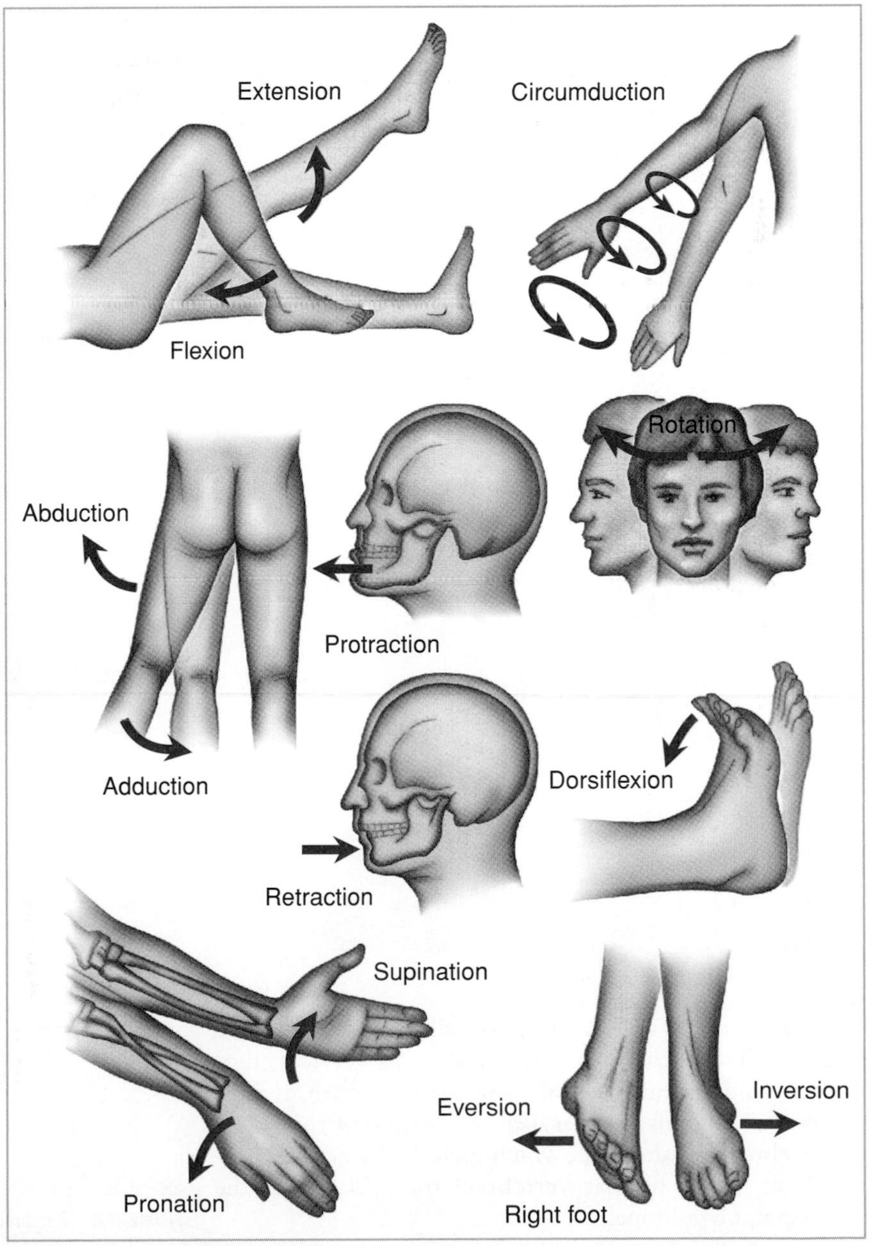

FIGURE 21-5 Types of body movements.

The Axial Skeleton

The axial skeleton is the central portion of the skeleton (see Figure 21-6). It consists of the skull, the sternum, the ribs, the vertebrae, the sacrum, and the coccyx. Twenty-two bones form the skull, 8 of which are located in the cranium and 14 that form the face (see Figure 21-7).

The vertebral column, which houses the spinal cord, consists of a series of vertebrae that are connected in

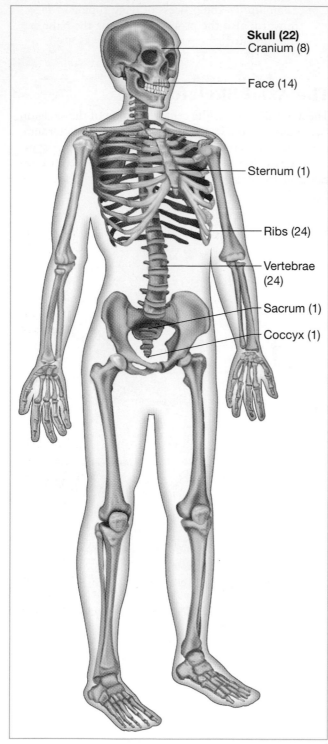

FIGURE 21-6   The axial skeleton.

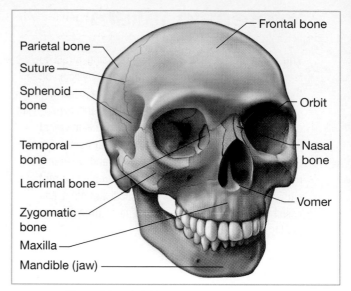

FIGURE 21-7   The cranial and facial bones.

The bones of the rib cage, which are also part of the axial skeleton and which can be seen in Figure 21-9, serve as protection for the vital organs, such as the heart and lungs. There are a total of 12 pairs of ribs.

such a way as to form four spinal curves (see Figure 21-8). These curves are referred to as cervical, thoracic, lumbar, and sacral. The vertebrae are divided into five regions: the cervical, consisting of the first 7 vertebrae; the thoracic, which include the next 12 vertebrae; the 5 lumbar vertebrae; the sacral, and the coccyx, or tailbone.

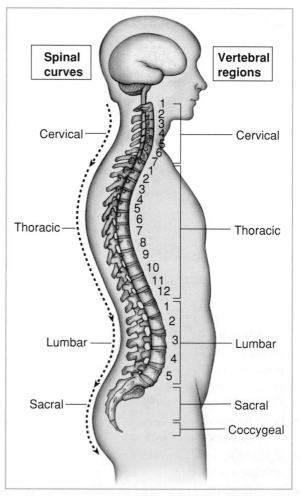

FIGURE 21-8   Vertebral regions showing the four spinal curves.

On the posterior, or back side, the ribs articulate with the thoracic vertebrae. Anteriorly, or in front, 10 pair of ribs articulate with the sternum, which consists of the manubrium, body, and xiphoid process. Two pairs of ribs are called the floating ribs because they are attached only to the spinal vertebrae. There are three pairs of false ribs. They are called false because their cartilages do not reach the sternum directly. Instead, the cartilages of the three false ribs, which are located above the floating ribs, join the cartilages attached to the seven pairs of true ribs above. The true ribs attach both to the sternum and to the spinal vertebrae, while the false and the floating ribs have no cartilaginous attachments to the sternum at all. The three pair of false ribs are joined together on the anterior side of the body with the costal cartilage.

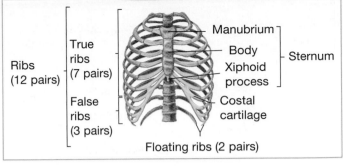

FIGURE 21-9   The rib cage.

The Appendicular Skeleton

The appendicular skeleton, which is responsible for body movement, consists of the upper and lower extremities, the pectoral girdle, and the pelvic girdle. The upper extremities include the pectoral girdle, consisting of the clavicles and the scapula. The bones of the upper extremities include the humerus, radius, ulna, carpals, metacarpals, and phalanges. The bones of the lower extremities include the femur, patella, tibia, fibula, tarsals, metatarsals, and phalanges (see Figure 21-10).

The pelvis, which is also part of the appendicular skeleton, forms the lower portion of the trunk of the body. It is easy to visualize the pelvis as a basin, with the posterior being formed by the sacrum and coccyx, and the hipbones forming the sides and front. The hipbones that help to form the bony pelvis are the ileum, the pubis, and the ischium (Figure 21-10C). In childhood, these bones are separate, but they fuse in adulthood.

The male pelvis (see Figure 21-11A) is shaped like a funnel, with the inferior outlet being significantly more narrow than seen in the female. It is stronger and heav-

ier, and is more suited for lifting and running than is the female pelvis, which is shaped more like a basin than is the male pelvis. It may be oval to round and is wider than the male pelvis. The female pelvis, which can be seen in Figure 21-11B, is constructed to accommodate a fetus during pregnancy and then facilitate its downward passage through the pelvic cavity during the birth process. The female pelvis is lighter and broader than the male pelvis.

Common Disorders Associated with the Skeletal System

Various pathological conditions are associated with the skeletal system (see Table 21-2). (See Patient Education for information about teaching patients how to maintain bone health and prevent bone loss.)

Abnormal Curvature of the Spine

There are three common abnormal curvatures of the spine: scoliosis, lordosis, and kyphosis (see Figure 21-12). Scoliosis is an abnormal lateral curvature of the spine. This condition usually appears during adolescence, during periods of rapid growth. Treatment modalities may include the application of a brace or cast, traction, electrical stimulation, or surgery.

Patient Education

Medical assistants teach patients how to maintain bone health and prevent bone loss. Education can include information about dietary supplementation, exercise, lifestyle modification, and hormone replacement. When adults have healthy bones, they stand a smaller chance of developing bone fractures. Exercise and healthy nutrition can also help children to develop healthy bones and healthy habits to help prevent bone disease later in life. Any patient, regardless of his or her current state of bone health, can benefit from education and simple lifestyle changes.

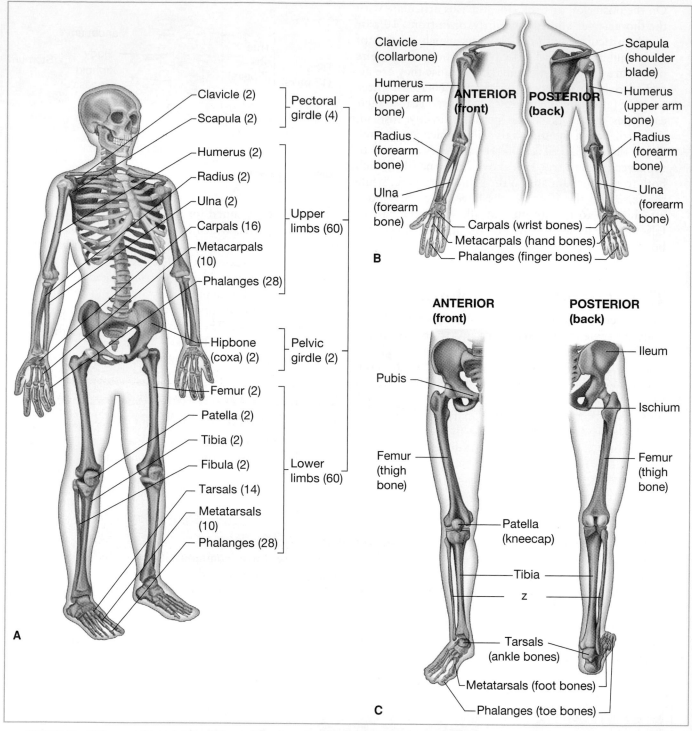

FIGURE 21-10 (A) The appendicular skeleton. (B) Bones of the upper extremities. (C) Bones of the lower extremities.

Lordosis, also known as "swayback," is a condition in which the abdomen and buttocks protrude due to an exaggerated lumbar curvature. Lordosis is most commonly treated with physical therapy activities. Finally, kyphosis, sometimes referred to as "humpback," is a result of the normal thoracic curvature becoming exaggerated due to a congenital defect, disease process (such as tuberculosis, syphilis, or malignancy), compression fracture, faulty posture, osteoarthritis, rheumatoid arthritis, rickets, osteoporosis, or other conditions.

Arthritis

Arthritis is the inflammation of one or more joint. Various disease processes cause arthritis, including joint injury, autoimmune disorders, and wear and tear

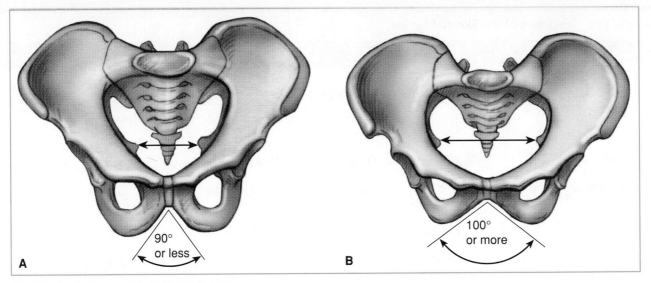

FIGURE 21-11   (A) The male pelvis; (B) the female pelvis.

on the joints. It is a condition that can occur in any individual of any age, although it most commonly occurs in older adults. Symptoms of arthritis include joint pain and swelling, morning stiffness, warmth and redness around a joint, and decreased ability to move the joint.

The treatment for arthritis varies, depending on the cause, the severity of the disease, the joints affected, and the age, occupation, and daily activities of the patient. Treatment is aimed at pain reduction and preventing further disability. Simple modifications in daily activities, including adequate rest and appropriate forms of exercise, may help to reduce the symptoms. Low-impact aerobic exercise (such as swimming) may relieve joint strain. Other times, more extensive therapies, including the application of heat or cold, joint protection, medications, and surgery, may be used. Medications to reduce joint pain and swelling include acetaminophen, aspirin, nonsteroidal anti-inflammatory drugs (NSAIDs), corticosteroids, and other immuno-suppressive drugs. There are also "antibiologic" drugs, still fairly new, which can help reduce inflammation. These medications are administered by injection or intravenously.

Osteoarthritis

Osteoarthritis is the most common type of arthritis resulting from years of wear and tear on joints (see Figure 21-13). It most frequently occurs in the elderly in the hips, knees, and finger joints. Obesity, a history of trauma, and various genetic and metabolic diseases increase the risk of osteoarthritis.

Rheumatoid Arthritis

Rheumatoid arthritis is an autoimmune disorder in which the joints may actually become deformed due to the inflammation (see Figure 21-14). This formation can be typically seen in the hands; however, rheumatoid arthritis may affect other parts of the body.

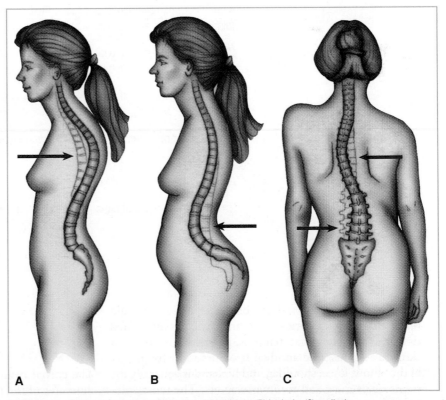

FIGURE 21-12   Abnormal curvatures of the spine: (A) kyphosis; (B) lordosis; (C) scoliosis.

TABLE 21-2 Disorders of the Skeletal System

Disorder	Description
Arthritis	Inflammation of the bone joints
Bunion	Enlargement of the joint at the base of the great toe caused by inflammation of the bursa of the great toe
Bursitis	Inflammation of the bursa, the connective tissue surrounding a joint
Carpal tunnel syndrome	Pain caused by compression of the nerve as it passes between the bones and tendons of the wrist
Gout	Inflammation of the joints caused by excessive uric acid
Kyphosis	Abnormal increase in the outward curvature of the thoracic spine; also known as hunchback or humpback
Lordosis	Abnormal increase in the forward curvature of the lumbar spine; also known as swayback
Osteoarthritis	Noninflammatory type of arthritis resulting in degeneration of the bones and joints, especially those bearing weight
Osteomalacia	Softening of the bones caused by a deficiency of phosphorus or calcium; it is thought that in children the cause is insufficient sunlight and vitamin D
Osteomyelitis	Inflammation of the bone and bone marrow due to infection; can be difficult to treat
Osteoporosis	Decrease in bone mass that results in a thinning and weakening of the bone with resulting fractures; the bones become more porous, especially in the spine and pelvis
Paget's disease	A fairly common metabolic disease of the bone from unknown causes; it usually attacks middle-aged and elderly people and is characterized by bone destruction and deformity
Rheumatoid arthritis	Chronic form of arthritis with inflammation of the joints, swelling, stiffness, pain, and changes in the cartilage that can result in crippling deformities
Rickets	Deficiency in calcium and vitamin D in early childhood that results in bone deformities, especially bowed legs
Ruptured intervertebral disk	Herniation or outpouching of a disk between two vertebrae; also called a slipped or herniated disk
Scoliosis	Abnormal lateral curvature of the spine
Spinal stenosis	Narrowing of the spinal canal causing pressure on the cord and nerves

Bursitis

Bursitis is inflammation of the bursa, a small sac of fluid that cushions and lubricates an area where joint-related tissues, including bones, tendons, ligaments, muscles, or skin, rub against one another. It occurs most frequently in the elbow, knee, shoulder, and hip, and is generally the result of overuse and trauma to joints. The most common signs and symptoms include joint pain, swelling, and tenderness surrounding the joint. Treatment usually involves rest, pain medication, steroid injections, aspiration of excess fluid from the bursa, and antibiotics.

Carpal Tunnel Syndrome

The carpal tunnel is a narrow passageway about the diameter of the thumb located on the palm side of the wrist. The tunnel protects the main nerve to the hand

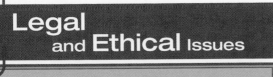
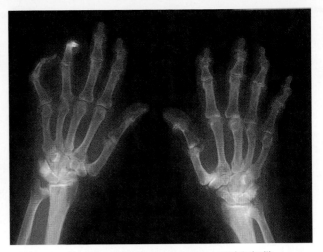

FIGURE 21-13 X-ray showing typical joint changes associated with osteoarthritis.

and the nine tendons that bend the fingers. When pressure is placed on this nerve (the median nerve), pain is produced along with numbness and hand weakness.

Injury or trauma to the areas, including repetitive movement of the wrists, can cause swelling of the tissues that surround the nerve, causing the known symptoms of carpal tunnel syndrome. Repetitive movements might be caused by sports such as racquetball or tennis, or activities such as sewing, keyboarding, driving, assembly-line work, painting, writing, the use of hand tools or vibrating tools, or other similar activities.

The most common age of occurrence of carpal tunnel syndrome is between ages 30 and 60. It occurs more commonly in women than men. Certain conditions increase the risk of carpal tunnel syndrome, including obesity, diabetes, and rheumatoid arthritis. Proper treatment can alleviate the symptoms of pain and numbness, and can restore the normal use of the wrists. Treatment can include the application of wrist splints at night for several weeks. Hot and cold compresses may also be used. Another important treatment is the evaluation of the working environment. Individuals should ensure that their wrists are held relatively straight during keyboarding and other activities. If the wrists are hyperextended (bent backwards), the chance for carpal tunnel syndrome increases. Many other specialized tools are available that can be used to decrease wrist stress.

Medications used in the treatment of carpal tunnel syndrome include the use of NSAIDs such as ibuprofen or naproxen. Injections of corticosteroids can also help decrease the symptoms. If these measures do not provide significant relief, then a surgical procedure that decreases the pressure on the median nerve is about 85 percent effective in relieving carpal tunnel symptoms. The healing process from the surgery may take several months, so the results are not immediately seen.

Fractures

Fractures or bone breaks, are classified based on their external appearance, the site of the fracture, and the nature of the crack or break in the bone. The different types of fractures, some of which are illustrated in Figure 21-15, include:

- Closed: Also known as a simple fracture, this type of fracture does not involve a break in the skin. It is completely internal.

- Open (compound): These are more dangerous fractures because of the projection of the fracture through the skin. Because the integrity of the skin and other tissues is damaged in this type of fracture, there is a greater risk of infection or hemorrhage than with a closed fracture.

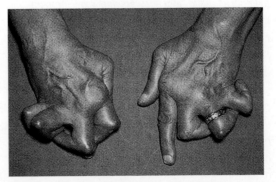

FIGURE 21-14 Typical hand deformities associated with rheumatoid arthritis.

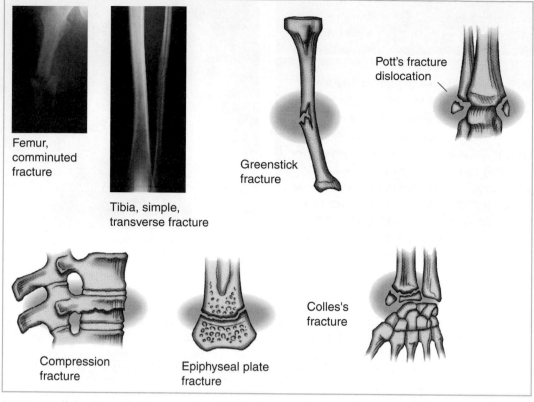

FIGURE 21-15 Various types of fractures.

- Comminuted: In this type of fracture, part of the bone is shattered into a multitude of bony fragments.

- Transverse: These fractures break the shaft of the bone across its longitudinal access.

- Greenstick: This type of fracture usually occurs in young children, whose bones are still relatively soft. In a greenstick fracture, only one side of the shaft is broken; the other side is bent, similar to breaking a green stick.

- Spiral: Spiral fractures are spread along the length of a bone, and are produced by twisting stresses.

- Colles's: Colles's fracture is frequently the result of reaching forward to stop or cushion a fall. This fracture is exemplified by a break in the distal portion of the radius. Colles's fractures are most frequently seen in children and the elderly.

- Pott's: These are fractures that occur in the ankle and affect both bones of the lower leg (the tibia and fibula).

- Compression: Compression fractures occur in the vertebrae after severe stress, such as when someone falls and "sits down" with a significant amount of force.

- Epiphyseal: These fractures are commonly seen in children in areas where the matrix is undergoing calcification and the chondrocytes are dying.

Dislocations

As discussed earlier, joints are areas where two or more bones come together. If a sudden impact injures a joint, the bones that meet at that joint may become dislocated, or not connected. That means the bones are no longer in their normal position. Usually the

Preparing for
Externship

The medical assistant an externship who begins may be intimidated by feeling like he or she needs to know all of the right answers and know them immediately. However, it is impossible to know everything. Instead, the medical assistant should know how to ask questions and should not be afraid to ask questions. The medical assistant should keep a small notebook handy to write down the answers to questions, along with procedures, medication doses, important phone numbers, and other information learned to prevent the need to ask the same question over again. This notebook should be updated regularly.

joint capsule and ligaments tear when a joint becomes dislocated, and often the nerves are injured.

Dislocations usually occur following a blow, fall, or other trauma. The dislocated joint may be visibly out of place, discolored, or misshapen, limited in movement, swollen or bruised, and intensely painful, especially if the person tries to use the joint or bear weight on it.

Gout

Gout is a disease caused by the formation of crystals in the joints, leading to inflammation. It is most commonly seen in men over the age of 40, and the most frequent joint affected is the great toe. Medications are available to treat gout, and a diet rich in colorful fruits and vegetables helps to decrease the symptoms of gout.

Osteoporosis

Osteoporosis is characterized by the progression of loss of bone density and the thinning of bone tissue. This condition is seen most commonly in older adults, especially postmenopausal women and in individuals who do not consume enough calcium. If there is not enough calcium in the diet, then the body appropriates calcium from the bones to continue the many chemical reactions requiring calcium. Vitamin D is required for the processing of calcium.

Osteoporosis affects more than 25 million Americans, mostly women ages 50 to 70 years old. Individuals with osteoporosis are subject to increased fracture potential, especially in the hips, vertebrae, and wrists.

Individuals are at a higher risk of this disease if they have a family history of osteoporosis. Others who may also be at risk include people who tend not to do weight-bearing exercises as part of their lifestyle, Cau-

Cultural Considerations

Although Caucasian women have a higher risk of osteoporosis, the disease also affects other races. It is important to teach all women, and men, the risk factors for osteoporosis and the prevention of osteoporosis. Any individual who is slender is at a greater risk for osteoporosis, but larger individuals may also be at risk. It is also important to double check the patient's past medical history. Any individual who has taken steroids over a long period of time is at risk, and the physician should be alerted.

casian females who have never been pregnant and are experiencing early menopause, individuals who have a history of frequent corticosteroid use, and those people who smoke, drink alcohol, have a diet high in salt, caffeine, or fat, or have an insufficient intake of calcium or vitamin D (Cultural Considerations). The risk in these populations can be decreased by increasing calcium and vitamin D intake, decreasing risk-increasing behaviors, and engaging in daily weight-bearing exercise.

Diagnosis of osteoporosis is done by bone density testing. Treatments include calcium and vitamin D supplementation, medications to help preserve calcium, hormone replacement, and exercise.

SUMMARY

The skeletal system makes up the framework of the human body. Consisting of 206 bones and cartilage and ligaments this system is responsible for providing shape and support, protecting internal organs, and serving as a storage place for mineral salts, calcium, and phosphorus. The skeletal system also plays an important role in the formation of blood cells and in providing an area for the attachment of skeletal muscles.

Chapter Review

COMPETENCY REVIEW

1. Define and spell the terms to learn for this chapter.
2. Name the two main divisions of the skeletal system.
3. Name the five classifications of bone and give an example of each.
4. Discuss the six main functions of the skeletal system.

5. Name the three classifications of joints.
6. What is abduction?
7. What is adduction?
8. What is extension?
9. What is the medical term for lying face down?
10. What is arthritis?

PREPARING FOR THE CERTIFICATION EXAM

1. Which of the following bones is NOT one of the lower extremity bones?
   A. femur
   B. patella
   C. tibia
   D. ulna
   E. tarsal

2. A wrist fracture is
   A. comminuted
   B. compound
   C. transverse
   D. greenstick
   E. Colles's

3. Backward bending movement at a joint is called
   A. circumduction
   B. inversion
   C. dorsiflexion
   D. supination
   E. plantar flexion

4. Which of the following bones is NOT one of the bones of the upper extremities?
   A. fibula
   B. clavicle
   C. scapula
   D. humerus
   E. radius

5. Which of the following bones is NOT one of the cranial bones?
   A. temporal
   B. vomer
   C. occipital
   D. parietal
   E. sphenoid

6. The cheekbones are the
   A. mandibular bones
   B. maxillary bones
   C. palatine bones
   D. zygomatic bones
   E. lacrimal bones

7. How many bones are in the lumbar vertebrae?
   A. 1
   B. 3
   C. 5
   D. 7
   E. 12

8. The end of a long bone is called the
   A. epiphysis
   B. diaphysis
   C. periosteum
   D. mediastinum
   E. cartilage

9. What is the name of the membrane that forms the covering of bones, except at their articular surfaces?
   A. epiphysis
   B. diaphysis
   C. periosteum
   D. mediastinum
   E. cartilage

10. Which of the following is NOT a division of the spine?
    A. lumbar
    B. thoracic
    C. parietal
    D. cervical
    E. sacral

CRITICAL THINKING

1. If Josephine has broken her wrist, what is the most likely type of fracture she sustained?
2. Why did the physician order physical therapy?
3. What other lifestyle changes could Josephine make to slow the development of her osteoporosis?

INTERNET ACTIVITY

Do an internet search to look up the National Osteoporosis Association. Research the association to see what information they provide for both patients and health care providers. Utilize this information to learn how to teach a patient about osteoporosis.

MediaLink More on the skeletal system, including interactive resources, can be found on the Student CD-ROM accompanying this textbook.

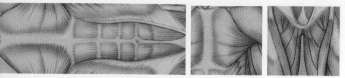

Medical Assistant Role Delineation Chart

HIGHLIGHT indicates material covered in this chapter.

ADMINISTRATIVE

Administrative Procedures

- Perform basic administrative medical assisting functions
- Schedule, coordinate and monitor appointments
- Schedule inpatient/outpatient admissions and procedures
- Understand and apply third-party guidelines
- Obtain reimbursement through accurate claims submission
- Monitor third-party reimbursement
- Understand and adhere to managed care policies and procedures
- *Negotiate managed care contracts*

Practice Finances

- Perform procedural and diagnostic coding
- Apply bookkeeping principles

- Manage accounts receivable
- *Manage accounts payable*
- *Process payroll*
- *Document and maintain accounting and banking records*
- *Develop and maintain fee schedules*
- *Manage renewals of business and professional insurance policies*
- *Manage personnel benefits and maintain records*
- *Perform marketing, financial, and strategic planning*

CLINICAL

Fundamental Principles

- Apply principles of aseptic technique and infection control
- Comply with quality assurance practices
- Screen and follow up patient test results

Diagnostic Orders

- Collect and process specimens
- Perform diagnostic tests

Patient Care

- Adhere to established patient screening procedures
- Obtain patient history and vital signs
- Prepare and maintain examination and treatment areas
- Prepare patient for examinations, procedures and treatments

- Assist with examinations, procedures and treatments
- Prepare and administer medications and immunizations
- Maintain medication and immunization records
- Recognize and respond to emergencies
- Coordinate patient care information with other health care providers
- Initiate IV and administer IV medications with appropriate training and as permitted by state law

GENERAL

Professionalism

- Display a professional manner and image
- Demonstrate initiative and responsibility
- Work as a member of the health care team
- Prioritize and perform multiple tasks
- Adapt to change
- Promote the CMA credential
- Enhance skills through continuing education
- Treat all patients with compassion and empathy
- Promote the practice through positive public relations

Communication Skills

- Recognize and respect cultural diversity
- Adapt communications to individual's ability to understand
- Use professional telephone technique

- Recognize and respond effectively to verbal, nonverbal, and written communications
- Use medical terminology appropriately
- Utilize electronic technology to receive, organize, prioritize and transmit information
- Serve as liaison

Legal Concepts

- Perform within legal and ethical boundaries
- Prepare and maintain medical records
- Document accurately
- Follow employer's established policies dealing with the health care contract
- Implement and maintain federal and state health care legislation and regulations
- Comply with established risk management and safety procedures
- Recognize professional credentialing criteria
- *Develop and maintain personnel, policy and procedure manuals*

Instruction

- Instruct individuals according to their needs
- Explain office policies and procedures
- Teach methods of health promotion and disease prevention
- Locate community resources and disseminate information
- *Develop educational materials*
- *Conduct continuing education activities*

Operational Functions

- Perform inventory of supplies and equipment
- Perform routine maintenance of administrative and clinical equipment
- Apply computer techniques to support office operations
- *Perform personnel management functions*
- *Negotiate leases and prices for equipment and supply contracts*

- *Denotes advanced skills.*

SOURCE: Reprinted by permission of the American Association of Medical Assistants from the AAMA Role Delineation Study: Occupational Analysis of the Medical Assisting Profession.

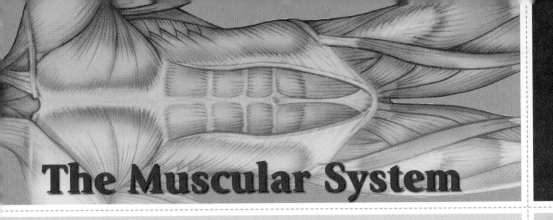

The Muscular System

chapter 22

Learning Objectives

After completing this chapter, you should be able to:

- Define and spell the terms to learn for this chapter.
- Describe the muscular system of the body.
- Explain the functions of muscle.
- Identify and discuss types of muscle tissue.
- Explain the structure of skeletal muscles
- Discuss attachments to skeletal muscles.
- Identify the major muscles of the body.
- Identify and explain common disorders of the muscular system.

Terms to Learn

antagonist	insertion	skeletal muscle
aponeurosis	muscle cramps	smooth muscle
atrophy	muscular dystrophy (MD)	sprain
cardiac muscle	myasthenia gravis (MG)	strain
endomysium	origin	synergist
epimysium	oxygen debt	tendonitis
fascia	perimysium	tendons
fascicles	prime mover	tetanus
fibromyalgia		

Case Study

ROBERT HERLY IS A 3-YEAR-OLD CHILD seen by Dr. Kikkawa. Robert's mother states that Robert has been falling a lot and seems to be very clumsy. He has a waddling gait, runs and climbs slowly, and walks on his toes. He has a family history of muscular dystrophy. Dr. Kikkawa takes a complete family history and orders a muscle biopsy, an EMG, and blood work, including a serum creatinine kinase.

Dr. Kikkawa diagnoses Robert with Duchenne's muscular dystrophy. Treatment will include physical therapy, deep breathing exercises, and occupational therapy for Robert, and genetic counseling and referral services for Robert's parents.

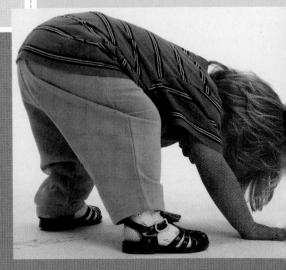

The muscular system (see Figure 22-1), is composed of specialized cells called muscle fibers. These fibers, which are made of different lengths and shapes, and are differently colored from white to deep red, form and become muscles. Muscles make up about 42 percent of a person's total body weight. Each muscle consists of a group of fibers held together by connective tissue that are held together by a fibrous sheath called fascia. Each fiber within a muscle also has its own nervous system connection that has a stored supply of energy in the form of glycogen. Muscle must be supplied with proper nutrition and oxygen to perform properly.

The muscular system is well permeated by vessels from the circulatory system and the lymphatic system.

Functions of Muscle

The predominant function of the muscular system is contractibility. Muscles, where attached to bones or internal organs and blood vessels, are responsible for movement—and nearly all movement in the body is the result of muscle contraction.

In addition to movement, muscles have other functions, including tonicity, heat production, and stability. Tonicity is what helps us to maintain posture through a continual partial contraction of skeletal muscles. The

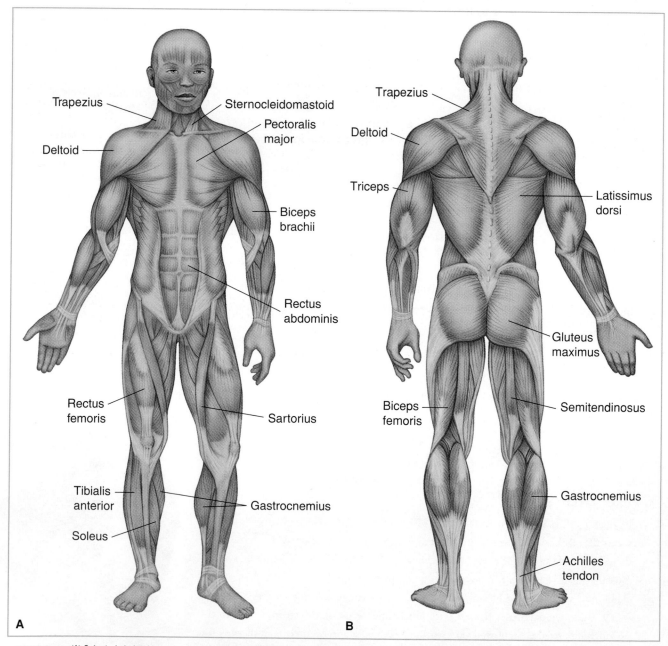

FIGURE 22-1   (A) Selected skeletal muscles (anterior view). (B) Selected skeletal muscles and the Achilles tendon (posterior view).

THE CHILD

- From the time of fetal development and as a child continues to develop, the muscles and bones continue to grow. And while the movements of a newborn are uncoordinated and random, muscular development continues to proceed from head to toe and from the center of the body to the periphery. The head and neck muscles are the first muscles that can be controlled, so a baby will hold his or her head upright before he or she can sit up. Babies need freedom of movement to help develop those muscles in the proper order.

THE OLDER ADULT

- The changes related to mobility are the most obvious in the older adult. There can be measurable differences in muscle strength, endurance, range of motion, coordination, elasticity, and flexibility of connective tissue.
- The prevention of decreases in strength is fully dependent on regular exercise. Thus, exercise helps to strengthen muscles and keeps joints, tendons, and ligaments more flexible, allowing for a more active lifestyle.

body alternates the muscle fibers that are contracted and those that are relaxed, so all muscles have a chance to maintain the posture (contraction) and rest between contractions. Muscles also produce heat through the chemical changes involved in muscular activity. This is what helps the body to maintain a normal temperature. Finally, muscles help the body to maintain stability, meaning that muscles are responsible for holding bones together so that the joints of the body remain stable.

Types of Muscle Tissue

A muscle is a tissue that performs different functions that cause some sort of movement to take place. The three different types of muscle cells are skeletal, smooth, and cardiac (see Figure 22-2). The various muscles of our bodies serve as the engines or powerhouses of the body and are so constructed to provide speed and power. Each muscle cell is designed for various functions that are needed by a certain area in the body. Muscle tissue has the ability to contract or to shorten, thus producing movement of internal and external body parts. Breathing, speaking, walking, talking, eating, and almost every other function require muscle tissue.

Smooth muscles are composed of elongated, spindle-shaped cells and

are commonly involved in involuntary motions. Involuntary muscle contractions or motions are those movements that cannot be consciously controlled. The nucleus is centrally located and there are no striations in smooth muscle cells. These types of cells are located

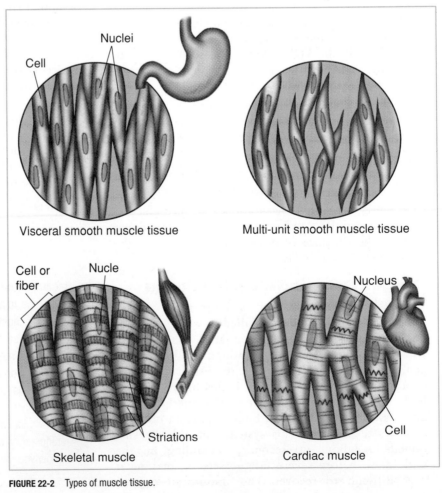

FIGURE 22-2 Types of muscle tissue.

throughout the body. Muscles made from these types of cells include those found in the walls of blood vessels, the urinary bladder, and the digestive system.

Skeletal muscles allow movement by being attached to bones in the body. Skeletal muscles control voluntary movements, which can be consciously controlled. Skeletal muscles are made up of cylindrical fibers that are found in the locomotive system. The nucleus of each cell tends to be toward the edge of each cell and the cells are striated.

Cardiac muscles are roughly quadrangular in shape and have a single central nucleus. The cells form a network of branching fibers. The muscles are cross striated and are involuntary. The muscles are found in the heart. Muscle tissues are supplied with nerve fibers that carry messages to and from the central nervous system (brain and spinal cord).

Finally, it is important to note that muscles are composed of about 75 percent water, 20 percent protein, and about 5 percent carbohydrates, lipids, inorganic salts, and nonprotein nitrogenous compounds. The composition does vary in the different muscles.

Energy Production for Muscle

Muscles use energy in the form of ATP (adenosine triphosphate), which is a type of chemical energy needed for sustained or repeated muscular contractions. To make the ATP, thus creating an atmosphere in which the muscle cells can make this energy, the muscle must do the following:

- Break down the creatine phosphate, which is a protein that stores extra phosphate groups. This is a very fast way for the muscles to produce energy.

- Carry out anaerobic respiration by which glucose is broken down to lactic acid, thus forming the ATP.

- Carry out aerobic respiration, by which glucose, glycogen, fats, and amino acids are broken down in the presence of oxygen, thus leading to the production of ATP.

Oxygen Debt and Muscle Fatigue

When skeletal muscles are used for more than a minute or two, a condition called **oxygen debt** may occur. Simply put, this means that if your body is working hard, and you are breathing in a lot of oxygen, your body may not be able to absorb enough to cope with the level of activity. If this happens, your body is mainly utilizing the anaerobic energy system and, as a result, lactic acid builds up as an undesirable waste product. This system can only be sustained for about 60 seconds, depending on the individual, before severe fatigue sets in, making it very difficult to recover. The amount of oxygen

"owed" to the body in order to recover is called the oxygen debt.

Muscle fatigue, which is often accompanied by muscle cramps, occurs when a muscle has lost its ability to contract. Like oxygen debt, it usually develops as a result of an accumulation of lactic acid. It may also occur if the blood supply to a muscle is stopped or interrupted, or if a motor neuron loses its ability to release acetylcholine into the muscle fibers.

Structure of Skeletal Muscles

Skeletal muscle is also known as striated muscle or voluntary muscle (see Figure 22-3). Skeletal muscle is controlled by the conscious part of the brain, and each of these muscles attaches to bones. There are 600 different skeletal muscles that are responsible for the movement of the body through contractility, extensibility, and elasticity. When viewed under a microscope, skeletal muscle has a cross-striped appearance, which is the reason why skeletal muscle is also known as striated muscle. Various sizes, shapes, and fiber arrangements create a variety of muscles that can each perform a specific function for its use in the body.

Several coverings made up of connective tissue are associated with skeletal muscle. The **fascia** is the structure covering the entire skeletal muscle and separating the muscles from one another. Muscles, which are surrounded by a thin covering called the **epimysium**, are attached to bones by structures called **tendons**. The **aponeurosis** is a wide, thin, sheet-like tendon, made up of fibrous connective tissue, that typically attaches muscles to other muscles. The **perimysium**, also made up of connective tissue,

Professionalism

Because there are going to be unhappy patients, and physicians, in any medical practice, it is important to realize that most of the time, individuals who complain about service are not attacking the person responding to their call, but are instead venting their frustration, because they do not understand something. As a professional, it is important for you to understand that listening and learning go hand-in-hand. If a person is upset or concerned about his or her health, instead of getting angry, take the time to "listen," and try to focus on how you can best meet that person's needs.

is responsible for dividing a muscle into sections called **fascicles**. The **endomysium** is the covering made up of connective tissue that surrounds the individual muscle cell.

Attachments to Skeletal Muscles

The actions of the skeletal muscles depend greatly on what the skeletal muscles are attached to. The origins and insertions are the locations at which skeletal muscles attach. The **origin** is the attachment to the bone that is more fixed, or still, while the **insertion** is the attachment point on the bone that moves.

Muscles and nerves function together as a motor unit. Skeletal muscles require innervation to contract. To complete such a task, these muscles must move as a single unit. The three types of skeletal muscle units include:

- **Antagonist**—a muscle that counteracts, or opposes, the action of another muscle
- **Prime mover**—a muscle that is the primary actor in a given movement. This is the muscle that produces the movement in muscle contraction
- **Synergist**—a muscle that acts with another muscle to produce movement

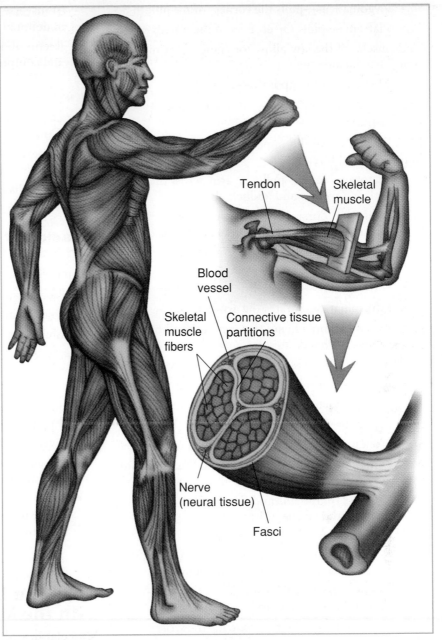

FIGURE 22-3 A skeletal muscle consists of a group of fibers held together by connective tissue. It is enclosed in a fibrous sheath (fascia).

Major Skeletal Muscles

When describing the major skeletal muscles, it is important to remember that these muscles are often identified according to their location, size, action, shape, or number of attachments of the muscle. They are usually listed in the following groups:

- Muscles of the head
- Muscles of the arm, wrist, hand, and fingers
- Respiratory muscles
- Abdominal muscles
- Muscles of the pectoral girdle
- Muscles of the leg, ankle, and foot.

Muscles of the Head

The muscles of the head include those that move the head, provide facial expressions, and move the jaw. They include the following muscles:

- Sternocleidomastoid—pulls the head from side to side and head to chest
- Splenulus capitis—rotates the head and allows it to bend to the side

The muscles that provide for facial expression include the following:

- Frontalis—raises the eyebrows
- Orbicularis oris—allows the lips to pucker
- Orbicularis oculi—allows the eyes to close

- Zygomaticus—pulls the corners of the mouth up
- Platysma—pulls the corners of the mouth down

The muscles of the jaw allow for chewing, or mastication. They include the following:

- Masseter and temporalis—close the jaw

Muscles of the Arm, Wrist, Hand, and Fingers

Muscles that move the upper extremity include those in the arm and forearm:

- Pectoralis major—pulls the arm across the chest and also rotates and adducts the arms
- Latissimus dorsi—provides for extension, adduction, and rotation of the arm inwardly
- Deltoid—provides for abduction and extension of the arm at the shoulder
- Subscapularis—rotates the arm medially
- Infraspinatus—rotates the arm laterally
- Biceps brachii—flexes the arm at the elbow and rotates the hand laterally
- Brachialis—flexes the arm at the elbow
- Brachioradialis—flexes the forearm at the elbow
- Triceps brachii—extends the arm at the elbow
- Supinator—rotates the forearm laterally
- Pronator teres—rotates the forearm medially

Muscles that move the wrist, hand, and fingers include the following:

- Flexor carpi radialis and flexor carpi ulnaris—flex and abduct the wrist
- Palmaris longus—flexes the wrist
- Flexor digitorum profundus—flexes the distal joints of the fingers, but not the thumb
- Extensor carpi radialis longae and brevis—extend the wrist and abduct the hand
- Extensor carpi ulnaris—extends the wrist
- Extensor digitorum—extends the fingers, but not the thumb

Respiratory Muscles

The muscles of respiration include the following:

- Diaphragm—separates the thoracic cavity from the abdominal cavity and its contraction causes the process of inspiration
- External and internal intercostals—contraction of these muscles expands and lowers the ribs during breathing

Abdominal Muscles

The muscles of the abdominal wall include the following:

- External and internal obliques—compress the abdominal wall
- Transverse abdominis—also compresses the abdominal wall
- Rectus abdominis—flexes the vertebral column and compresses the abdominal wall

Muscles of the Pectoral Girdle

The muscles that move the pectoral girdle, or shoulder, include the following:

- Trapezius—raises the arms and pulls the shoulders downward
- Pectoralis minor—pulls the scapula downward and raises the ribs

Muscles of the Leg, Ankle, and Foot

The muscles that move the leg include the following:

- Psoas major—flexes the thigh
- Iliacus—also flexes the thigh
- Gluteus maximus—extends the thigh

The muscles that move the ankle and foot include the following:

- Gastrocnemius—flexes the foot and aids in pushing the body forward
- Tibialis anterior—causes dorsiflexion and inversion of the foot
- Peroneus—everts the foot and helps bring about plantar flexion
- Flexor and extensor digitorum longus—flexes and extends the toes and assists in other movements of the feet

Common Disorders Associated with the Muscular System

Muscular disorders are characterized by abnormalities of muscle fibers. In addition, many neurological disorders, such as lesions of the central or peripheral nervous system and abnormalities of neuromuscular transmission, can also produce symptoms that are primarily muscular. Other systemic disorders, including those that are frequently seen in conditions of the cardiovascular, respiratory, and endocrine systems, frequently mimic muscular disorders but do not directly affect muscular function. These systemic disorders account for more than half of muscular complaints.

Difficulty in walking, unsteadiness with occasional falls, and joint stiffness with leg pains, especially at night, may also be due to conditions affecting the skeletal system, such as degenerative joint disease and rheumatoid arthritis. Significant degenerative joint disease can limit mobility by producing structural spinal

Medical assistants teach patients how to maintain good posture and a healthy attitude toward exercise. Education can include information about dietary supplementation, exercise, and lifestyle modification. When adults maintain a healthy attitude toward exercise, they stand less chance of developing disorders that will negatively affect them and their muscular system in later life.

Exercise and healthy nutrition can also help children to develop healthy habits to prevent muscle weakness and other disorders later in life. Expectant parents can also prevent pain and hardships by testing their unborn infants for possible congenital and neuromuscular diseases prior to birth.

changes and joint symptoms in the limbs and occasionally by damaging the spinal cord, nerve roots, and peripheral nerves.

Atrophy

Atrophy occurs with the disuse of muscles over a long period of time. Oftentimes, atrophy is caused by bed rest and immobility, which cause a loss of muscle mass and strength. If the atrophy is caused by a specific treatment (such as a cast or traction), some atrophy can be minimized by the practice of isometric exercises of the immobilized limb. Isometric exercise uses active muscle contractions performed against stable resistance—for example, tightening the muscles of the thighs or the buttocks. Active exercise of uninjured limbs helps prevent atrophy.

Lipoatrophy, which is a type of atrophy that can occur at a site of insulin or corticosteroid injections, is the atrophy of fat tissue. It is also known as lipodystrophy.

Fibromyalgia

Fibromyalgia is a widespread musculoskeletal pain and fatigue disorder affecting an estimated 3 million individuals in the United States, generally women more than men. Symptoms include mild to severe muscle pain and fatigue, sleep disorders, irritable bowel syndrome, depression, and chronic headaches. There is no obvious known cause of fibromyalgia, but there is evidence pointing to a genetic predisposition that creates a neuromuscular/neuroendocrine abnormality that disturbs the usual sensory perception, especially to pain signals.

The American College of Rheumatology (ACR) has identified specific criteria for fibromyalgia. The ACR states that a patient must show pain at 11 of 18 trigger points to be considered for a diagnosis of fibromyalgia. The patient must also have a history of widespread pain lasting at least 3 months.

Treatment is geared toward improving the quality of sleep and reducing pain. Sleep is important for many body functions, including tissue repair and antibody

production, so the disruption of sleep will directly affect the quality of life in a patient with fibromyalgia. Frequently, the medications prescribed for fibromyalgia include muscle relaxants, antidepressants, antianxiety medications, and anti-inflammatories. Other treatments frequently employed include chiropracty, acupuncture, acupressure, relaxation techniques, and massage.

Muscle Cramps and Pain

Muscle cramps or pain in the absence of electrolyte or pH disturbance commonly indicates a peripheral nerve disorder and less commonly an abnormality in muscle fibers. Intense pain that is most prominent in proximal muscles in the morning may indicate polymyalgia rheumatica. Pain in localized muscle regions may indicate fibromyalgia. Pain largely restricted to muscle groups and periarticular tissue may indicate diffuse arthritic disease with limited muscle function.

Muscular Dystrophy

Muscular dystrophy (MD) is one of a group of genetic diseases characterized by progressive weakness and degeneration of the skeletal or voluntary muscles that

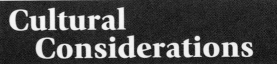

Cultural Considerations

Some cultures, such as those seen in the Far East, include exercise and holistic health as a way of life. Hence, many of the citizens of those countries may experience fewer problems affecting the muscular system. It is important for the medical assistant to be sensitive to the beliefs of patients from different cultures and to gain an understanding of how culture may play a role in their daily lives.

control movement. The muscles of the heart and some other involuntary muscles are also affected in some forms of muscular dystrophy, and a few forms involve other organs as well. The major forms of muscular dystrophy include:

- Duchenne's muscular dystrophy
- Becker's muscular dystrophy
- Limb-girdle muscular dystrophy
- Facioscapulohumeral muscular dystrophy
- Congenital muscular dystrophy
- Oculopharyngeal muscular dystrophy
- Distal muscular dystrophy
- Emery-Dreifuss muscular dystrophy
- Myotonic dystrophy

Muscular dystrophy can affect people of all ages. Although some forms first become apparent in infancy or childhood, others may not appear until middle age or later. Duchenne's muscular dystrophy is the most common kind of muscular dystrophy affecting children. Myotonic dystrophy is the most common of these diseases in adults.

There is no specific treatment for any of the forms of muscular dystrophy. Physical therapy to prevent contractures (a condition in which shortened muscles around joints cause abnormal and sometimes painful positioning of the joints), orthoses (orthopedic appliances used for support), and corrective orthopedic surgery may be needed to improve the quality of life in some cases. The cardiac problems that occur with Emery-Dreifuss muscular dystrophy and myotonic dystrophy may require a pacemaker. The myotonia (delayed relaxation of a muscle after a strong contraction) occurring in myotonic dystrophy may be treated with medications such as phenytoin or quinine.

The prognosis (outlook) with muscular dystrophy varies according to the type of muscular dystrophy and the progression of the disorder. Some cases may be mild and very slowly progressive with normal life span, while other cases may have more marked progression of muscle weakness, functional disability, and loss of ambulation. Life expectancy depends on the degree of progression and late respiratory deficit. In Duchenne's muscular dystrophy, death usually occurs in the late teens to early 20s.

Myasthenia Gravis

Myasthenia gravis (MG) is a chronic neuromuscular disease characterized by varying degrees of weakness of the skeletal or voluntary muscles of the body. The muscle weakness increases during periods of activity and improves after periods of rest. MG most commonly occurs in young adult women and older men but can occur at any age. Although MG may affect any voluntary muscle, certain muscles, including those that control eye movements, eyelids, chewing, swallowing, coughing, and facial expressions, are more often affected. Weakness may also occur in the muscles that control breathing and arm and leg movements. The muscles involved in MG vary from one individual to the next.

Today, MG is well controlled. Therapies include medications such as anticholinesterase agents, prednisone, cyclosporine, and azathioprine; thymectomy, which is the surgical removal of the thymus gland; plasmapheresis, a procedure in which abnormal antibodies are removed from blood plasma; and high-dose intravenous immunoglobulin, which modifies the immune system. A physician will determine which treatment option is best for each patient depending on the severity of the weakness, which muscles are affected, and the patient's age and other associated medical problems.

With treatment, most MG patients will have excellent improvement of their muscle weakness. In some patients, MG may go into remission and muscle weakness may disappear completely. In a few cases, MG may cause severe weakness resulting in acute respiratory failure; however, most patients can expect to lead normal or nearly normal lives.

Sprains and Strains

A sprain is an injury to a ligament—a stretching or a tearing—whereas a strain is an injury to either a muscle or a tendon. Depending on the severity of the injury, a strain may be a simple overstretching of the muscle or tendon, or it can result in a partial or complete tear.

Sprains

Typically, sprains occur when people fall and land on an outstretched arm, slide into base, land on the side of their foot, or twist a knee with the foot planted firmly on the ground. This results in an overstretching or tearing of the ligament supporting that joint.

Although sprains can occur in both the upper and lower parts of the body, the most common site is the ankle. Ankle sprains are the most common injury in the United States and often occur during sports or recreational activities.

The usual signs and symptoms include pain, swelling, bruising, and loss of the ability to move and use the joint (called functional ability). However, these signs and symptoms can vary in intensity, depending on the severity of the sprain. Sometimes people feel a pop or tear when the injury happens. In general, a grade I or mild sprain causes overstretching or slight tearing of the ligaments with no joint instability. A person with a mild sprain usually experiences minimal pain, swelling, and little or no loss of functional ability. Bruising is absent or slight, and the person is usually able to put weight on the affected joint. A grade II or moderate sprain causes partial tearing of the ligament and is characterized by bruising, moderate pain, and swelling. A person with a moderate sprain usually has some difficulty putting weight on the affected joint and experiences some loss of function. An x-ray or MRI may be needed.

People who sustain a grade III or severe sprain completely tear or rupture a ligament. Pain, swelling, and bruising are usually severe, and the patient is unable to put weight on the joint. An x-ray is usually taken to rule out a broken bone.

When diagnosing any sprain, the doctor will ask the patient to explain how the injury happened. The doctor will examine the affected joint and check its stability and its ability to move and bear weight.

Strains

A **strain** is caused by twisting or pulling a muscle or tendon. Strains can be acute or chronic. An acute strain is caused by trauma or an injury such as a blow to the body; it can also be caused by improperly lifting heavy objects or overstressing the muscles. Chronic strains are usually the result of overuse—prolonged, repetitive movement of the muscles and tendons.

Two common sites for a strain are the back and the hamstring muscle (located in the back of the thigh). Contact sports such as soccer, football, hockey, boxing, and wrestling put people at risk for strains. Gymnastics, tennis, rowing, golf, and other sports that require extensive gripping can increase the risk of hand and forearm strains. Elbow strains sometimes occur in people who participate in racquet sports, throwing, and contact sports.

Typically, people with a strain experience pain, muscle spasm, and muscle weakness. They can also have localized swelling, cramping, or inflammation and, with a minor or moderate strain, usually some loss of muscle function.

Tendonitis

A tendon is the end part of a muscle that attaches the muscle to the bone. The normally very elastic and soft muscle tapers off at the end to form the much more dense and stiff tendon. While this density makes the tendons stronger, the lack of elasticity of the tendon and the constant pulling on its attachment to the bone with movement make it much more susceptible to a low level of tearing at a microscopic level. This tearing will produce the inflammation and irritation known as **tendonitis**. Often spelled *tendinitis*, either spelling is correct for this condition. Tendonitis is usually seen after excessive repetitive movement with which the tendon gradually becomes tighter until the fibers start to tear. For example, a person who plays tennis may overuse the muscles of the elbow through hitting the ball repetitively and cause tendonitis, or inflammation, to the area.

The most common tendon areas that become inflamed are the elbow, wrist, biceps, shoulder (including rotator cuff attachments), leg, knee (patellar), ankle, hip, and Achilles. Of course, tendonitis varies with each person, because it strikes the areas used most. The symptoms can also vary from an achy pain and stiffness in the local area of the tendon, to a burning that surrounds the whole joint around the inflamed tendon. With this condition, the pain is usually worse during and after activity, and the tendon and joint area can become stiffer the following day.

With proper care for the area, the pain in the tendon should lessen over 3 weeks, but it should be noted that the healing of the area continues and does not peak until at least 6 weeks following the initial injury. This is due to scar tissue formation, which initially acts like the glue to bond the tissue back together. Scar tissue will continue to form past 6 weeks in some cases and as long as a year in severe cases. After 6 months this condition is considered chronic and much more difficult to treat. The initial approach to treating tendonitis is to support and protect the tendons by bracing any areas of the tendon that are being pulled on during use. It is important to loosen up the tendon, reduce the pain, and minimize any inflammation.

Tetanus

Tetanus is an often fatal infectious disease caused by the bacteria *Clostridium tetani,* which usually enters the body through a puncture, cut, or open wound. It is characterized by profoundly painful spasms of muscles, including "locking" of the jaw so that the mouth cannot open (*lockjaw*). *Clostridium tetani* releases a toxin that affects the motor nerves (the nerves that stimulate the muscles).

Prevention of tetanus is aided by immediately cleaning and covering any open wound and by vaccination. All children should be immunized against tetanus by receiving a full series of 5 DPT vaccinations ("baby

Preparing for
Externship

One hallmark of a professional is the ability to seek the cause of problems and solve problems for patients without ever fixing blame on any specific individual. Frustrated patients are not interested in who is responsible for something that has gone wrong, but are instead concerned about having their problem resolved. Because humans work in the medical field, mistakes will happen. Be sure to focus on defining the problem and a remedy to the problem rather than trying to place the blame.

shots"), which generally are started at 2 months of age and completed at about 5 years of age. Tetanus and diphtheria toxoid (Td) is now recommended at 11 to 12 years of age if at least 5 years have elapsed since the last dose of tetanus and diphtheria toxoid-containing vaccine.

Follow-up booster vaccination is recommended every 10 years thereafter (i.e., 21 years old, 31 years old, etc.). Although a 10-year period of protection exists after the basic childhood series is completed (at age 11 to 12), should a potentially contaminated wound occur during the second half of this block of time (i.e., at ages 5 to 12), an "early" booster may be given and the 10-year "clock" is then reset. It is important to remember that unvaccinated people who get a puncture wound or cut should get tetanus immunoglobulin and a series of tetanus shots immediately. People who have been immunized but are unsure of when their last tetanus shot was should get a booster.

SUMMARY

The muscular system is composed of specialized cells called muscle fibers. These fibers, when brought together, form muscle, which makes up about 42 percent of a person's total body weight. In order for our muscles to perform properly, which is to create movement, maintain posture and stability, and aid in heat production, they must be supplied with proper nutrition and oxygen.

Chapter Review

COMPETENCY REVIEW

1. Define and spell the terms to learn for this chapter.
2. Name the three types of muscle tissue.
3. What are the two points of attachment for muscles.
4. What are the other names for skeletal muscle?
5. What are the three parts of muscle?
6. What are other names for smooth muscle?
7. Give examples of internal organs with smooth muscle.
8. What is the name of heart muscle?
9. What is a special property of cardiac muscle?
10. What are the three primary functions of muscle?

PREPARING FOR THE CERTIFICATION EXAM

1. Aponeuroses are
   A. flattened tendons attaching muscles
   B. striated muscles
   C. smooth muscles
   D. bones of the lower extremities
   E. bones of the upper extremities

2. Which of the following is NOT a type of muscle tissue?
   A. clavicle
   B. smooth
   C. visceral
   D. striated
   E. cardiac

3. The muscle that separates the thoracic and abdominal cavities is the
   A. psoas major
   B. psoas minor
   C. diaphragm
   D. epiglottis
   E. biceps

4. The predominant function of the muscular system is
   A. heat production
   B. contractibility
   C. elasticity
   D. posture
   E. stability

continued on next page

5. The term used to describe the muscle's maintenance of posture through contraction is
   A. tonicity
   B. movement
   C. elasticity
   D. contractibility
   E. movability

6. A condition that occurs due to the disuse of muscles over a long period of time is called
   A. fibromyalgia
   B. myasthenia gravis
   C. atrophy
   D. muscular dystrophy
   E. tendonitis

7. How many types of muscle tissues are there?
   A. two
   B. three
   C. four
   D. five
   E. six

8. The structure covering the entire skeletal muscle and separating them from one another is called the
   A. perimysium
   B. endomysium
   C. fascicle
   D. fascia
   E. epimysium

9. What form of muscular dystrophy usually leads to death between the late teens and the early 20s?
   A. Duchenne's muscular dystrophy
   B. Becker's muscular dystrophy
   C. limb-girdle muscular dystrophy
   D. facioscapulohumeral muscular dystrophy
   E. congenital muscular dystrophy

10. What is the name of the chronic neuromuscular disease characterized by varying degrees of weakness of the skeletal or voluntary muscles of the body?
    A. fibromyalgia
    B. myasthenia gravis
    C. muscular dystrophy
    D. atrophy
    E. melanoma

CRITICAL THINKING

1. What were the symptoms that clued the doctor in to a diagnosis of Duchenne's muscular dystrophy?

2. Why will Robert benefit from physical therapy?

INTERNET ACTIVITY

Do an Internet search to learn about resources for families who have members with muscular dystrophy.

MediaLink More on the muscular system, including interactive resources, can be found on the Student CD-ROM accompanying this textbook.

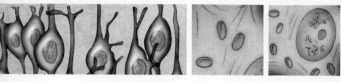

Medical Assistant Role Delineation Chart

HIGHLIGHT indicates material covered in this chapter.

ADMINISTRATIVE

Administrative Procedures

- Perform basic administrative medical assisting functions
- Schedule, coordinate and monitor appointments
- Schedule inpatient/outpatient admissions and procedures
- Understand and apply third-party guidelines
- Obtain reimbursement through accurate claims submission
- Monitor third-party reimbursement
- Understand and adhere to managed care policies and procedures
- *Negotiate managed care contracts*

Practice Finances

- Perform procedural and diagnostic coding
- Apply bookkeeping principles

- Manage accounts receivable
- *Manage accounts payable*
- *Process payroll*
- *Document and maintain accounting and banking records*
- *Develop and maintain fee schedules*
- *Manage renewals of business and professional insurance policies*
- *Manage personnel benefits and maintain records*
- *Perform marketing, financial, and strategic planning*

CLINICAL

Fundamental Principles

- Apply principles of aseptic technique and infection control
- Comply with quality assurance practices
- Screen and follow up patient test results

Diagnostic Orders

- Collect and process specimens
- Perform diagnostic tests

Patient Care

- Adhere to established patient screening procedures
- Obtain patient history and vital signs
- Prepare and maintain examination and treatment areas
- Prepare patient for examinations, procedures and treatments

- Assist with examinations, procedures and treatments
- Prepare and administer medications and immunizations
- Maintain medication and immunization records
- Recognize and respond to emergencies
- Coordinate patient care information with other health care providers
- Initiate IV and administer IV medications with appropriate training and as permitted by state law

GENERAL

Professionalism

- Display a professional manner and image
- Demonstrate initiative and responsibility
- Work as a member of the health care team
- Prioritize and perform multiple tasks
- Adapt to change
- Promote the CMA credential
- Enhance skills through continuing education
- Treat all patients with compassion and empathy
- Promote the practice through positive public relations

Communication Skills

- Recognize and respect cultural diversity
- Adapt communications to individual's ability to understand
- Use professional telephone technique

- Recognize and respond effectively to verbal, nonverbal, and written communications
- Use medical terminology appropriately
- Utilize electronic technology to receive, organize, prioritize and transmit information
- Serve as liaison

Legal Concepts

- Perform within legal and ethical boundaries
- Prepare and maintain medical records
- Document accurately
- Follow employer's established policies dealing with the health care contract
- Implement and maintain federal and state health care legislation and regulations
- Comply with established risk management and safety procedures
- Recognize professional credentialing criteria
- *Develop and maintain personnel, policy and procedure manuals*

Instruction

- Instruct individuals according to their needs
- Explain office policies and procedures
- Teach methods of health promotion and disease prevention
- Locate community resources and disseminate information
- *Develop educational materials*
- *Conduct continuing education activities*

Operational Functions

- Perform inventory of supplies and equipment
- Perform routine maintenance of administrative and clinical equipment
- Apply computer techniques to support office operations
- *Perform personnel management functions*
- *Negotiate leases and prices for equipment and supply contracts*

- *Denotes advanced skills.*

SOURCE: Reprinted by permission of the American Association of Medical Assistants from the AAMA Role Delineation Study: Occupational Analysis of the Medical Assisting Profession.

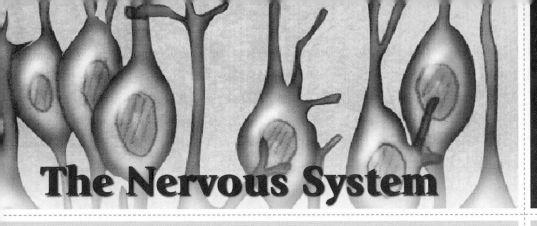

The Nervous System

Learning Objectives

After completing this chapter, you should be able to:

- Define and spell the terms to learn in this chapter.
- Identify and discuss the structures that make up the nervous system.
- Explain how nerve impulses are transmitted.
- State the functions of the central nervous system, the peripheral nervous system, and the autonomic nervous system, and distinguish the differences between each.
- Identify and explain common disorders associated with the nervous system.

Terms to Learn

Alzheimer's disease
amyotrophic lateral sclerosis (ALS)
Bell's palsy
cerebrospinal fluid
encephalitis

epilepsy
headache
meningitis
multiple sclerosis (MS)
neuralgia
paraplegia

Parkinson's disease
quadriplegia
sciatica
seizure
spina bifida
stroke

Case Study

EMILY MONTERO IS A 73-YEAR-OLD FEMALE who presents at Dr. Esso's office complaining of a new onset of left-sided weakness and drooping of the side of her face. This started about 2 hours ago with a headache, and she is experiencing progressively worsening symptoms. Her blood pressure is 172/108, and her pulse is rapid and thready. She denies pain other than her headache.

Dr. Esso immediately has his medical assistant call 911 and arrange for transport to the emergency room. Mrs. Montero receives a CT scan that shows a thrombus in her brain with no other acute abnormalities seen. She is given thrombolytics (clot-busters) and is admitted to the ICU. Eventually, she is put on a rehabilitation service, and returns to Dr. Esso's office 12 weeks later with a slight limp and no other difficulties.

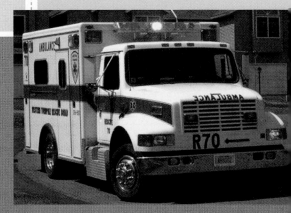

he nervous system is the body's information gatherer, storage center, and control system (see Figure 23-1). Its overall function is to collect information about external conditions in relation to the body's external state, to analyze this information, and to initiate appropriate responses to satisfy certain needs. The most powerful of these needs is survival. The nerves do not form one single system, but several systems that are interrelated. Some of these are physically separate, others are different in function only. The brain and spinal cord make up the central nervous system. The peripheral nervous system is responsible for the body functions that are not under conscious control, such as the heartbeat or the digestive system. The

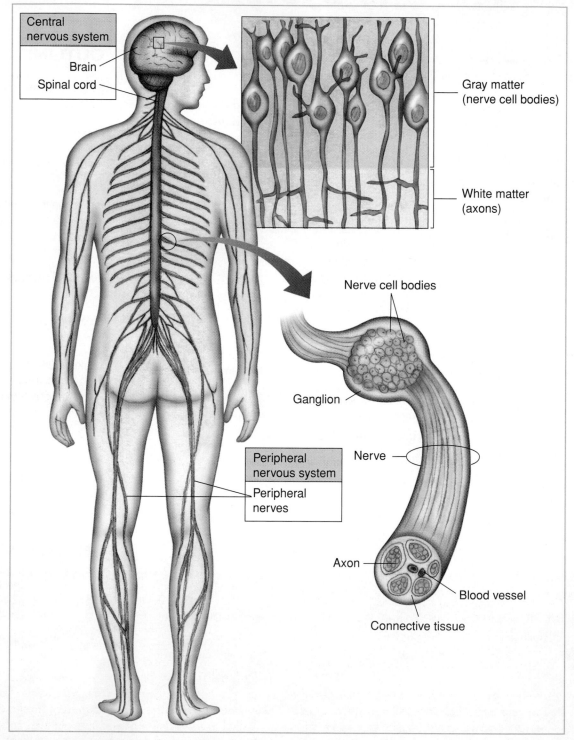

FIGURE 23-1 The nervous system.

smooth operation of the peripheral nervous system is achieved by dividing it into sympathetic and parasympathetic systems. These systems have opposing actions and check on each other to provide a balance. The nervous system uses electrical impulses, which travel along the length of the cells. The cell processes information from the sensory nerves and initiates an action within milliseconds. These impulses travel at up to 250 miles per hour, while other systems such as the endocrine system may take many hours to respond with hormones.

Functions of the Nervous System

The nervous system is responsible for three separate functions: (1) It detects and interprets sensory information. (2) It then takes that information and makes decisions about how it is being received. (3) Finally, it carries out a motor function based on the decisions made.

Neurons

All nervous system tissues are made of up neurons, or nerve cells, and their supporting tissues, called neuroglia. The neuron (see Figure 23-2) is the structural and functional unit of the nervous system. These cells are specialized conductors of impulses that enable the body to interact with its internal and external environments. There are three types of neurons: motor neurons, sensory neurons and interneurons. (For development of the nervous system in children and changes with aging, see Lifespan Considerations).

The motor neurons cause the muscles to contract and the glands to secrete their products and organs to perform their functions. They also inhibit the actions of glands and organs, controlling most of the body's functions. Motor neurons are called *efferent*, meaning that they transmit messages away from the cell body to the muscles and organs. Motor nerves have a nucleated cell body with processes extending away from the cell body. The processes, or "nerve fibers," are called the axon and dendrites. Neurons typically have several dendrites and one axon. The dendrites carry impulses to the cell body, and the axon carries impulses away from it. Most axons are covered with a fatty insulating substance called the myelin sheath. Axons with an intact myelin sheath transmit faster than those without. The axons and dendrites, along with the membrane of the cell body, provide the main receptive surfaces of the neuron to which processes from other neurons communicate.

Sensory neurons differ from motor neurons in that they do not have dendrites. They process and transmit sensory information to the cell body with sheathed, axon-resembling peripheral processes. They

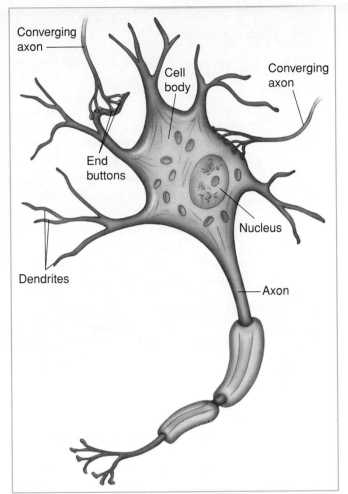

FIGURE 23-2 A neuron (nerve cell) with two converging axons.

are attached to sensor receptors and transmit impulses to the central nervous system. As a result, the central nervous system will stimulate motor neurons in response, causing movement. Sensory neurons are often called *afferent* neurons, since they carry impulses to the cell body and the central nervous system.

Interneurons are also known as associative neurons and are housed entirely within the central nervous system. They mediate impulses between the motor and sensory neurons.

Nerve Fibers, Nerves, and Tracts

A nerve fiber is a single elongated process, usually an axon or peripheral process. Each nerve fiber is wrapped in a protective membrane called a *sheath*. Schwann cells create the myelin sheath. Not all nerve cells have myelin sheaths. Damage to nerve cells without a myelin sheath is permanent, because regeneration of the nerve cell can only happen when Schwann cells are present. Cells without the Schwann cells and the myelin sheath are called unmyelinated cells. Unmyelinated cells have a very thin sheath that provides minimal protection.

Typically, the nerves in the peripheral nervous system are myelinated, and those in the central nervous system are not.

A nerve is a bundle of nerve fibers, located outside the brain and spinal cord, connecting various parts of the body. Afferent, or sensory, nerves carry messages to the central nervous system, and efferent, or motor, nerves carry messages from the central nervous system. There are also mixed nerves, which can be both afferent and efferent (sensory and motor).

Groups of nerve fibers within the central nervous system are referred to as *tracts*. To be a tract, all of the nerves included must have the same origin, function, and termination. The spinal cord contains afferent (sensory) tracts ascending to the brain and efferent (motor) tracts descending from the brain. The brain contains numerous tracts, including the *corpus callosum*, which is the largest, and which joins the right and left hemispheres of the brain.

Nerve Impulses and Synapses

A receptor is the point where a stimulation of the nerve occurs. There are many types of sensory receptors, starting from the very simple nerves that receive pain to very complex receptors, including those in the retina of the eye, which collect all the input necessary for sight. Receptors are typically function specific (pain, heat, cold, sharp), and they react by initiating a chemical change, or impulse. The transmission of an impulse by a nerve fiber is based on the "all or none" principle, meaning, that either there is a response or there isn't. The receptor must receive sufficient stimulation to send the impulse, or the impulse is not transmitted to the brain. Each receptor has its own threshold at which it will react to a stimulus, and each will only respond when its threshold is reached. Impulses travel from the receptors down the dendrites to the cell body, and then down the axon of the nerve to the synapse. The end of the axon is knob shaped, and there are specialized cells at that knob which secrete neurotransmitters (nerve system chemicals) that travel across the synapse to the dendrites of the next nerve, where the entire process repeats itself until the synapse ends at a motor plate attached to a muscle, creating movement. The space at the end of the synapse is called the *synaptic cleft*. The neurotransmitters reach the synaptic cleft, where they cause another chemical–electrical change, causing the next nerve cell to react.

Central Nervous System

The central nervous system (CNS) (Figure 23-3) encompasses the brain and spinal cord (see Figure 23-1). The CNS receives impulses from the entire body, processes the information, and responds with the appropriate action. Activity may be conscious or unconscious, depending on the source of the sensory stimulus. Both the brain and the spinal cord are divided into gray matter and white matter. Gray matter is the unsheathed cell bodies and true dendrites. The white matter consists of the myelinated nerve fibers. In the spinal cord, the arrangement of the gray and white matter is in an H-shaped fashion, with the gray matter forming the core of the spinal cord, surrounded by the white matter. In the brain, the reverse arrangement is true; the white matter forms the core of the brain with the gray matter surrounding the cortex (surface layer).

Brain

Millions of nerve cells and fibers make up the brain. It is the largest mass of nervous tissue in the body, weighing about 1,380 grams in males, and 1,250 grams in females. When fully developed, the brain fills the cranial cavity and is enclosed by three membranes, or meninges. The meninges, from the inside moving outward, are the pia mater, the arachnoid, and the dura mater. The major divisions of the brain are the cerebrum, the diencephalon, the brainstem, which consists of the midbrain and the hindbrain. The hindbrain includes the cerebellum, the pons, the medulla oblongata, and the reticular formation (see Figure 23-4).

Cerebrum

The cerebrum, which develops from the front portion of the forebrain, is the largest part of the mature brain. It consists of two large masses, called *cerebral hemispheres,* that are almost mirror images of each other. They are connected by a deep bridge of nerve fibers called the *corpus callosum* and are separated by a layer called the *falx cerebri.* The surface of the cerebrum is marked by numerous ridges or *convolutions,* called *gyri,* that are separated by grooves. A shallow groove is called a *sulcus,* and a very deep one is a *fissure.* A *longitudinal* fissure separates the right and left hemispheres of the cerebrum, and a *transverse* fissure separates the cerebrum from the cerebellum. Various sulci divide each hemisphere into *lobes* (sometimes called *poles*). The four lobes are named for the skull bones under which they rest: the frontal lobe, the parietal lobe, the temporal lobe, the occipital lobe, and the insula. The cerebrum is concerned with the higher brain functions of interpreting sensory impulses and initiating muscle movement. It stores information and uses it to process reasoning. It also functions in determining intelligence and personality.

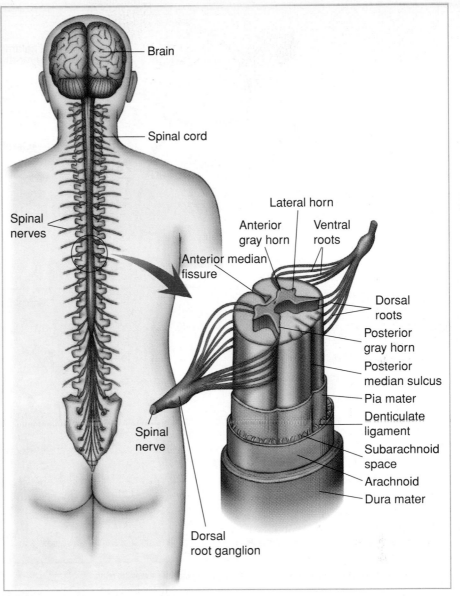

FIGURE 23-3 The central nervous system.

LOBES OF THE CEREBRUM   As previously stated, there are four lobes located in the cerebrum. The frontal lobe is located in front of the central sulcus and is concerned with reasoning, planning, parts of speech and movement, emotions, and problem solving. The parietal lobe is located behind the central sulcus and is concerned with perception of stimuli related to touch, pressure, temperature, and pain. The temporal lobe is located below the lateral fissure and it is concerned with perception and recognition of auditory stimuli (hearing) and memory. The occipital lobe, which is located at the back of the brain, behind the parietal lobe and temporal lobe, is concerned with many aspects of vision.

CORTEX AND VENTRICLES   The outermost layer that surrounds the cerebrum is called the cerebral cortex. Composed of gray matter and containing neuron cell bodies and dendrites, the cortex contains nearly

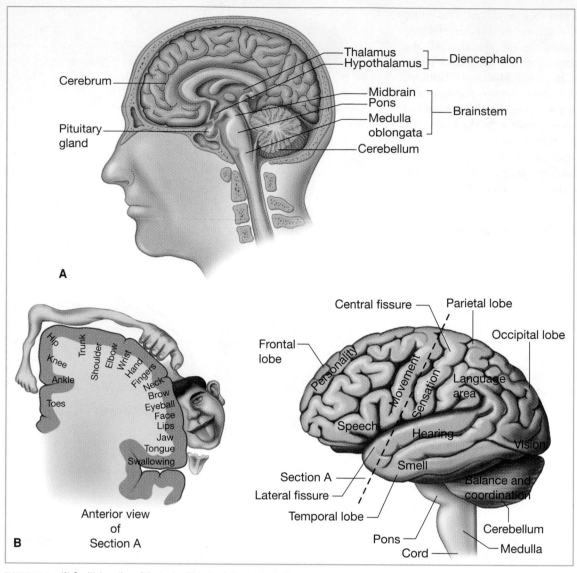

FIGURE 23-4 (A) Sagittal section of the brain. (B) Lateral view of the brain.

75 percent of all neurons in the entire nervous system. Just below the cerebral cortex is white matter. In addition to interpreting sensory information and initiating body movements, the cerebral cortex is also responsible for storing memories and creating emotions.

Within the cerebral hemispheres and brainstem are a series of cavities called *ventricles*. These spaces are contiguous with the central canal of the spinal cord and, like the spinal cord, they are filled with cerebrospinal fluid. The largest of the ventricles are the first and second (lateral) ventricles, which extend into the cerebral hemispheres and occupy portions of the frontal, temporal, and occipital lobes. The third ventricle is in a narrow space in the midline of the brain and connects with the lateral ventricles through openings in the front of it, which are called interventricular foramina. The fourth ventricle is located in the brainstem, just in front of the cerebellum. It is connected to the third ventricle by a narrow canal, the *cerebral aqueduct* (aqueduct of Sylvius), which passes lengthwise through the brainstem. This ventricle is contiguous with the central canal of the spinal cord and has openings in its roof that lead into the meninges (membranes that cover the brain and spinal cord).

Diencephalon

The diencephalon contains the thalamus and hypothalamus. The thalamus, which is the largest of the two divisions of the diencephalon, acts as a telephone line of sorts, allowing information to get through to the cerebral cortex. It also relays motor impulses from the cerebellum and the basal ganglia to the motor areas of the cortex. Some impulses related to emotional behavior are also passed through the thalamus to the cerebral cortex.

The hypothalamus is important for regulating hormones, hunger, thirst, and arousal. Located inferior to the thalamus, it functions as a regulator of autonomic nervous activity associated with behavior and emotional expression. The hypothalamus also produces neurosecretions to control water balance, glucose and fat metabolism, the regulation of body temperature, and other metabolic activities. It also produces hormones for the posterior pituitary gland and manages secretions from the anterior and posterior pituitary glands. The pituitary gland is attached to the inferior side of the hypothalamus by the infundibulum.

Brainstem

The brainstem consists of the midbrain and the hindbrain. Just as the name suggests, the brainstem resembles the stem of a branch. The midbrain is the upper part of the branch that is connected to the forebrain. This region of the brain sends and receives information. Data from our senses, such as the eyes and ears, are sent to this area and then directed to the forebrain.

The hindbrain makes up the lower portion of the brainstem and consists of four units. The medulla oblongata controls involuntary functions such as digestion and breathing. The second unit of the hindbrain, the pons, also assists in controlling these functions. The third unit, the cerebellum, is responsible for the coordination of movement. The fourth unit is the reticular form action, which is responsible for sleep.

MEDULLA OBLONGATA The medulla oblongata connects the brain and the spinal cord. This area is also known as the brainstem and all afferent and efferent nerve tracts from the spinal cord either pass through or terminate in the medulla oblongata. The medulla's functions are the control of breathing, swallowing, coughing, sneezing, and vomiting. Centers in the medulla are responsible for regulating arterial blood pressure and contributing to the control of the circulation of blood.

PONS The pons is a broad band of white matter anterior to the cerebellum and between the midbrain and medulla oblongata. The pons has fiber tracks that link the cerebellum and medulla to higher cortical areas.

CEREBELLUM The cerebellum, which is located in the back of the skull below the cerebrum and behind the pons and medulla oblongata, is the largest part of the hindbrain. The surface of the cerebellum has a large cortex of gray cell bodies with nerve fibers and white matter on its interior. The cerebellum functions in balance and coordination of voluntary movement.

RETICULAR FORMATION The reticular formation is a diffuse network of small groups of cells bodies and their processes located in and around the brainstem. The reticular formation is responsible for sleep, wakefulness, and some reflex activities of the spinal nerves.

Spinal Cord

The spinal cord extends from the medulla oblongata down past the vertebrae and the tailbone, terminating at the cauda equine (which means "horse's tail"), infe-rior to the spine. The spinal cord has an H-shaped central portion of gray matter surrounded by white matter. The white matter consists of nerve tracts and fibers that send sensory input to the brain and conduct motor impulses from the brain back to the body. Other fibers connect nerve cells from one area of the cord to other areas of the cord. The function of the spinal cord is to conduct sensory impulses from the body to the brain and send motor impulses from the brain to the body. The spinal cord also serves as a reflex center for nerve impulses that do not need to pass through the brain.

Cerebrospinal Fluid

Although it is colorless in appearance, cerebrospinal fluid is often considered to be the "blood" of the nervous system. Produced by the choroid plexus, which is located in the ventricles of the brain, the cerebrospinal fluid moves from the ventricles into the connecting canal, and then through the spinal canal and the subarachnoid space that surround the brain. Cerebrospinal fluid has several functions, including serving as a cushion to protect the brain and spinal cord floating in the fluid, and nourishing the brain and spinal cord with oxygen and glucose. It also contains several neurotransmitters, including monoamines, acetylcholine, and neuropeptides.

Peripheral Nervous System

The peripheral nervous system (PNS), which also includes the somatic nervous system, is one of the two major divisions of the nervous system. The other is the central nervous system which is made up of the brain and spinal cord. The nerves in the peripheral nervous system connect the central nervous system to sensory organs (such as the eye and ear), other organs of the body, muscles, blood vessels, and glands.

The somatic nervous system is the part of the PNS that is associated with the voluntary control of body movements through the action of skeletal muscles. It consists of afferent fibers, which receive information from external sources, and efferent fibers, which are responsible for muscle contraction. It is the part of the peripheral nervous system that is made up of 12 cranial nerves from the brain, 31 pairs of spinal nerves from the spinal cord, and all of their branches.

The 12 cranial nerves and the spinal nerves and roots are called the autonomic nerves. The autonomic nerves are concerned with automatic functions of the body. Specifically, autonomic nerves are involved with the regulation of the heart muscle, the tiny muscles lining the walls of blood vessels, and glands.

Cranial Nerves

The cranial nerves are composed of 12 pairs of nerves that emanate from the nervous tissue of the brain (see Figure 23-5). To reach their targets, they must

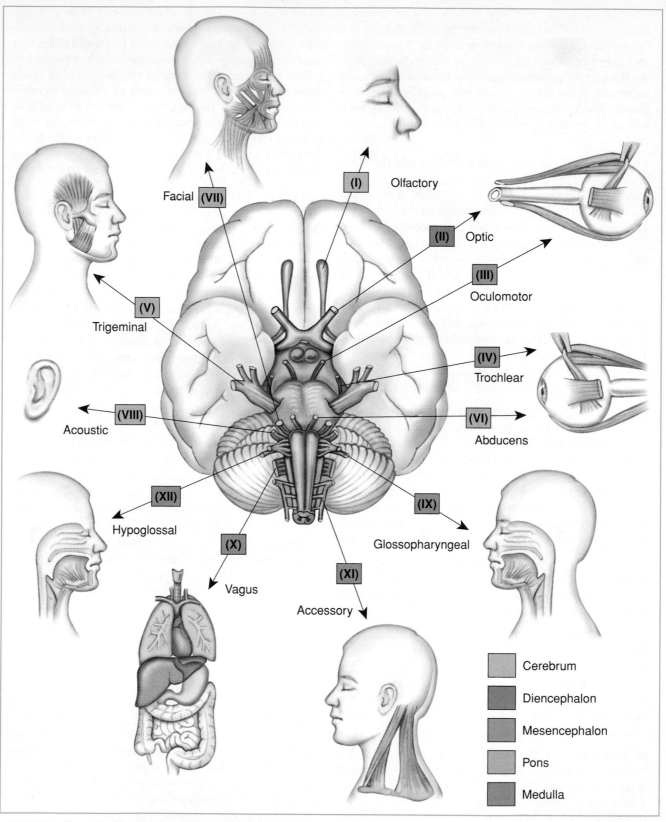

FIGURE 23-5 The relationship of the 12 cranial nerves to specific regions of the brain.

Legend (right side):
- Cerebrum
- Diencephalon
- Mesencephalon
- Pons
- Medulla

Labels:
- Facial (VII)
- (I) Olfactory
- (II) Optic
- (III) Oculomotor
- (IV) Trochlear
- (V) Trigeminal
- (VI) Abducens
- (VIII) Acoustic
- (XII) Hypoglossal
- (X) Vagus
- (XI) Accessory
- (IX) Glossopharyngeal

TABLE 23-1   The 12 Pairs of Cranial Nerves

Brain Region	Cranial Nerve Number	Cranial Nerve Name	General Function
Telencephalon	I	Olfactory	Olfaction (smell)
Diencephalon	II	Optic	Vision
Midbrain	III	Oculomotor	Eye movement (most of our eye movements are commanded through this nerve)
	IV	Trochlear	Eye movement (only one eyeball muscle, the trochlear muscle, is controlled through this nerve)
	V	Trigeminal	Sensation of face and mouth Mastication (chewing) commands
Pons	VI	Abducens	Eye movement (only one eyeball muscle, the lateral rectus muscle, is controlled through this nerve)
	VII	Facial	Facial muscle contraction Some taste sensation Some glandular innervation
	VIII	Acoustic or vestibulocochlear	Senses from our ears: hearing and balance
	IX	Glossopharyngeal	Some taste Some swallowing muscles
Medulla (and spinal cord for CN XI)	X	Vagus	Involuntary functions, it has a role in heart rate and breathing rate Some taste Some swallowing muscles and laryngeal muscles
	XI	Spinal accessory	Some laryngeal muscles Some muscles of the back and neck
	XII	Hypoglossal	Movement of tongue

ultimately exit and enter the cranium through openings in the skull. Hence, their name is derived from their association with the cranium. The function (see Table 23-1) of the cranial nerves is for the most part similar to the spinal nerves, the nerves that are associated with the spinal cord. The motor components of the cranial nerves are derived from cells that are located in the brain. These cells send their axons out of the cranium where they will ultimately control muscle, such as eye movements; glandular tissue, as in the salivary glands; or specialized muscle, like that found in the heart or stomach. The sensory components of cranial nerves originate from collections of cells that are located outside the brain. These collections of nerve cell bodies are called *sensory ganglia*. They are essentially the same functionally and anatomically as the dorsal root ganglia that are associated with the spinal cord. In general, sensory ganglia of the cranial nerves send out a branch that divides into two branches: a branch that enters the brain and one that is connected to a sensory organ. Examples of sensory organs are pressure or pain sensors in the skin and more specialized ones such as taste receptors of the tongue. Electrical impulses are transmitted from the sensory organ through the ganglia and into the brain via the sensory branch that enters the brain. In summary, the motor components of cranial nerves transmit nerve impulses from the brain to target tissue outside of the brain, while components transmit nerve impulses from sensory organs to the brain.

Spinal Nerves

Thirty-one pairs of spinal nerves originate from the spinal cord. They are all mixed nerves, and they provide a two-way communication system between the spinal cord and parts of the arms, legs, neck, and trunk of the body. Although spinal nerves do not have individual names, they are grouped according to the level from which they stem, and each nerve is numbered in sequence. Hence, there are 8 pairs of *cervical nerves* (numbered C1–C8), 12 pairs of *thoracic nerves* (T1–T12), 5 pairs of *lumbar nerves* (L1–L5), 5 pairs of *sacral nerves* (S1–S5), and 1 pair of *coccygeal nerves*. The nerves coming from the upper part of the spinal cord pass outward nearly horizontally, while those from the lower regions descend at sharp angles. This is derived from the consequence of growth. In early life, the spinal cord extends the entire length of the vertebral column, but with age, the column grows faster than the cord. As a result, the adult spinal cord ends at the level between the first and second lumbar vertebrae, so the lumbar, sacral, and coccygeal nerves descend to their exits beyond the end of the cord.

Autonomic Nervous System

The autonomic nervous system (ANS) is a regulatory structure that helps people adapt to changes in their environment. It adjusts or modifies some functions in response to stress. It also helps to regulate the size of blood vessels and blood pressure, the heart's electrical activity and ability to contract, and the flow of air in the lungs. The ANS also regulates the movement and work of the stomach, intestine and salivary glands, the secretion of insulin, and the urinary and sexual functions. The ANS acts through a balance of its two components, the sympathetic nervous system and the parasympathetic nervous system.

Sympathetic and Parasympathetic Nervous Systems

As we have already stated, the autonomic nervous system is divided into two subsystems, the sympathetic and the parasympathetic, which work in tandem, either in a synergistic or an antagonistic way. The sympathetic system is responsible for providing the responses and energy needed to cope with stressful situations such as fear or extremes of physical activity. In response to such stress, the sympathetic system raises blood pressure, heart rate, and the blood supply to the skeletal muscles at the expense of the gastrointestinal tract, kidneys, and skin; dilates both the pupils and the bronchioles, providing improved vision and oxygenation; and generates needed energy by stimulating glycogenolysis in the liver and lipolysis in adipose tissue. In general, it serves to stimulate organs and to mobilize energy.

Between stressful situations, the body needs to rest, recover, and gain new energy. These tasks are under the control of the parasympathetic system, which lowers the heart rate and blood pressure, diverts blood back to the skin and the gastrointestinal tract, contracts the pupils and bronchioles, stimulates salivary gland secretion, and accelerates peristalsis. The parasympathetic system influences organs toward restoration and the saving of energy. Table 23-2 provides a summary of some of

TABLE 23-2 Summary of the Effects of the Sympathetic and Parasympathetic Nervous Systems

Sympathetic	Structure	Parasympathetic
Rate increased	Heart	Rate decreased
Force increased	Heart	Force decreased
Bronchial muscle relaxed	Lungs	Bronchial muscle contracted
Pupil dilation	Eye	Pupil constriction
Motility reduced	Intestine	Digestion increased
Sphincter closed	Bladder	Sphincter relaxed
Decreased urine secretion	Kidneys	Increased urine secretion

the effects of both the sympathetic and the parasympathetic nervous system.

Common Disorders Associated with the Nervous System

The nervous system involves a complex interaction between special elements designed to originate or to carry unique electrochemical charges to and from the various organs within the body. Like its endocrine counterpart, the nervous system initiates and regulates body functions and ensures its owner of an awareness of his or her surrounding environment.

Alzheimer's Disease

Alzheimer's disease is a progressive, degenerative disease of the brain characterized by loss of memory and other cognitive functions. Alzheimer's affects an individual's ability to carry out daily activity. It affects the parts of the brain that control thought, memory, and language. Alzheimer's is not a normal part of aging, although it does affect over 4 million people. The symptoms start slowly, with the first signs typically being mild forgetfulness, especially about more recent events. Such difficulties may not be serious and the patient and family may write them off as the normal consequences of growing older. However, as the disease progresses, the symptoms are more easily noticed by family members and the individual. They lose the ability to think clearly and may begin to forget how to do basic tasks such as brushing their teeth or combing their hair. They may begin to have problems being able to speak clearly, understand, read, or write. As the disease progresses, they may being to wander and change their behavior, becoming aggressive, agitated, or depressed, or have more difficulty swallowing. As the disease destroys the nervous system, they will eventually be unable to speak, walk, sit or swallow and will require complete and total care.

At this time, there is no definitive known cause of Alzheimer's, or the other related dementias. Family history plays a role, as does age and activity. There are medications that are used for patients in early Alzheimer's (those who can function, but are impaired). These medications can slow the progression of the disease, but stopping the medications will restart the previous speed at which the disease was progressing.

Amyotrophic Lateral Sclerosis

Amyotrophic lateral sclerosis (ALS) is a disease of unknown cause, that breaks down tissues in the nervous system, and affects the nerves responsible for movement. It is also known as motor neuron disease and Lou Gehrig's disease, after the baseball player whose career

Professionalism

It is the responsibility of the medical assistant to be courteous, professional, and understanding while providing the neurological patient with care. Each office should have a routine for determining what type of care and treatment is necessary for patients afflicted with neurological disorders. Knowing what these tasks are and what is expected of you prior to the patient coming into the office is paramount to the medical assistant's role.

it ended. It is a disease of the motor neurons, that is, those nerve cells reaching from the brain to the spinal cord (upper motor neurons) and the spinal cord to the peripheral nerves (lower motor neurons) that control muscle movement. In ALS, for unknown reasons, these neurons die, leading to a progressive loss of the ability to move virtually any of the muscles in the body. ALS affects "voluntary" muscles, those controlled by conscious thought, such as the arm, leg, and trunk muscles. ALS, in and of itself, does not affect sensation, thought processes, the heart muscle, or the "smooth" muscle of the digestive system, bladder, and other internal organs. Most people with ALS retain function of their eye muscles as well. However, various forms of ALS may be associated with a loss of intellectual function (dementia) or sensory symptoms.

Bell's Palsy

Bell's palsy is a weakness or paralysis of the muscles that control expression on one side of your face. The disorder results from damage to a facial nerve, one of which runs beneath each ear to the muscles on the same side of your face. The condition may result in a droopy appearance of your face, which can be a blow to your self-esteem. Most often, Bell's palsy isn't serious. The disorder clears up on its own within weeks or months for most people. In some cases, doctors prescribe a corticosteroid medication within the first few days, hoping to increase the likelihood of a good recovery. Bell's palsy, also called facial palsy, is named for Dr. Charles Bell, of Edinburgh, Scotland, who first described the condition in 1882. About 40,000 people in the United States experience Bell's palsy each year. The problem can occur at any age.

Encephalitis

Encephalitis is an inflammation in the brain. The most common causes of encephalitis are viral infections. Symptoms include fever, headache, vomiting, photophobia (sensitivity to light), stiff neck and back, confusion, drowsiness, clumsiness, and irritability. If there is a loss of consciousness, poor responsiveness, seizures, muscle weakness, or impaired judgment, emergency care is required, because these symptoms indicate a life-threatening turn in the disease. There are approximately 1,500 cases per year in the United States, with the most frequently affected individuals being the elderly and infants. Treatment for encephalitis includes antiviral medications, antibiotics, anticonvulsants for seizures, steroids to decrease inflammation, and sedatives for irritability and agitation. Fever may be treated with over-the-counter medications. Typically, individuals with encephalitis or meningitis are hospitalized.

Epilepsy and Seizure Disorders

Epilepsy is a common neurological disorder that results when something interferes with electrical impulses in the brain. In this disorder, the nervous system produces intense, abnormal bursts of electrical activity in the brain, which can lead to seizures. Seizures temporarily interfere with muscle control, movement, speech, vision, or awareness. Having seizures can be terrifying, especially if they are severe. Fortunately, treatment is available to reduce the abnormal electrical impulses in your brain and control seizures. Epilepsy is not a form of mental retardation or mental illness and is not contagious. The cause of epilepsy is not always clear. Less than one-half of people with epilepsy have an identifiable, primary cause. Epilepsy is sometimes the result of another condition, such as head injury, brain tumor, brain infection, or stroke.

Seizure disorders can affect about one-half of a percent of the population. Seizures can also accompany epilepsy, which can affect people of all ages. Some individuals only have one seizure, while others may have repeated episodes. The most common test used to diagnose seizures is an electroencephalogram (EEG). Brain scans (CT scans) are also used to rule out anomalies in brain structure. For most individuals with epilepsy, the seizures are controlled by medications. These medications are typically taken for life, and the control of the seizures will be compromised if they stop taking the medications. More severe cases might require surgical intervention.

Headaches

Recurring headache may be the most common reason for seeking medical care. **Headaches** account for about 10 million visits to physicians' offices each year—not counting visits to nonphysicians, chiropractors, hypnotists, or other health care providers who offer headache relief. But as common as the condition is, it is still in many respects a mystery. Researchers are not exactly sure what causes headaches or which people are more susceptible, though they believe a biological predisposition may be responsible and that overuse of pain-relievers and caffeine can make them worse. Likewise, doctors cannot always tell what kind of headache an individual has and therefore what kind of medicine would be best. Headaches are described in various ways, including the use of such terms as tension headache, muscle contraction headache, stress headache, daily chronic headache, migraine headache, and cluster headache. Specialists also deal with post-traumatic headache and disease-related headache.

Types of Headaches

In 1988, the International Headache Society (IHS) developed the criteria most often used to differentiate the verious type of headaches from one another. They are based on clinical features of the headache, including the number of attacks per month, length of time per attack, pain characteristics, and accompanying symptoms. The types of headaches include migraine, tension, cluster, and post-traumatic.

MIGRAINE HEADACHES In the United States, it is estimated that 17.6 percent of women and 5.7 percent of men have one or more migraine headaches a year, with half of all the 8.7 million women who suffer from mild to moderate migraines saying they have more than one migraine each month. It is thought that hormones cause the higher frequency of migraines in women. The characteristic that usually distinguishes migraine from other types of headache is pain experienced on one side of the head behind the eye.

TENSION HEADACHES Muscle contraction headache, stress headache, ordinary headache, psychomyogenic headache, and idiopathic headache are some of the many other names for tension headache. A mild to moderate squeezing or pressing pain that is steady and nonthrobbing on both sides of the head, back of the neck, and possibly the facial area characterizes a typical attack. It can last from an hour to several hours or more and may occur once or twice a week. They can either be an episodic tension headache or a chronic tension headache. The problem is considered episodic if 10 such headaches have occurred any time previously. Sensitivity to light or sound may also be part of this kind of headache. To be labeled chronic the headache must occur more than 15 times a month. It is important to note that a tension headache can occur at any age. It is often hereditary. Sore and contracted neck, shoulder, and/or back muscles usually accompany it. As with both migraine and tension headache, people suffering from daily chronic headache often overuse painkillers like aspirin or prescription drugs. The overuse of medication, and of caffeine, is believed to be a major causative factor in daily chronic headache.

CLUSTER HEADACHES Unlike migraine, which primarily affects women, cluster headache mainly affects men. Although the exact U.S. incidence is not known, an estimated 500,000 to 2 million Americans experience cluster headaches. These excruciatingly painful headaches occur in bursts every year or two, seemingly more often in the spring and autumn than any other time. The cluster period usually lasts between 2 and 3 months. The penetrating and mostly nonthrobbing pain is often felt behind the eyes or in the temples. Attacks can last from 45 minutes to 2 hours and tend to occur at night. Individuals who smoke cigarettes or drink alcohol excessively are more likely to suffer cluster headaches. Many cluster headache sufferers also have peptic ulcers. Women who have cluster headaches may also have a history of migraine.

POST-TRAUMATIC HEADACHES As many as half of all people who suffer a head or neck injury will develop one or more headache patterns after the primary injury has healed. Symptoms are the same as those of migraine or tension headache. Certain areas of the head may also be sensitive to touch. The condition seems to be unrelated to the amount or severity of damage caused by the primary injury. Symptoms usually develop 24 to 48 hours after the trauma, but can develop later.

Meningitis

Meningitis is an infection of the meninges that surround and protect the brain and spinal cord. Symptoms, which may occur without warning, include high fever, severe and persistent headache, neck stiffness, and nausea and vomiting. Changes in behavior, sleepiness, and difficulty waking indicate an emergency situation requiring immediate medical involvement. Typically, meningitis is caused by a bacterial or viral infection, and lasts about 10 days. Meningitis can be fatal, so medical intervention is mandatory.

Multiple Sclerosis

Multiple Sclerosis (MS) is a chronic, potentially debilitating disease that affects the brain and spinal cord, and there is no known cure. MS is an autoimmune disease, in which the body actually attacks itself. In MS, the body directs the antibodies and white cells to attack the myelin sheath surrounding the nerves in the brain and spinal

Cultural Considerations

There are many cultural stereotypes about neurological diseases. Some individuals may consider these diseases as a "curse" or a weakness" and may not volunteer a lot of information about such disorders. Respect their beliefs, and focus on supporting your patients and their families. Be very careful about asking questions, and make sure that questions are focused on the disease and may not be construed as being judgmental.

cord. This causes inflammation and injury to the sheath and the nerves, and later on, scarring may result. Because of these effects, the transmission of nerve impulses is impeded, resulting in difficulty with movement, vision, or sensation. Symptoms, which may vary with each attack, include weakness, paralysis, or tremor of one or more extremities; muscle spasticity; numbness, decreased, or abnormal sensation in any area; and urinary hesitancy, urgency, or frequency. Fever can also worsen attacks, as can hot baths, sun exposure and stress.

Neuralgia

Neuralgia is an intense burning or stabbing pain caused by irritation of or damage to a nerve. The pain is usually brief but may be severe. It often feels as if it is shooting along the course of the affected nerve. The causes of neuralgia are varied. Chemical irritation, inflammation, trauma (including surgery), compression by nearby structures such as tumors, and infections may all lead to neuralgia. In many cases, however, the cause is unknown or unidentifiable.

Treatment of neuralgia is aimed at reversing or controlling the cause of the nerve problem (if identified) as well as providing pain relief. Therefore, the treatment varies depending on the cause, location, and severity of the pain and other factors. Even if the cause of the neuralgia is never identified, the condition may improve spontaneously or disappear with time. The cause, if known, should be treated. This may include surgical removal of tumors, or surgical separation of the nerve from blood vessels or other structures that compress it.

Preparing for
Externship

In preparing for externship, the medical assistant should focus on learning how to respond to individuals who don't appear "normal." Different patient presentations are seen in neurological practices, especially patients who may have a history of strokes, epilepsy, dementia, or brain trauma. It is especially important to realize that just because an individual is unable to speak clearly or make sense, inside, his or her brain may work perfectly, and it is only the outward expression that is compromised. Never speak poorly of an individual who has a different presentation, especially in his or her presence or that of the family. There is no way for the medical assistant to know exactly what is going on inside the patient's mind.

Mild over-the-counter analgesics such as aspirin, acetaminophen, or ibuprofen may be helpful for mild pain. Narcotic analgesics such as codeine may be needed for a short time to control severe pain. These traditional painkillers, however, often have disappointing results. Other treatments may include nerve blocks, local injections of anesthetic agents, or surgical procedures to decrease sensitivity of the nerve. Some procedures involve the ablation (surgical destruction) of the affected nerve using different methods, such as local radio-frequency, heat, balloon compression, and injection of chemicals.

Paraplegia and Quadriplegia

A lesion of the spinal cord can result in paralysis of certain areas of the body, along with the corresponding loss of sensation. Paraplegia refers to paralysis from approximately the waist down, and quadriplegia refers to paralysis from approximately the shoulders down. Most spinal cord injuries result in loss of sensation and function below the level of injury, including loss of controlled function of the bladder and bowel. Due to the decreased movement and inability to walk, paraplegia may cause numerous medical complications, many of which can be prevented with good nursing care. Complications include pressure sores (decubitus), thrombosis, and pneumonia. Physiotherapy, apart from in assisting in movement, may aid in preventing these complications.

Parkinson's Disease

Parkinson's disease is a progressive disorder, with no known cure, caused by degeneration of the nerve cells in the parts of the brain that control movement. Because of the degeneration, there is a shortage of the neurotransmitter dopamine, causing the movement impairments that characterize the disease.

Parkinson's typically presents as a tremor of a limb, especially when the body is at rest. The tremor usually begins on one side, is localized to one limb, and is usually seen in the hand. Other common symptoms include (slow movement) (bradykinesia) or an inability to move (akinesia) rigid limbs, a shuffling gait, and a stooped posture. Other frequent signs of Parkinson's include reduced facial expression (the "mask") and a soft voice. The disease may also cause depression, personality change, dementia, sleep disturbances, speech impairment, and sexual difficulties. Parkinson's tends to worsen over time.

Sciatica

Sciatica, or pain along the large sciatic nerve that runs from the lower back down the back of each leg, is a relatively common form of low back pain and leg pain. This pain along the sciatic nerve can be caused when a root that helps form the sciatic nerve is pinched or irritated. It is usually caused by pressure on the sciatic nerve from a herniated disk (also referred to as a ruptured disk, pinched nerve, slipped disk, etc.). The problem is often diagnosed as a *radiculopathy,* meaning that a disk has protruded from its normal position in the vertebral column and is putting pressure on the radicular nerve (nerve root) in the lower back, which forms part of the sciatic nerve. Sciatica occurs most frequently in people between 30 and 50 years of age. Often a particular event or injury does not cause sciatica; instead, it may develop as a result of general wear and tear on the structures of the lower spine. The vast majority of people who experience sciatica get better with time (usually a few weeks or months) and find pain relief with nonsurgical treatments.

Spina Bifida

Spina bifida is the most frequently occurring, permanently disabling, and devastating of all birth defects. It affects approximately 1 out of every 1,000 newborns in the United States. More children have spina bifida than have muscular dystrophy, multiple sclerosis, and cystic fibrosis combined. It results from the failure of the spine to close properly during the first month of pregnancy. In severe cases, the spinal cord protrudes through the back and may be covered by skin or a thin membrane. Surgery to close a newborn's back is generally performed within 24 hours after birth to minimize the risk of infection and to preserve existing function in the spinal cord. Because of the paralysis resulting from the damage to the spinal cord, people born with spina bifida may need surgeries and other extensive medical care. The condition can also cause bowel and bladder complications. A large percentage of children born with spina bifida also have hydrocephalus, the accumulation of fluid in the brain. Hydrocephalus is controlled by a surgical procedure called *shunting* that relieves the fluid buildup in the brain by redirecting it into the abdominal area. Most children born with spina bifida live well into adulthood as a result of today's sophisticated medical techniques.

Stroke

A **stroke** known in medicine as a cerebrovascular accident (CVA), is the third leading cause of death in the United States. Death occurs to brain tissue when the blood supply to a part of the brain is decreased, either by a clot or by hemorrhage. Brain cells can die when their oxygen supply is interrupted for more than a few minutes, so speed in diagnosis and treatment is extremely important. One common cause of stroke is atherosclerosis, or narrowing of the arteries by fatty plaques. At other times, the flow of blood over the plaque causes the release of clotting factors, which leads to a blood clot that can block the flow of blood to a specific part of the brain, causing a stroke.

SUMMARY

The nervous system is a very complex communication system that affects all functions in the body. The structure and function of the nervous system, while initially seeming complex, provides for an efficient system of stimulus recognition and motor reaction for the entire body. The brain and the central nervous system collect, interpret, and coordinates all sensory input and responses performed by the peripheral nervous system. The destruction of the myelin sheath is detrimental to the functioning of the entire system. Neurological disorders must be recognized and reported to the appropriate professionals in a very timely manner to prevent long-lasting disability.

Chapter Review

COMPETENCY REVIEW

1. Define and spell the terms to learn for this chapter.
2. What are the two divisions of the nervous system?
3. What are the structural and functional units of the nervous system?
4. What is an axon?
5. What is a neuron?

6. What are the parts of the central nervous system?
7. What are the functions of the hypothalamus?
8. What are the functions of the medulla oblongata?
9. What are three functions of the spinal cord?
10. What are three functions of the central nervous system?

PREPARING FOR THE CERTIFICATION EXAM

1. The first cranial nerve (olfactory) is concerned with
   A. sense of taste
   B. sense of smell
   C. sense of hearing and equilibrium
   D. chief sensory nerve of face and head
   E. sense of sight

2. The cerebrum is the largest part of the mature brain. Which of the following is NOT a part of the cerebrum?
   A. frontal lobe
   B. parietal lobe
   C. cerebellar hemisphere
   D. temporal lobe
   E. occipital lobe

3. The junction between two nerve endings that permits the transmission of a nerve impulse to continue is the
   A. gap
   B. synapse
   C. connectors
   D. receptors
   E. sensors

4. The cranial nerve that supplies most of the organs in the abdominal cavity and the thoracic cavity is the
   A. acoustic
   B. glossopharyngeal
   C. vagus
   D. spinal accessory
   E. hypoglossal

5. Afferent neurons
   A. carry impulses away from the brain and spinal cord
   B. carry impulses to the brain and spinal cord
   C. carry sensory impulses
   D. exist only in the central nervous system
   E. are stimulated only as part of the sympathetic nervous system

6. What chemicals are found in the synapse of the nerves?
   A. endorphins
   B. efferent transmitters
   C. afferent transmitters
   D. neurotransmitters
   E. adrenalin

7. The 12 cranial nerves are located within what part of the nervous system?
   A. central nervous system
   B. peripheral nervous system
   C. autonomic nervous system
   D. voluntary nervous system
   E. sympathetic nervous system

8. The membrane surrounding the brain and spinal cord is called the
   A. vertebrae
   B. cranium
   C. cranial nerves
   D. meninges
   E. pons

9. Which portion of the brain controls respiration, heart rate, and blood pressure?
   A. thalamus
   B. hypothalamus
   C. medulla oblongata
   D. brainstem
   E. cerebrum

10. The portion of the brain controlling motor function is the
    A. frontal lobe
    B. parietal lobe
    C. occipital lobe
    D. temporal lobe
    E. cerebellum

CRITICAL THINKING

1. Why did Dr. Esso send Mrs. Montero to the hospital via the 911 emergency number?

2. Why did Mrs. Montero receive clot-busting drugs?

3. What cardiovascular symptoms were present that led Dr. Esso to think that his patient may have suffered a stroke?

INTERNET ACTIVITY

Do an Internet search to learn about Alzheimer's support groups.

MediaLink More in the nervous system, including interactive resources, can be found on the Student CD-ROM accompanying this textbook.

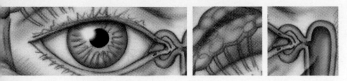

Medical Assistant Role Delineation Chart

HIGHLIGHT indicates material covered in this chapter.

ADMINISTRATIVE

Administrative Procedures

- Perform basic administrative medical assisting functions
- Schedule, coordinate and monitor appointments
- Schedule inpatient/outpatient admissions and procedures
- Understand and apply third-party guidelines
- Obtain reimbursement through accurate claims submission
- Monitor third-party reimbursement
- Understand and adhere to managed care policies and procedures
- *Negotiate managed care contracts*

Practice Finances

- Perform procedural and diagnostic coding
- Apply bookkeeping principles

- Manage accounts receivable
- *Manage accounts payable*
- *Process payroll*
- *Document and maintain accounting and banking records*
- *Develop and maintain fee schedules*
- *Manage renewals of business and professional insurance policies*
- *Manage personnel benefits and maintain records*
- *Perform marketing, financial, and strategic planning*

CLINICAL

Fundamental Principles

- Apply principles of aseptic technique and infection control
- Comply with quality assurance practices
- Screen and follow up patient test results

Diagnostic Orders

- Collect and process specimens
- Perform diagnostic tests

Patient Care

- Adhere to established patient screening procedures
- Obtain patient history and vital signs
- Prepare and maintain examination and treatment areas
- Prepare patient for examinations, procedures and treatments

- Assist with examinations, procedures and treatments
- Prepare and administer medications and immunizations
- Maintain medication and immunization records
- Recognize and respond to emergencies
- Coordinate patient care information with other health care providers
- Initiate IV and administer IV medications with appropriate training and as permitted by state law

GENERAL

Professionalism

- Display a professional manner and image
- Demonstrate initiative and responsibility
- Work as a member of the health care team
- Prioritize and perform multiple tasks
- Adapt to change
- Promote the CMA credential
- Enhance skills through continuing education
- Treat all patients with compassion and empathy
- Promote the practice through positive public relations

Communication Skills

- Recognize and respect cultural diversity
- Adapt communications to individual's ability to understand
- Use professional telephone technique

- Recognize and respond effectively to verbal, nonverbal, and written communications
- Use medical terminology appropriately
- Utilize electronic technology to receive, organize, prioritize and transmit information
- Serve as liaison

Legal Concepts

- Perform within legal and ethical boundaries
- Prepare and maintain medical records
- Document accurately
- Follow employer's established policies dealing with the health care contract
- Implement and maintain federal and state health care legislation and regulations
- Comply with established risk management and safety procedures
- Recognize professional credentialing criteria
- *Develop and maintain personnel, policy and procedure manuals*

Instruction

- Instruct individuals according to their needs
- Explain office policies and procedures
- Teach methods of health promotion and disease prevention
- Locate community resources and disseminate information
- *Develop educational materials*
- *Conduct continuing education activities*

Operational Functions

- Perform inventory of supplies and equipment
- Perform routine maintenance of administrative and clinical equipment
- Apply computer techniques to support office operations
- *Perform personnel management functions*
- *Negotiate leases and prices for equipment and supply contracts*

- *Denotes advanced skills.*

SOURCE: Reprinted by permission of the American Association of Medical Assistants from the AAMA Role Delineation Study: Occupational Analysis of the Medical Assisting Profession.

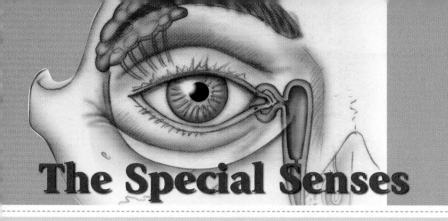

The Special Senses

chapter 24

Learning Objectives

After completing this chapter, you should be able to:

- Define and spell the terms to learn for this chapter.
- Identify the structures that make up the special senses.
- State the anatomy of the eye and briefly explain the function of each structure.
- Discuss common disorders associated with the eye.
- Cite the anatomy of the ear and briefly explain the function of each structure.
- Explain common disorders associated with the ear.
- Identify the anatomy of the nose and explain how the sense of smell occurs.
- Discuss the sense of taste and briefly explain the function of the taste buds.

Terms to Learn

amblyopia	hearing loss	otosclerosis
astigmatism	hordeolum	presbycusis
audiology	hyperopia	presbyopia
cataract	impacted cerumen	retinal detachment
conjunctivitis	macular degeneration	strabismus
corneal abrasion	Ménière's disease	tinnitus
glaucoma	otitis media	

Case Study

CELIA THOMPSON HAS BROUGHT 2-YEAR-OLD DESIREE to see Doctor Gammage, complaining of irritability that has lasted for several days. According to the patient's mother, Desiree has also been running a fever and continues to "pull" on her ears. She does not want to eat, and cries when lying down. Doctor Gammage examines Desiree and determines that she has otitis media. He gives the patient oral antibiotics and aural anesthetics. He also prescribes acetaminophen (Tylenol) as needed.

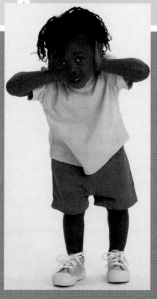

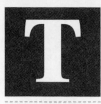his chapter discusses the special senses, which include the structures and organs that make it possible for us to see, hear, smell, taste, and feel different sensations.

The Eye and the Sense of Vision

The eye is a fluid-filled and spherical-shaped organ, composed of special anatomical structures that work together in order to facilitate sight. Light passes through the cornea, pupil, lens, and the vitreous body to stimulate sensory receptors on the retina. Vision is made possible by the coordinated actions of the nerves that control the movement of the eyeball, the amount of light admitted by the pupil, the focusing of the light on the retina by the lens, and the transmission of the resulting impulses to the brain.

Anatomy of the Eye

The eye may be broken down into three separate compartments. The first section includes the cavity, which houses the eyeball. Each eyeball has both a front, or anterior, cavity that is filled with a watery fluid called the aqueous humor, and a posterior, or back, section, which is located behind the lens and is filled with a very thick fluid called the vitreous humor (see Figure 24-1).

The eye is also composed of a wall that has three separate layers. The outer layer houses two structures that play a key role in allowing light to enter the eye. These include the sclera, or "white" part of the eye,

and the cornea, frequently referred to as the "window" of the eye, because it allows the light to enter.

The middle layer of the eye is composed of those structures that are primarily concerned with supplying rich blood to the eye. These include the choroids, which line the sclera and absorb extra light entering the eye; the ciliary body, the structure responsible for holding and moving the lens; and the iris, which contains the pupil, or "hole" in the iris, and which is responsible for controlling the amount of light entering the eye. The pigment or eye color is also located in the middle layer.

The third, or inner, layer of the eye is the retina. This structure is concerned with allowing a person to see visual images through the use of rods and cones that act as visual receptors. The lens focuses and sharpens the light onto the retina. The function of the lens is to sharpen the focus of the light on the retina. This process is called *accommodation*. This is a reflexive function of the body and is combined with the changes in the size of the pupil, the curvature of the lens, and the convergence of the optic axis to maintain the image in the same area on both retinae. The eye also accommodates for distance and depth perception.

The second section of the eye is concerned with those structures that help to protect the eye and provide for visual acuity. These structures include the eyelids, the conjunctiva, the lacrimal apparatus, and the extrinsic eye muscles.

The eyelids close over the eyeball, protecting the eye from intense light, foreign matter, and impacts. They also keep the eye moist by preventing the tears from evaporating. The margins (or the edges) of the superior and inferior palpebrae (the moving parts of the eyelids) have eyelashes that protect the eye from foreign matter. The opening between the eyelids is called the palpebral fissure, which allows light to reach the inner eye. The canthus is the place where the superior and inferior palpebrae meet, also known as the corner of the eye.

The tissue located on the underside of the eyelid and the anterior, or front, portion of the eyeball is a mucous membrane called the conjunctiva. This membrane acts as a protective covering for the exposed surface of the eyeball.

The lacrimal apparatus includes all of the structures that produce, store, and remove the tears that cleanse and lubricate the eye. They include the lacrimal gland located above the outer corner of the eye, which secretes tears through lacrimal

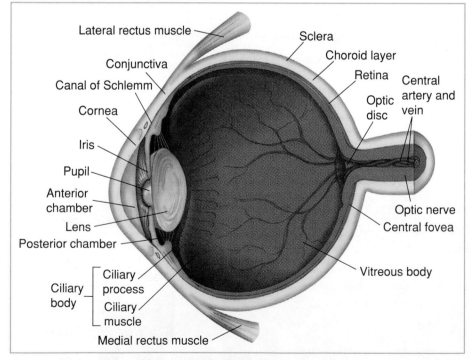

Lateral rectus muscle
Conjunctiva
Canal of Schlemm
Cornea
Iris
Pupil
Anterior chamber
Lens
Posterior chamber
Ciliary body — Ciliary process / Ciliary muscle
Medial rectus muscle
Sclera
Choroid layer
Retina
Optic disc
Central artery and vein
Optic nerve
Central fovea
Vitreous body

FIGURE 24-1   *The eyeball and its anatomical structures.*

As with all of the body systems, the process of aging also affects our senses of sight, hearing, smell, taste, and touch. As such, specific developmental changes begin from the time of early embryonic development and continue throughout one's life.

- Special sense organs are formed early in embryonic development. Maternal infections during the first 5 or 6 weeks of pregnancy may cause visual abnormalities, such as strabismus, as well as sensorineural deafness and other congenital ear problems, in the developing child.
- The developing infant has poor visual acuity, is often farsighted, and lacks color vision and depth perception at birth. The eye continues to grow and mature until the eighth or ninth year of life.
- The newborn infant can hear sounds, but initial responses are reflexive. By the toddler stage, the child is listening critically and beginning to imitate sounds as language development begins.
- Taste and smell are most acute at birth and decrease in sensitivity after the age of 40 as the number of olfactory and gustatory receptors decreases.
- Problems of aging associated with vision include presbyopia; glaucoma, which is the main cause of blindness in the United States; cataracts; and arteriosclerosis of the eye's blood vessels.
- Sensorineural deafness, or presbycusis, is a normal consequence of aging.

ducts found on the surface of the conjunctiva of the upper lid, and the lacrimal canaliculi, which are located at the inner corner of each eye and are responsible for collecting tears and then draining them into the lacrimal sac. The lacrimal sac empties into the nasolacrimal duct, which empties the tears into the nasal cavity (see Figure 24-2).

The six short extrinsic eye muscles connect the eyeball to the orbital cavity, providing it with support and rotary movement. Four of these muscles are straight, called rectus muscles, and two are oblique, or slanted, muscles.

The third section of the eye is primarily concerned with the path that is taken in order for an image to be seen by the person. Visual receptors are activated, thus allowing information to be sent by way of the optic nerve. Parts of this nerve are located at the base of the brain, the area of the brain responsible for vision. Vision occurs when the image is focused on the optic disc, which transfers the image to the optic chiasm and then to the optic nerve to the brain for interpretation of the image's impulses.

Common Disorders Associated with the Eye

Several different types of disorders can affect the eye. These conditions range from an inability to focus correctly on an object to irregularities found in the actual structures that make up the eye. These conditions include refractive errors, age-related disorders, and infections.

Refractive Errors

The most common disorders of the eye are refractive errors, which are caused as a result of the eye no longer being able to focus effectively on an object.

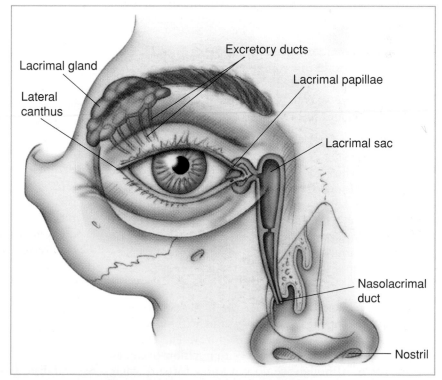

FIGURE 24-2 The lacrimal apparatus and its anatomical structure.

When preparing for a procedure, carefully plan the steps you will take. Make sure that you not only do exactly what you have been asked to do or prepare for, but be ready to take the next step. Always think ahead. Ask yourself what the physician might need next, whether it is having paperwork for labs ready to go or a prescription pad or being ready for a follow-up procedure. If the physician will be performing a minor surgical procedure, be sure that all the necessary supplies, including dressings, are ready for use.

The majority of refractive errors can be corrected by adding a corrective lens (glasses or contact lenses) to help refocus the light correctly on the retina. Other options for correction of refractive errors include radial keratotomy (RK) and the Lasik procedure (laser surgery that reshapes the cornea of the eye and corrects imperfections in the cornea). The three most common refractive errors include myopia, or nearsightedness, which occurs when the lens focuses the light in front of the retina; **hyperopia**, or farsightedness, caused by the lens focusing behind the retina; and **presbyopia**, a disorder that causes the loss of lens elasticity as a result of aging. Treatments for these refractive errors generally include contact lenses and eyeglasses.

Another common disorder of the eyes is **strabismus**, or crossed eyes. In this condition, the eyes are not able to focus on the same image. Treatment usually includes eyeglasses, eye exercises, wearing a patch over the stronger eye, and surgery to realign the eyes.

Astigmatism and Amblyopia

Astigmatism is a condition caused by irregularities of the cornea, thus leading to blurred images during near or distant vision. Treatment generally includes corrective lenses or surgery to reshape the cornea. **Amblyopia**, or "lazy eye," is a disorder seen in children that is caused by the eye muscles being weaker in one eye. The primary treatment is to wear a patch over the stronger eye to strengthen the muscles of the weaker eye.

Cataracts

A **cataract** is a clouding over the lens that prevents light from entering. Over time, and without proper treatment, images begin to look fuzzy. The cataract may cloud the lens so severely that vision becomes impossible. Although we do not know for sure what causes cataracts to occur, physicians believe there may be a correlation between their incidence and smoking, diabetes, and excessive exposure to sunlight. For early or immature cataracts, the use of eyeglasses, magnifying lenses, or stronger lighting is frequently used to aid vision. However, if these measures do not improve vision, surgery is the recommended treatment. Cataract removal is one of the most common surgeries performed in the United States. It is also one of the safest and most effective, with a complete cure rate of 90 percent in most cases.

Conjunctivitis

Conjunctivitis, commonly referred to as "pink eye," is an inflammation of the conjunctiva, the tissue that lines the inside of the eyelid. It is frequently caused by a virus, bacteria, irritating substances, such as shampoos, dirt, or smoke, or sexually transmitted infections (STIs). It is one of the most common and treatable eye infections seen in both children and adults. Conjunctivitis is highly contagious and can be easily spread from person to person. Early recognition of the symptoms is extremely important. Some of the most commonly seen symptoms include redness in the sclera of the eye, an increase in the amount of tears being produced, the presence of a thick yellow discharge that crusts over the eyelashes, itchy eyes, burning in the eyes, blurred vision, and an increased sensitivity to light.

Early recognition of the symptoms and early treatment, including administration of antihistamines or antibiotics by an ophthalmologist or family physician, are important. Cure is almost always 100 percent.

Glaucoma

Glaucoma is a condition caused by an increase in the amount of pressure being built up in the eye, which leads to an excessive amount of aqueous humor. If left untreated, the pressure can lead to damage of the optic nerve, resulting in blindness.

There are two basic types of glaucoma. In open-angle glaucoma, pressure builds up very slowly, causing a slow drainage of aqueous humor from the anterior segment of the eye. However, in acute-angle closure glaucoma, which is considered much more serious, the space between the iris and the cornea decreases, causing a greater degree of pressure to build.

Glaucoma affects people of all ages and all races. There are no symptoms of glaucoma, so it must be diagnosed by pressure testing in a doctor's office. About 80,000 people are totally blind, another 250,000 are blind in one eye, and over 1.2 million people have some degree of visual loss as a result of glaucoma.

Disorders Affecting the Retina

Several disorders affect the retina, but two of the most severe include **retinal detachment** and **macular degen-**

cration. While considered fairly rare and primarily affecting people as they age, a detached retina occurs when the retina separates from the underlying choroid layer. When such a separation occurs, vision becomes damaged. However, if the detachment is detected early, the separation can be repaired and the vision spared. In cases where the retina has already separated and become detached, vision can frequently be restored by surgery and laser therapy.

Macular degeneration, which is caused by a deterioration of the central portion of the retina, is an incurable disease of the eye that affects more than 10 million Americans, and is considered one of the leading causes of blindness in Americans over the age of 55.

There are two types of macular degeneration: dry and wet. Of these, 85 to 90 percent are the dry (atrophic) type. In the dry type of macular degeneration, small yellow deposits (*drusen*) form under the macula. This phenomena leads to a thinning and drying out of the macula. The amount of loss of central vision is directly related to the location and the amount of retinal thinning caused by the drusen. This form of macular degeneration has a slower progression than does the wet type. Sometimes, however, dry macular degeneration will turn into wet degeneration. There is no known treatment or cure for dry macular degeneration.

In the 10 percent of the cases of wet macular degeneration, abnormal new blood vessels, called subretinal neovascularizations, grow underneath the retina and the macula. These new blood vessels may then bleed and leak fluid, causing the macula to bulge or lift up, distorting or destroying the central vision. Vision loss may be rapid and severe. If performed early, laser surgery may halt the progression of wet macular degeneration, thus preventing a total loss of vision. There is no guarantee, however, that this will preserve vision, but it is the best treatment.

Corneal Abrasion

The cornea, which is located at the front of the eye, may become the site of lesions or abrasions. These can be a direct result of an injury, an infection, or sometimes both. A **corneal abrasion** is a very painful condition. The patient will be very sensitive to light and will have difficulty opening the affected eye. The usual treatment is visual rest and mild analgesic. If the abrasion becomes infected, treatment generally consists of antibiotics in the form of drops or ointment and the use of an eye patch.

Hordeolums

Also known as a "sty," **hordeolums** are considered very common and frequently contagious. Structurally, they appear as a pus-filled swelling located near the roots of the eyelash. They are often caused by a bacterial infection and are generally predisposed by blocked or infected eyelid glands or inflammation of the eyelids. Contaminated fingers that touch the eye area may also cause the infection. Painful hordeolums can also occur internally within the eyelids, usually in association with a blocked gland that provides lubrication for the eyelid. Hordeolums may resolve on their own; however, a warm, wet compress applied to the area may help relieve the pain. Antibiotics may be taken orally or antibiotic ointments applied topically to aid in the healing.

The Ear and the Sense of Hearing

The ear is the site of hearing and equilibrium. There are specialized anatomical structures that receive the vibration of sound and are also sensitive to gravity and the movements of the head. These structures are connected to the eighth cranial nerve by special nerve fibers.

Anatomy of the Ear

The ear consists of three separate sections: the external ear, the part visible to the outside; the middle ear, the part responsible for transmitting sounds to the inner ear; and the inner ear, which houses the receptors responsible for providing hearing and equilibrium, or balance (see Figure 24-3).

The External Ear

The external ear is the visible portion of the ear. The appendage on the side of the head consists of the pinna (auricle), the auditory canal (the auditory meatus), and the tympanic membrane (eardrum). The auricle collects sounds waves and then directs them through the auditory canal to the tympanic membrane. The auditory canal is about 2.5 cm long and is S shaped. The tympanic membrane separates the external ear from the middle ear.

The Middle Ear

The function of the middle ear is to transmit sound vibrations, provide equalization of air pressure on both sides of the tympanic membrane, and protect the ossicles from potentially damaging loud sounds. It is a tiny cavity of the temporal bone of the skill, located inside the tympanic membrane. This structure contains three small bones, or ossicles, that are necessary for hearing. The three bones are the malleus (hammer), the incus (anvil), and the stapes (stirrup). The names are indicative of their shapes. These bones react to the vibrations of the sound waves and mechanically transmit the vibrations from the tympanic membrane to the bones in the order presented. The oval window is a small opening on the cochlea, which marks the beginning of the inner ear. During transmission, the tympanic vibrations may be amplified as much as 22 times their original force.

The Inner Ear

The inner ear consists of a membranous labyrinth (maze) located within a bony labyrinth. The bony labyrinth has three divisions: the cochlea, the vestibule, and the three semicircular canals. The perilymph separates the membranous labyrinth from the bony labyrinth. The cochlear duct is one membranous division, located inside the cochlea, and the semicircular ducts are other divisions, located inside the semicircular canals. The final divisions of the membranous labyrinth are the utricle and the saccule, small sac-like structures located in the vestibule. Tiny hair cells that sense movement are located inside the inner ear, functioning as the receptors for hearing and equilibrium (balance).

The Cochlea

The cochlea is a spiral-shaped bony structure that resembles a snail's shell (see Figure 24-4). The spiral cavity of the bony cochlea contains three tube-like channels that run the entire length of the spiral. The three channels are the scala vestibule, the scala tympani, and the cochlear duct. The organ of Corti contains the hair cell sensory receptors used for the sense of hearing. The organ of Corti is located in the cochlear duct on the floor, also known as the basilar membrane. The perilymph (a pale fluid) fills the scala tympani and the scala vestibule, helping to transmit wound waves. Endolymph fills the cochlear duct and protects the hair cells, while assisting with the sense of hearing.

Common Disorders Associated with the Middle Ear

Many of the disorders affecting our hearing are inflammatory and often occur in the middle ear where sounds are transmitted and in the inner ear, at the point where balance

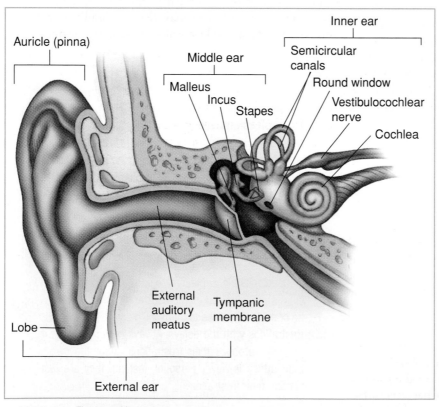

FIGURE 24-3 The ear and its anatomical structures.

and equilibrium take place. The most common inflammatory disorder affecting the middle ear is otitis media, and the most frequently encountered condition affecting the inner ear is Ménière's disease.

Otitis Media

Otitis is an inflammation of the ear. Otitis externa is an inflammation of the outer ear (swimmer's ear). **Otitis media** is inflammation of the middle ear. This inflammation can be caused by viral or bacterial infections, some related to sore throats, colds, or breathing problems.

Children suffer from otitis media more frequently than do adults. This is due to the size of the eustachian tube leading from the ear to the pharynx. If there is any swelling in the tissues that surround this tube, it can close, decreasing the ability of the ear to drain. If the naturally occurring fluids remain in ear, they can become a source of infection. The eustachian tube in children is also straighter than that of an adult, so a child drinking a bottle while lying down stands a greater chance of the fluids flowing backwards up the tube and into the middle ear.

The main goal of treating otitis media is to rid the middle ear of infection before more serious complications set in. Treatment usually involves eliminating the causes of the infection, killing any invading bacteria, boosting the immune system, and reducing swelling in the eustachian tubes. This is frequently accomplished through the introduction of oral antibiotics and decongestants, such as pseudoephedrine. In cases where the otitis media is more acute and there is thick effusion and poor eustachian tube function, daily or every other day tubal insufflation may be in order. Persistent serous fluid may be removed by needle aspiration, but thick mucoid or organized blood must be removed by myringotomy if it has not cleared after 2 or 3 weeks of intensive therapy.

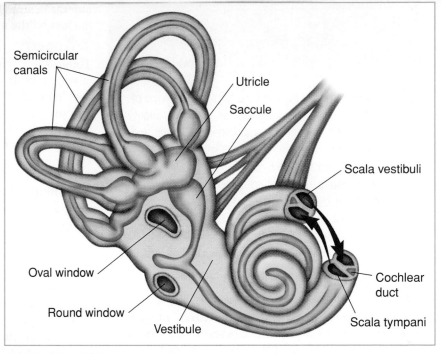

FIGURE 24-4 The cochlea.

Otosclerosis

Otosclerosis, which is frequently hereditary, is a condition that occurs when the tissue surrounding the bone of the stapes grows abnormally around it. When this happens, the overgrowth of the tissue prevents the stapes from transmitting sound vibrations to the inner ear. The result is profound hearing loss involving one or both ears.

Common Disorders Associated with the Inner Ear

The inner ear, as we have previously discussed, is most responsible for helping us to maintain our equilibrium and balance. Because of that, many of the disorders inherent to the inner ear are often accompanied by severe dizziness, ringing in the ears, and a loss of balance.

Ménière's Disease

Ménière's disease is a condition of the inner ear that causes a host of symptoms including vertigo (severe

---

Patient ⬧ Education

The parents of small children should be instructed to never allow their children to lie down while drinking a bottle. When a child drinks while supine the chances of getting middle ear infections increase. Instead, the child should be at a 30-degree angle at least while drinking a bottle and left in that position for a few minutes after drinking.

dizziness), tinnitus (ringing in the ears), fluctuating hearing loss, and a possible sensation of pressure or pain in the affected ear. The disease is named after the French physician Prosper Ménière, who first described the syndrome in 1861.

Symptoms of Ménière's disease, which often occur suddenly and can arise daily or infrequently, are associated with a change in fluid volume within the labyrinth portion of the inner ear. Many experts on Ménière's disease think that a rupture of the membranous labyrinth allows the endolymph and the perilymph to mix. This mixing may be the cause of the symptoms. There are other possible causes, including bacterial or viral infections, environmental factors, and noise pollution.

Although there is no known cure for Ménière's disease, symptoms of the disease can be controlled by reducing the body's retention of fluids, eating a low-salt diet, with no caffeine or alcohol, and possibly using diuretic drugs. Other medication changes that may be beneficial include those that control allergies and improve the blood circulation in the inner ear. Eliminating tobacco use and reducing stress levels are additional ways to reduce the severity of these symptoms.

Presbycusis

Presbycusis is a type of hearing loss involving the gradual deterioration of the sensory receptors located in the cochlea. Seen most frequently in older adults—and affecting approximately 25 percent of people by the time they reach the age of 60 to 70—it affects more men than women. It generally occurs in both ears, causing the patient to have problems hearing high-pitched tones as well as the normal verbal sounds heard during conversation and talking. Factors that lead to presbycusis include long exposures to loud noises, infection, injury, and, in some cases, side effects caused by certain medications. Treatment is generally to assist hearing loss by the use of a hearing aid.

Tinnitus

Tinnitus is a symptom associated with many forms of hearing loss. It can also be a symptom of other health problems. According to estimates by the American Tinnitus Association, at least 12 million Americans have tinnitus. Of these, at least 1 million experience it so severely that it interferes with their daily activities. People with severe cases of tinnitus may find it difficult to hear, work, or even sleep.

Tinnitus is frequently caused by hearing loss, loud noises, medicines, and other health problems, such as allergies, tumors, and problems arising from the cardiovascular system. If a physician suspects tinnitus, he or she may refer the patient to an otolaryngologist for diagnosis or an audiologist who will test the patient's hearing. Although there is no cure for tinnitus, scientists and doctors have discovered several treatments that may provide some relief. The most common of these include the use of hearing aids, maskers, or small electronic devices that are worn by the patient to help mask the sounds, and medications, such as antiarrhythmics and antidepressants.

Impacted Cerumen

Cerumen is a complex mixture of lipids, including waxy compounds produced by the sebaceous glands of the external auditory meatus as a mean of protecting the epithelial lining of the tract. **Impacted cerumen,** or wax, in the ear is a frequent occurrence in which the wax becomes so hard that it obstructs the auditory canal. It generally affects older adults and is frequently exacerbated by their use of cotton-tipped swabs to clean their ears. Treatment includes "softening" the wax, so that it may be removed by an ear syringe. If left untreated, impacted cerumen can lead to hearing loss or tinnitus.

Audiology and Hearing Loss

Audiology is the study of hearing disorders. Sustained noise over 85 decibels can cause permanent **hearing loss,** and the risk doubles with each 5-decibel increase.

The two most common types of hearing loss are conductive hearing loss, which may develop when sound waves have no way of being conducted through the ear and are often temporary, and sensorineural hearing loss, which occurs when neural structures of the ear become damaged, eventually leading to permanent deafness.

The Senses of Taste and Smell

Our sense of smell is dependent on olfactory cells, which are located high in the roof of the nasal cavity. This means that they respond to changes in chemical concentrations. Once a smell receptor is activated, it then sends information to the olfactory nerves, located in different areas of the brain (see Figure 24-5).

The sense of taste and the sense of smell work close together to create a combined effect that is interpreted by the brain. Therefore, when you smell something, some of the tiny molecules move from the nose down into the mouth region, thus stimulating the taste buds. In actuality, part of what we refer to as smell is really taste.

Taste buds, which are tiny bumps located on the tongue, are microscopic, so they cannot be seen by the naked eye (see Figure 24-6). Some can be found on the roof of the mouth, while others are located in the walls of the throat. Each of these buds is made up of cells that function as taste receptors. There are four types of taste cells, with each one of them functioning as an individual group of chemicals that ultimately provides us with different tastes. They include the sweet taste cells, located on the tip of the tongue; the sour taste cells, located on the sides of the tongue; the salty taste cells, located on the tip and sides of the tongue; and the bitter taste cells, located at the back of the tongue.

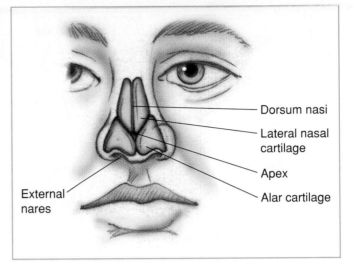

FIGURE 24-5 Nasal cartilages and external structures.

endings that are very sensitive to pain. However, the tongue is not as good at sensing hot or cold. That's why it seems so easy to burn the mouth when something is eaten that is really hot.

The Sense of Touch

Touch is our oldest, most primitive and pervasive sense. It is the first sense we experience in the womb and the last one we lose before death. And while the other four senses (sight, hearing, smell, and taste) are located in specific parts of the body, the sense of touch is found all over. This is because touch originates in the bottom layer of the skin, called the dermis. The dermis is filled with many tiny nerve endings called receptors that provide information about the things with which the body comes in contact (see Figure 24-7). They do this by carrying touch information to the spinal cord, which, in turn, sends messages to the brain where the feeling is registered.

Some areas of the body are more sensitive than others because they have more nerve endings. A good example of this is the pain that is felt when you accidentally bite down on your tongue. The pain occurs because the sides of the tongue have a lot of nerve

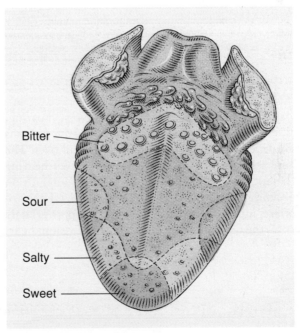

FIGURE 24-6 Tongue and taste buds.

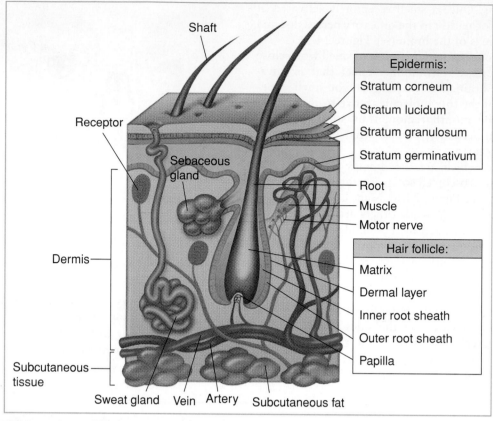

FIGURE 24-7 Layers of the skin showing receptors.

SUMMARY

The special senses, which include vision, hearing, smell, and taste, are special extensions of the nervous system, while the sense of touch is found all over. The eyes are responsible for vision and the ears for hearing and balance, and both systems require the integration of specialized cells that collaborate and provide the appropriate input so that the brain can appropriately interpret the data it receives. The senses of vision, hear-ing, taste, and smell are all activated through the brain and the nervous system. The sense of touch originates in the dermis, where nerve endings process and trans-fer information to the spinal cord, which sends mes-sages to the brain where the feeling is registered. During the aging process, all of these systems can de-cline significantly, greatly affecting the activities and quality of life.

Chapter Review

COMPETENCY REVIEW

1. Define and spell the terms to learn for this chapter.
2. What structures are contained in the middle layer of the eye?
3. What are the external structures of the ear?
4. What are the functions of the muscles of the eye?
5. What is the inner layer of the eye called?
6. What are the functions of the ear?
7. What are the three ossicles of the ear?
8. What is the bony labyrinth?
9. What is the most common "waxy" fluid found in the ear?
10. How many different types of taste cells are located on the tongue?

PREPARING FOR THE CERTIFICATION EXAM

1. What is the name of the substance that fills the anterior cavity that houses the eyeball?
   A. vitreous humor
   B. nasolacrimal fluids
   C. aqueous humor
   D. lacrimal glands
   E. lacrimal fluids

2. The structure of the eye that lines the sclera and absorbs extra light entering the eye is called the
   A. pupil
   B. aqueous humor
   C. retina
   D. ciliary body
   E. choroid

3. Refractive errors are defects in visual acuity. The eye has lost its ability to effectively focus light on the surface of the retina. Which of the following is NOT a refractive error?
   A. hyperopia (farsightedness)
   B. astigmatism
   C. presbyopia
   D. myopia (nearsightedness)
   E. glaucoma

4. A condition of the eye with excessive intraocular pressure that can damage the retina and the optic nerve, often causing blindness, is
   A. glaucoma
   B. cataracts
   C. retinal detachment
   D. astigmatism
   E. corneal ulcers

5. A highly contagious condition of the eye, often caused by a bacterial infection and generally predisposed by blocked or infected eyelid glands, is called
   A. corneal abrasion
   B. astigmatism
   C. hordeolum
   D. conjunctivitis
   E. macular degeneration

6. The mucous membranes that line the inner surfaces of the eyelids are called the
   A. retina
   B. sclera
   C. lens
   D. conjunctiva
   E. iris

7. A condition that is frequently hereditary, and occurs as a result of bone tissue growing abnormally around the stapes is called
   A. otitis externa
   B. otitis media
   C. otosclerosis
   D. Ménière's disease
   E. swimmer's ear

8. Symptoms of Ménière's disease include all of the following EXCEPT
   A. nausea and vomiting
   B. vertigo
   C. pain and pressure in the affected ear
   D. tinnitus
   E. eustachian tube dysfunction

9. All of the following are ossicles of the ear are EXCEPT
   A. cochlea
   B. malleus
   C. incus
   D. stapes
   E. anvil

10. Which taste cell is located on the tip of the tongue?
    A. bitter
    B. sour
    C. sweet
    D. salty
    E. bittersweet

CRITICAL THINKING

1. Why do young children get otitis media more frequently than adults?
2. Why do you think this patient refuses to eat when her ears hurt?
3. Why would acetaminophen (Tylenol) be prescribed for this patient?

INTERNET ACTIVITY

Do an Internet search on Lasik surgery to learn more about the procedure.

MediaLink More on the special senses, including interactive resources, can be found on the Student CD-ROM accompanying this textbook.

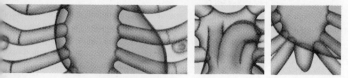

Medical Assistant Role Delineation Chart

HIGHLIGHT indicates material covered in this chapter.

ADMINISTRATIVE

Administrative Procedures

- Perform basic administrative medical assisting functions
- Schedule, coordinate and monitor appointments
- Schedule inpatient/outpatient admissions and procedures
- Understand and apply third-party guidelines
- Obtain reimbursement through accurate claims submission
- Monitor third-party reimbursement
- Understand and adhere to managed care policies and procedures
- *Negotiate managed care contracts*

Practice Finances

- Perform procedural and diagnostic coding
- Apply bookkeeping principles

- Manage accounts receivable
- *Manage accounts payable*
- *Process payroll*
- *Document and maintain accounting and banking records*
- *Develop and maintain fee schedules*
- *Manage renewals of business and professional insurance policies*
- *Manage personnel benefits and maintain records*
- *Perform marketing, financial, and strategic planning*

CLINICAL

Fundamental Principles

- Apply principles of aseptic technique and infection control
- Comply with quality assurance practices
- Screen and follow up patient test results

Diagnostic Orders

- Collect and process specimens
- Perform diagnostic tests

Patient Care

- Adhere to established patient screening procedures
- Obtain patient history and vital signs
- Prepare and maintain examination and treatment areas
- Prepare patient for examinations, procedures and treatments

- Assist with examinations, procedures and treatments
- Prepare and administer medications and immunizations
- Maintain medication and immunization records
- Recognize and respond to emergencies
- Coordinate patient care information with other health care providers
- Initiate IV and administer IV medications with appropriate training and as permitted by state law

GENERAL

Professionalism

- Display a professional manner and image
- Demonstrate initiative and responsibility
- Work as a member of the health care team
- Prioritize and perform multiple tasks
- Adapt to change
- Promote the CMA credential
- Enhance skills through continuing education
- Treat all patients with compassion and empathy
- Promote the practice through positive public relations

Communication Skills

- Recognize and respect cultural diversity
- Adapt communications to individual's ability to understand
- Use professional telephone technique

- Recognize and respond effectively to verbal, nonverbal, and written communications
- Use medical terminology appropriately
- Utilize electronic technology to receive, organize, prioritize and transmit information
- Serve as liaison

Legal Concepts

- Perform within legal and ethical boundaries
- Prepare and maintain medical records
- Document accurately
- Follow employer's established policies dealing with the health care contract
- Implement and maintain federal and state health care legislation and regulations
- Comply with established risk management and safety procedures
- Recognize professional credentialing criteria
- *Develop and maintain personnel, policy and procedure manuals*

Instruction

- Instruct individuals according to their needs
- Explain office policies and procedures
- Teach methods of health promotion and disease prevention
- Locate community resources and disseminate information
- *Develop educational materials*
- *Conduct continuing education activities*

Operational Functions

- Perform inventory of supplies and equipment
- Perform routine maintenance of administrative and clinical equipment
- Apply computer techniques to support office operations
- *Perform personnel management functions*
- *Negotiate leases and prices for equipment and supply contracts*

- *Denotes advanced skills.*

SOURCE: Reprinted by permission of the American Association of Medical Assistants from the AAMA Role Delineation Study: Occupational Analysis of the Medical Assisting Profession.

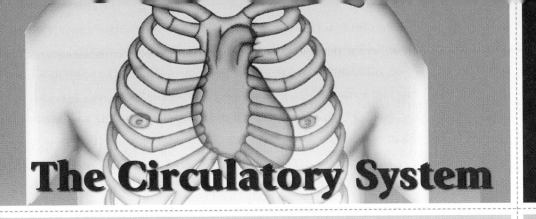

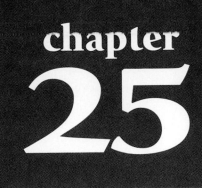

chapter 25

The Circulatory System

Learning Objectives

After completing this chapter, you should be able to:

- Define and spell the terms to learn for this chapter.
- Identify the organs that make up the circulatory system.
- Identify the structures that make up the heart and briefly explain the function of each.
- Explain the conduction system of the heart.
- Explain the functions of the arteries, veins, and capillaries.
- List and describe the components of blood.

- State the difference between Rh-positive blood and Rh-negative blood.
- Discuss the importance of blood typing and cite which blood types are compatible.
- Identify the organs of the lymphatic system and cite the location and function of each.
- Define lymph and explain how it is circulated throughout the body.
- Identify and explain common disorders associated with the circulatory system.

Terms to Learn

anemia	coronary heart disease	myocardial infarction
aneurysm	diastolic blood pressure	myocardium
angioplasty	dyspnea	pericardium
arrhythmia	endocardium	platelets
arteriosclerosis	erythrocytes	Purkinje fibers
atherosclerosis	heart murmur	RhoGAM
atria	hemostasis	sinoatrial node
atrioventricular node	hypertension	systolic blood pressure
bicuspid valve	hypotension	tachycardia
bradycardia	leukemia	thrombophlebitis
bundle of His	leukocytes	tricuspid valve
congestive heart failure	lymph	ventricles

Case Study

JOE FRANCISCO IS A 79-YEAR-OLD who comes to Dr. Schaffer's office complaining of chest pain. Joe has a history of multiple cardiac issues including hypertension and hyperlipidemia. Mr. Francisco is 85 pounds overweight. Dr. Schaffer asks his medical assistant to give Joe one sublingual nitroglycerin and to do an electrocardiogram. His vital signs are blood pressure 150/95; pulse 88; respirations 18. Oxygen is started at 2 liters per minute.

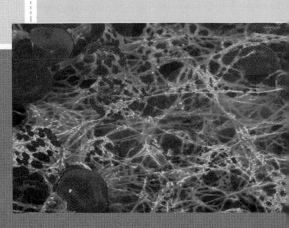

Overview of the Circulatory System

The circulatory system consists of the heart, the blood vessels, the blood, and the structures that make up the lymphatic system. The heart is responsible for the movement of blood through the arterial and vascular system throughout the entire body, providing oxygenation and the removal of waste for the entire body, while the lymphatic system, which is a subsystem of the circulatory system, acts as the body's transportation system. The lymphatic system is also responsible for defending the body against disease-causing agents, called pathogens.

The Heart

The heart is a four-chambered muscular pump lying just left of the midline of the chest (mediastinum), beneath the sternum (see Figure 25-1), and consisting of three linings: the outer lining, called the **pericardium**; the middle layer, or heart muscle, called the **myocardium**; and the innermost lining, called the **endocardium** (see Figure 25-2). Most of the heart is made of cardiac muscle, which is the only muscle with automaticity, meaning that the contractions are controlled by the autonomic nervous system.

The human heart is about the size of a fist and weighs approximately 9 ounces. It is cone shaped, with the apex at the most inferior point and the wider portion of the cone shape at the top.

Four chambers make up the heart, with the right side working to move blood from the body to the lungs, and the left side of the heart pumping the blood back to the body (see Figure 25-3).

The left and right sides of the heart are separated by a wall called the septum. The two upper chambers are called the **atria** (singular is *atrium*) and are receiving chambers. The lower two chambers pump blood out of the heart and are called the **ventricles**.

Blood Flow through the Heart

The right atrium is the first chamber that blood comes into as it enters the heart. This is the smallest chamber with the thinnest wall, and it is responsible for receiving all of the blood from the body via the superior vena cava and the inferior vena cava. The valve (or entryway) from the right atrium to the right ventricle is called the **tricuspid valve**.

After going through the tricuspid valve, the blood enters the right ventricle. This chamber is more muscular

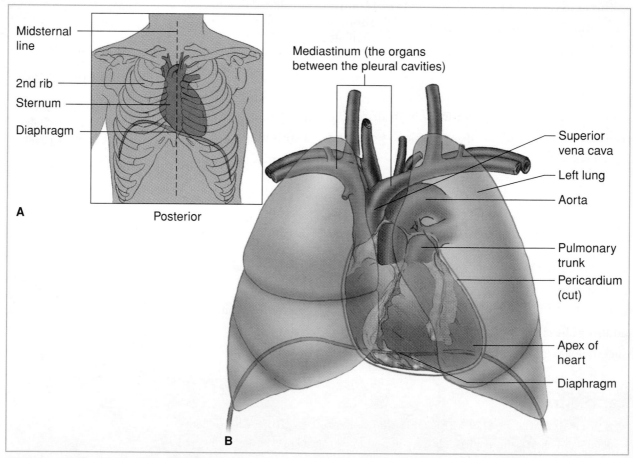

Midsternal line
2nd rib
Sternum
Diaphragm

A Posterior

Mediastinum (the organs between the pleural cavities)

Superior vena cava
Left lung
Aorta
Pulmonary trunk
Pericardium (cut)
Apex of heart
Diaphragm

B

FIGURE 25-1 Location of the heart in the chest cavity.

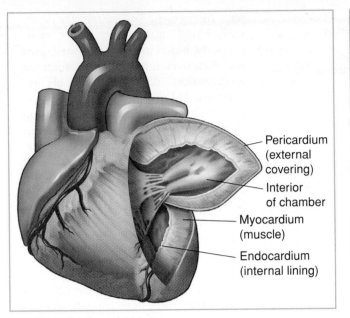

FIGURE 25-2 Linings of the heart.

Pericardium (external covering)

Interior of chamber

Myocardium (muscle)

Endocardium (internal lining)

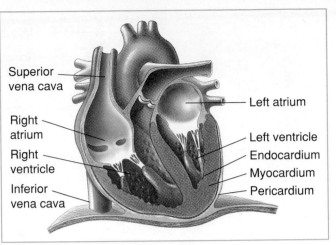

FIGURE 25-3 The heart: interior view of the heart chambers.

Superior vena cava

Right atrium

Right ventricle

Inferior vena cava

Left atrium

Left ventricle

Endocardium

Myocardium

Pericardium

than the right atrium. Blood leaves the right ventricle through the pulmonary valve to go to the lungs, via the pulmonary artery, where the carbon dioxide and waste material from the blood are exchanged for oxygen.

On its return from the lungs, blood enters the left atrium via the pulmonary vein. This atrium is more heavily muscled than is the right atrium. The blood leaves the left atrium through the mitral, or **bicuspid valve.**

The final stop within the heart for the blood is the powerhouse chamber, the left ventricle. The walls of this chamber are highly muscular, so they can pump blood out from the heart to the farthest reaches of the body. When the blood leaves the left ventricle through the aortic valve, it enters the aorta, to begin its journey to the body. The aorta is the largest artery in the body. Figure 25-4 shows the flow of blood through the heart.

It is important to note that during the time the blood is making its way through the heart, the valves are functioning as "doorways" for the blood to move through the chamber, thus never allowing the blood to flow backward (see Figure 25-5). A damaged or diseased valve can allow blood to escape and moves backward through the valves and is known as a **heart murmur.**

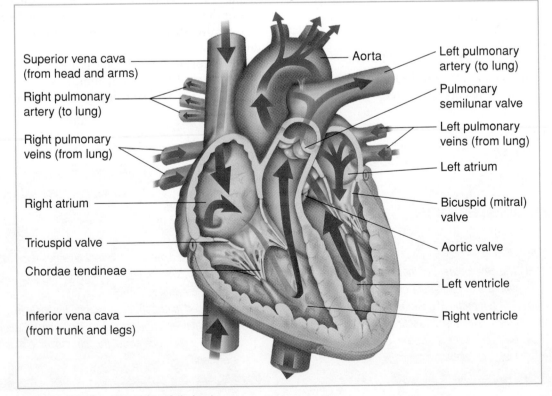

Superior vena cava (from head and arms)

Right pulmonary artery (to lung)

Right pulmonary veins (from lung)

Right atrium

Tricuspid valve

Chordae tendineae

Inferior vena cava (from trunk and legs)

Aorta

Left pulmonary artery (to lung)

Pulmonary semilunar valve

Left pulmonary veins (from lung)

Left atrium

Bicuspid (mitral) valve

Aortic valve

Left ventricle

Right ventricle

FIGURE 25-4 The flow of blood through the heart.

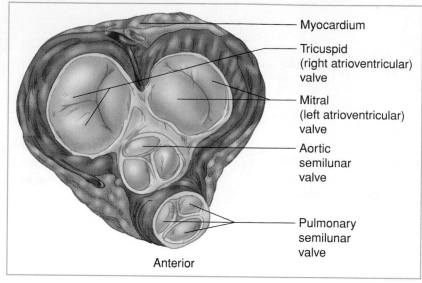

Myocardium

Tricuspid
(right atrioventricular)
valve

Mitral
(left atrioventricular)
valve

Aortic
semilunar
valve

Pulmonary
semilunar
valve

Anterior

FIGURE 25-5 The valves of the heart.

Physiology of the Heart

The heart is a strong muscle, moving blood out from the left ventricle to the entire body with very little obvious effort. The opening of the valves allows the chambers to pump the blood out and receive the next flow of blood into the chamber between contractions. The mechanical, or pump, action of the heart is the cardiac muscle contraction. When the chamber is full, the valves close, prohibiting backflow of blood into the previous chamber. The sounds heard when listening to the heart, auscultation, are made by the valves as they snap shut.

Vascular System of the Heart

The dense muscularity of the heart requires its own vascular system. The coronary arteries, which can be seen in Figure 25-6, supply the heart with blood, and the coronary veins drain the blood into the coronary sinus and then back into the right atrium for oxygenation. When these vessels are occluded (blocked), the heart muscle can be starved for oxygen, causing chest pain, and if the lack of oxygen occurs over a long period of time, then heart muscle damage or death will occur.

Conduction System of the Heart

Cardiac muscle has the property of automaticity. This means that the heart is able to determine its rate and rhythm by way of the autonomic nervous system. Three areas have specialized neuromuscular tissues that initiate the heartbeat. They are the **sinoatrial node** (SA node), the **atrioventricular node** (AV node), and the atrioventricular bundle, also known as the **bundle of His.** Figure 25-7 shows the conduction system of the heart.

The sinoatrial node is also called the "pacemaker." It is located in the upper wall of the right atrium, just blow the opening of the superior vena cava. The SA node is responsible for initiating the heartbeat. The electrical impulses discharged by the SA node are distributed to the right and left atria, causing contractions of the atria. Heart rates initiated by the SA node are typically 60 to 80 beats per minute in a healthy adult at rest.

The atrioventricular node is located beneath the endocardium of the right atrium. It is a "gatekeeper," responsible for transmitting impulses from the SA

Lifespan
Considerations

THE CHILD
- The development of the circulatory system begins with the development of the fetal heart during the first 2 months of gestation, and the newborn's circulation begins to function just after birth.
- Children have a smaller circulatory system, and their vital signs are typically different than those of adults. Their blood pressure will typically be higher than that of an adult, as will their pulse and respiratory rates.

THE OLDER ADULT
- Cardiac and other circulatory changes once attributed to aging may be minimized with appropriate lifestyle modifications.
- Reduced blood flow, elevated blood lipids, and defective endothelial repair that can be seen in aging may accelerate the course of circulatory disease.

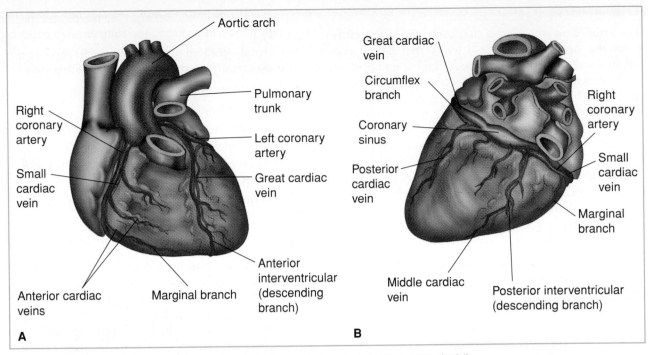

FIGURE 25-6   Coronary circulation. (A) Coronary vessels portraying the complexity and extent of the coronary circulation; (B) coronary vessels that supply the anterior surface of the heart.

node to the inferior portions of the heart. The **Purkinje fibers** are specialized conductive fibers located within the walls of the ventricles. They are responsible for relaying cardiac impulses to the cells of the ventricles, which allow the ventricles to contract.

The final part of the electrical system of the heart is the AV bundle or the bundle of His. The AV bundle extends from the AV node into the intraventricular septum (the wall separating the right and left ventricles), where it branches off, sending a branch to each ventricle. The Purkinje system includes the bundle of His and the peripheral fibers. These fibers end in the ventricular muscles where they cause the strong ventricular muscle contractions.

The Cardiac Cycle

The cardiac cycle includes all of the events that occur during one complete heartbeat. On the average, the heart beats about 70 times per minute, although adult heart rates can vary from 60 to 110 beats per minutes.

The cardiac cycle has three phases. Phase 1, called *atrial systole,* takes about 0.15 second. During this phase, both atria are contracted, while the ventricles are relaxed. Phase 2 is called *ventricular systole.* It takes about 0.30 second to complete. During this phase, both ventricles are contracted, while the atria are relaxed. The third phase of the cycle is called *atrial and ventricular diastole*. It is the longest phase, taking about 0.40 second to complete. During this phase, both atria and ventricles are relaxed and the pressure in the heart chambers is low. Blood returning to the heart from the superior and inferior venae cavae and the pulmonary veins fills the right and left atria and flows passively into the ventricles.

Heart Sounds

A heartbeat produces the familiar "LUB-DUP" sounds as the chambers contract and the valves close. The first heart sound, "lub," is heard when the ventricles contract and the AV valves close. This sound lasts longest and has a lower pitch. The second heart sound, "dup," is heard when the relaxation of the ventricles allows the semilunar valves to close.

In some cases, the valves may become ineffective, causing a clicking or swishing sound after the "lub." This is called a heart murmur. These "leaky" valves do not close completely and allow blood to pass back into the atria or into the ventricles.

Blood Vessels

Blood vessels, which include arteries, arterioles, veins, venules, and capillaries, are responsible for forming a closed pathway that carries blood from the heart to all the cells of the body, and then back again.

The Arteries

The arteries are the vessels that carry the blood away from the heart. There are arteries that carry oxygenated and deoxygenated blood, making it important to remember that arteries always move away from the heart (see Figure 25-8). The arteries are elastic tubes that expand when there is pressure (during the contraction of the heart) and then relax between beats. Because of this expansion and recoil, arteries are an easy place to record the rate of the heart, by palpating the pulse. Some of the most common sites for palpating an artery to obtain an accurate pulse rate include the following locations (see Figure 25-9):

- Radial—found in the lateral wrist, just proximal to the thumb
- Brachial—located in the antecubital space of the elbow, commonly used for taking blood pressures.

It can also be found between the biceps and triceps muscle in pediatric and thinner adult patients

- Carotid—located in the lateral neck; this site is most commonly used in emergency situations
- Temporal—located in the temple area
- Femoral—found in the groin
- Popliteal—located behind the knee on the posteromedial aspect
- Dorsalis pedis—found on the upper surface of the foot
- Anterior tibial—located in the ankle medial to the Achilles tendon.

Veins

The vessels that transport blood from peripheral tissues to the heart are the veins (see Figure 25-10). Veins have thin walls that contain valves that force blood to flow toward the heart and prevent blood from pooling in the lower extremities. Veins have elastic walls, similar to the arteries, but the pressure in the veins is significantly lower than in the arteries. Veins are more superficial than arteries, and are used as phlebotomy sites for obtaining blood specimens, and as sites to administer intravenous (IV) medications.

Capillaries

Capillaries are microscopic blood vessels that have single-celled walls located in the tissues (see Figure 25-11). Oxygenated blood travels through the arterioles to capillaries and on to the tissue cells, where the oxygen is deposited and waste material is picked up. The capillaries transport carbon dioxide and waste material in the blood to the small venules and on to the veins returning to the heart.

Blood Pressure

Blood pressure is defined as the measurement of the force applied to the walls of the arteries. The pressure is determined by the force and amount of blood pumped and by the size and flexibility of the arteries.

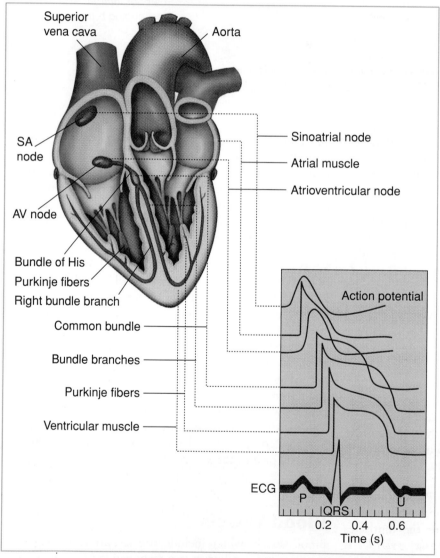

FIGURE 25-7 The conduction system of the heart. Action potentials for the SA and AV nodes, other parts of the conduction system, and the atrial and ventricular muscles are shown along with the correlation to recorded electrical activity (electrocardiogram ECG [EKG]).

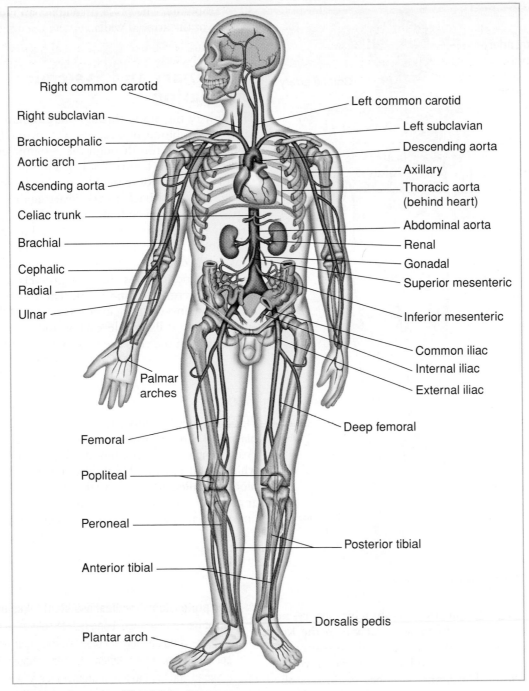

FIGURE 25-8 An overview of the arterial system.

Labels (clockwise/left side):
Right common carotid
Right subclavian
Brachiocephalic
Aortic arch
Ascending aorta
Celiac trunk
Brachial
Cephalic
Radial
Ulnar
Palmar arches
Femoral
Popliteal
Peroneal
Anterior tibial
Plantar arch

Labels (right side):
Left common carotid
Left subclavian
Descending aorta
Axillary
Thoracic aorta (behind heart)
Abdominal aorta
Renal
Gonadal
Superior mesenteric
Inferior mesenteric
Common iliac
Internal iliac
External iliac
Deep femoral
Posterior tibial
Dorsalis pedis

Blood pressure is continually changing depending on activity, temperature, diet, emotional state, posture, physical condition, and medication use.

Blood pressure is usually measured in the brachial artery with a sphygmomanometer, an instrument that records changes in terms of millimeters of mercury. A blood pressure cuff connected to the sphygmomanometer is wrapped around the patient's arm, and a stethoscope is placed over the brachial artery. The blood pressure cuff is inflated until no blood flows through it; thus, no sounds can be heard through the stethoscope. The cuff pressure is then gradually lowered. *Korotkoff sounds* are the sounds heard during the measurement of blood pressure, and up to five phases or sounds may be heard. The first phase heard is when the systolic pressure is recorded. As the pressure in the cuff is lowered still more, the Korotkoff sounds change tone and loudness. When the cuff

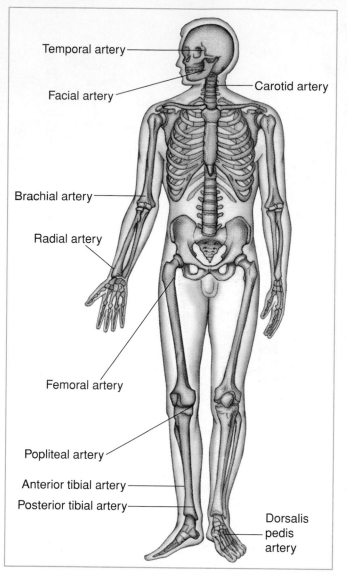

Temporal artery

Facial artery

Carotid artery

Brachial artery

Radial artery

Femoral artery

Popliteal artery

Anterior tibial artery

Posterior tibial artery

Dorsalis pedis artery

FIGURE 25-9 The primary pulse points of the body.

pressure no longer constricts the brachial artery, no sound is heard. The cuff pressure at which the Korotkoff sounds disappear is the diastolic pressure.

The average resting blood pressure for a young adult is 120/80. The higher number is the **systolic blood pressure**, that is, the pressure recorded in an artery when the left ventricle contracts. The lower number is the **diastolic blood pressure**, the pressure recorded in an artery when the left ventricle relaxes. The recorded measurement is written one above the other, with the systolic number on top and the diastolic number on the bottom. For example, a blood pressure measurement of 120/80 mmHg (millimeters of mercury) is expressed verbally as "120 over 80."

Pulse Pressure

The pulse pressure is the difference between the systolic and diastolic blood pressure. Normal pulse pressure is 30 to 50 points. The pulse pressure is an indication of the tone of the arterial walls.

Pulmonary and Systemic Circulation

The flow of the blood through the circulatory system involves the blood making its way through the pulmonary system and through the systemic circulation of the body (see Figure 25-12). Pulmonary circulation involves the route the blood takes from the heart to the lungs and back to the heart again. The function of pulmonary circulation is to oxygenate the blood while allowing for the carbon dioxide to leave the blood and enter the lungs to be exhaled.

Systemic circulation involves the route blood takes from the time it leaves the heart, travels through the body, and returns to the heart. The function of systemic circulation is to deliver oxygen and other nutrients to body cells, while carbon dioxide and waste products from the cells are picked up.

Blood

Blood is a type of connective tissue made up of cells and plasma. There are three types of blood cells; erythrocytes, which are the red blood cells, leukocytes are the white blood cells; and platelets. The fluid part of the blood is called *plasma*. While the average adult has approximately 5 liters of blood, a person's blood volume may vary depending on his or her size, the amount

Professionalism

The professional medical assistant takes pride in his or her appearance. Long hair should be tied back so there is no chance of contaminating hair with any specimens or other fluids. Jewelry should be restrained and kept at a minimum. Rings and bracelets especially should be kept at a minimum because of the issues of frequent hand washings and wearing latex gloves. Long sleeves should not hang off the arms where they could get wet with frequent hand washing or possibly touch specimens. If the clinic uniform is scrubs, the scrubs should be pressed and worn with pride. In a situation where the environment is cool, it is generally acceptable to wear a plain t-shirt underneath the scrub top for extra warmth. White lab coats should be bleached so as to remove stains.

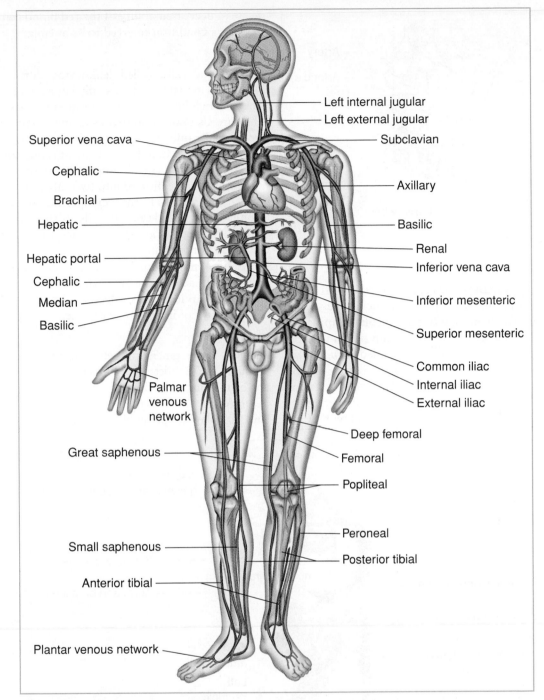

Left internal jugular
Left external jugular
Subclavian
Axillary
Basilic
Renal
Inferior vena cava
Inferior mesenteric
Superior mesenteric
Common iliac
Internal iliac
External iliac
Deep femoral
Femoral
Popliteal
Peroneal
Posterior tibial

Superior vena cava
Cephalic
Brachial
Hepatic
Hepatic portal
Cephalic
Median
Basilic
Palmar venous network
Great saphenous
Small saphenous
Anterior tibial
Plantar venous network

FIGURE 25-10 An overview of the venous circulation.

of adipose tissue, and hydration. The formation of blood cells (hematopoiesis) in adults primarily occurs in the bone marrow.

Composition of Blood

When a fresh blood sample is spun in a centrifuge tube, the blood separates into three layers. The lower layer in the tube is composed of red blood cells, the middle *buffy coat* layer contains the white blood cells and platelets, and the top layer is plasma. The percentage of blood attributed to red blood cells is called the *hematocrit*. Plasma contains a variety of inorganic and organic molecules dissolved or suspended in water. Plasma accounts for about 55 percent of the total volume of whole blood. Figure 25-13 shows the formed elements of blood, including erythrocytes, leukocytes (neutrophils, eosinophils, basophils, lymphocytes, and monocytes), and thrombocytes (platelets).

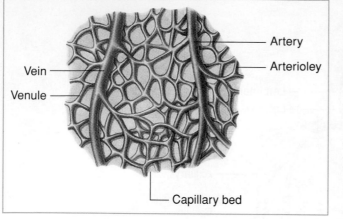

FIGURE 25-11 The capillaries.

Red Blood Cells

Red blood cells (RBCs), or **erythrocytes**, are produced in the red bone marrow. They are biconcave-shaped cells that are small enough to pass through capillaries. Mature red blood cells do not contain nuclei in order to make room for a red pigment called *hemoglobin*. The function of hemoglobin is to carry oxygen. A RBC count refers to the number of red blood cells in 1 cubic millimeter of blood. This count is normally between 4 million and 6.5 million red blood cells. A low RBC in-dicates a decreased ability of the red blood cell to carry oxygen, a condition referred to as anemia.

White Blood Cells

White blood cells, called **leukocytes**, differ from red blood cells in that they are usually larger, have a nucleus, lack hemoglobin, and are translucent unless stained. They are also not as numerous as red blood cells; there are normally only 5,000 to 11,000 per cubic millimeter of blood. White blood cells fight infection and in this way are important contributors to homeostasis.

Leukocytes are divided into two categories: *Granulocytes* have granules in their cytoplasm, are visible after staining, and include neutrophils, eosinophils, and basophils. Monocytes and lymphocytes are *agranulocytes*, which do not contain granules.

A differential white blood cell count allows the number of each of the five types of leukocytes to be measured. An increase or decrease in percentages may be indicative of infection or disease.

Blood Platelets

Platelets are fragments of cells (thrombocytes) that are found in the bloodstream. Thrombocytes control bleeding by forming a clot (coagulation) at the point of injury. A normal platelet count is between 130,000 and 360,000 platelets per cubic millimeter of blood.

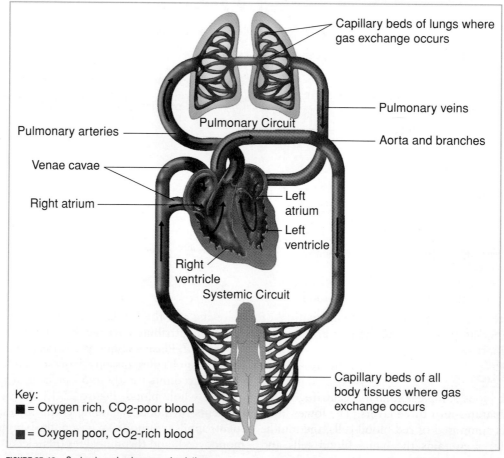

FIGURE 25-12 Systemic and pulmonary circulation.

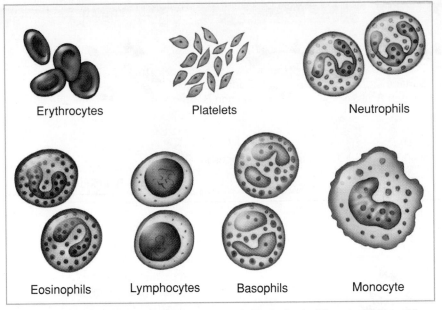

FIGURE 25-13 The formed elements of blood: erythrocytes, leukocytes (neutrophils, eosinophils, basophils, lymphocytes, and monocytes), and thrombocytes (platelets).

Blood Plasma

Plasma is the liquid portion of the blood consisting of 90 percent water. The other 10 percent is a mixture of proteins, nutrients, gases, electrolytes, fats, hormones, enzymes, and waste products. Albumin is the most abundant protein found in plasma and it functions to help maintain the fluid volume in the blood to control blood pressure. Fibrinogen, used in clot formation, and globulins, some of which are antibodies and some are molecule transporters, are the other proteins found in plasma.

Functions of Blood

Blood has three major functions: transportation, defense, and regulation.

Transportation

Blood moves from the heart to all the organs, where gas and nutrient exchange with the tissues takes place across thin capillary walls. Hemoglobin transports oxygen to the cells and picks up carbon dioxide. The blood then transports oxygen from the lungs and nutrients from the digestive tract and delivers these to the tissues. The waste material is removed from the blood and excreted by the kidneys. Various organs and tissues also secrete hormones into the blood, and the blood transports these to other organs and tissues, where they serve as signals that influence cellular metabolism.

Defense

Leukocytes defend the body against invasions by pathogens, microscopic infectious agents, such as bacteria and viruses. This is accomplished in several ways. Neutrophils and monocytes are capable of engulfing and destroying pathogens (*phagocytosis*). Lymphocytes are able to produce and secrete antibodies into the blood. Antibodies incapacitate the pathogens, making them vulnerable to destruction. Another method of defense has to do with blood clotting. When an injury occurs, platelets form a clot, thus preventing blood loss. Coagulation involves platelets and the plasma protein fibrinogen forming a barrier to seal the wound. Without the clotting of blood, we could bleed to death even from a tiny cut.

Regulation

Blood helps to regulate body temperature by picking up heat, mostly from active muscles and then distributing it throughout the body. If the blood is too warm, the heat dissipates from dilated blood vessels in the skin, and the

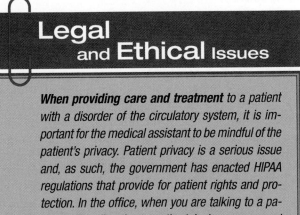

Legal and Ethical Issues

When providing care and treatment to a patient with a disorder of the circulatory system, it is important for the medical assistant to be mindful of the patient's privacy. Patient privacy is a serious issue and, as such, the government has enacted HIPAA regulations that provide for patient rights and protection. In the office, when you are talking to a patient either directly or on the telephone, you must ensure that other patients cannot hear your conversation. Charts should always be turned so that no one walking by can see any personal information on them. Never leave schedules or charts in a place where nonemployees might be able to see them.

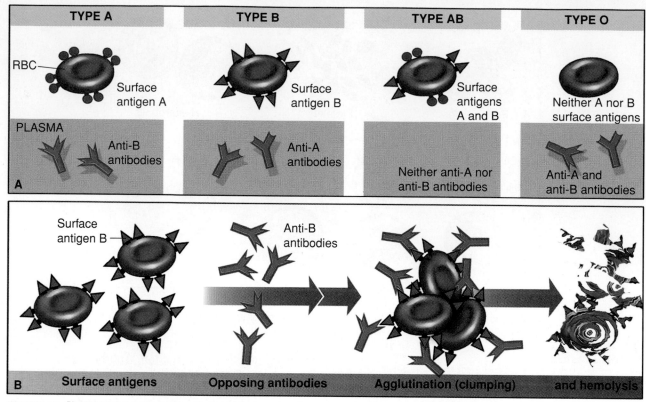

FIGURE 25-14 Blood typing and cross-reactions: The blood type depends on the presence of surface antigens (agglutinogens) on RBC surfaces. (A) The plasma antibodies (agglutinins) that will react with foreign surface antigens; (B) in a cross-reaction, antibodies that encounter their target antigens lead to agglutination and hemolysis of the affected RBCs.

skin becomes flushed as heat is released. The salts and plasma proteins found in the blood act to keep the liquid content of blood high. In this way, the blood plays a key role in helping the body to maintain its own water–salt balance. Because the blood contains buffers, it also helps to regulate the body's pH and keep it relatively constant.

Hemostasis and Bleeding Control

Hemostasis is a term used to describe the stoppage of bleeding. When a blood vessel breaks, the smooth muscle located at the site of the breakage causes the vessel wall to contract, which, in turn, causes the blood vessel to spasm. The spasm reduces the amount of blood lost through the vessel. When this occurs, platelets begin to attach themselves to the broken area and to each other in order to form a type of plug. The plug eventually stops the bleeding. After a period of time, the platelet plug is replaced by the formation of a blood clot. This process is called *coagulation*. During this process, the plasma protein fibrinogen is converted to fibrin. Once the fibrin forms, it sticks to the damaged area of the vessel, eventually creating a meshwork capable of entrapping blood cells and platelets. The end result is a mass,

the blood clot, which stops the bleeding until the vessel has had time to repair itself.

Blood Types

Blood type is determined by the presence or absence of two antigens called type A antigen and type B antigen, located on the surface of red blood cells (see Figure 25-14). Whether these antigens are present or not depends on the particular inherited genes of the individual. The ABO group consists of four blood types: A, B, AB, and O (see Table 25-1).

Agglutination, or clumping, occurs when an antigen protein on the surface of red blood-cells bind to antibodies in the plasma. A and B antibodies present in the plasma make it necessary to type and cross-match blood for transfusions. Blood typing is performed by adding anti-A and anti-B antiserum to drops of blood and observing for agglutination. Anti-A serum will react with type A antigens, but will not agglutinate with anti-B antibody. Anti-B serum will react with type B antigens, but will not agglutinate with anti-A antibody.

Type A

A person with type A antigen on the surface of the red blood cells has type A blood. They also have antibody B in their plasma.

TABLE 25-1 Blood Group Identification by Antigen and Antibody and Routine ABO Blood Typing

Blood Group Identification		
Blood Group	**Antigen**	**Antibody**
A	A	Anti-B
B	B	Anti-A
AB	A and B	Neither
O	Neither anti-A nor anti-B	Anti-A, B

A

Routine ABO Blood Typing					
Reaction of Cells Tested with Group		**Red Cell ABO**	**Reaction of Serum Tested against Group**		**Reverse ABO**
Anti-A	Anti-B		A_1 Cells	B Cells	
0	0	0	+	+	0
+	0	A	0	+	A
0	+	B	+	0	B
+	+	AB	0	0	AB

B

Type B

People who have type B blood have antigen B on the surface of their red blood cells. They also have antibody A in their plasma.

Type AB

A person with type AB blood has both antigens A and B on the surface of their red blood cells, and they have neither antibody A nor antibody B in their plasma. For that reason, people with type AB blood are called universal recipients, because the majority of them can receive all ABO blood types

Type O

Someone with type O blood has no antigens on the surface of the red blood cells. However, they do have both antibody A and antibody B in their plasma. For that reason, people with type O blood are referred to as universal donors because their blood can be administered to most people regardless of the recipients' blood type.

The Rh Factor

The Rh factor is based on an antigen first discovered on red blood cells of the Rhesus monkey. Thus, the name *Rh* came about. Someone who is Rh positive has the red blood cells that contain the Rh antigen. A person who is Rh negative does not contain the Rh antigen. If someone who is Rh negative is given Rh-positive blood, then the Rh-negative person's blood will form antibodies upon exposure to the Rh antigens. If the Rh-negative person is given Rh-positive blood on a second occasion, the antibodies will bind to the donor cells and agglutination will occur.

The Rh factor plays a big role during pregnancy (see Figure 25-15), making it vital for a woman to know her Rh type. If an Rh-negative female mates with an Rh positive male, there is a fifty–fifty chance that, should she become pregnant, the fetus will be Rh positive. When the blood of a developing fetus that is Rh positive mixes with the blood of a mother who is Rh negative, the mother will develop antibodies against the fetus's red blood cells. While the first Rh-positive

Patients with cardiac conditions should be taught the signs and symptoms of a heart attack. They must understand that chest pain that is not alleviated within 2 to 3 minutes is a sign of a possible heart attack, and they are losing precious minutes if they are waiting for the pain to "go away." Patients who have a nitroglycerin prescription should take their nitroglycerin as prescribed, but if the nitroglycerin does not relieve the pain, they should still seek emergency medical care, preferably by calling 911 emergency services.

fetus generally does not suffer from these antibodies due to the length of time it takes for the mother's body to generate them, if a second Rh-positive fetus is conceived, the fetus's blood will be attacked by the antibodies almost immediately. The main reason that this occurs is because the blood cells of the baby and mother do not mix until birth. Thus, the first child is not usually affected. When this occurs, it can lead to a serious condition called erythroblastosis fetalis in which the baby is born severely anemic. The condition can be prevented by administering the drug **RhoGAM** to the Rh-negative mother, which will inhibit the production of antibodies against the Rh antigen.

The Lymphatic System

The lymphatic system is a subsystem of both the circulatory system and the immune system. Its primary responsibility is to defend the body from foreign invasion by disease-causing agents such as viruses, bacteria, or

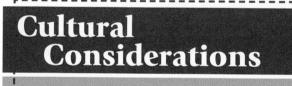

Cultural Considerations

When working with patients of different cultures, try to obtain information about cultural habits, especially those related to diet. Oftentimes, teaching for dietary adaptations is focused on a "traditional American" diet—one that not all patients follow. Ask the patient what types of foods they eat and how those foods are prepared. Then it is easier to assist the patient in making dietary modifications to create a more healthful diet without deviating from their own cultural norms. Other modifications include exercise, and it is important to help patients find activities that are appropriate for their cultural expectations.

fungi. It consists macroscopically of the bone marrow, spleen, thymus gland, lymph nodes, tonsils, appendix, and a few other organs.

The lymphatic system, which is seen in Figure 25-15, contains a network of vessels that assists in circulating body fluids. These vessels transport excess fluids away from interstitial spaces in body tissue and return it to the bloodstream. Lymphatic vessels prevent the backflow of the lymph fluid. They have specialized organs called lymph nodes that filter out destroyed microorganisms.

The function of the lymphatic system is seen most easily at the microscopic level. Blood cells are produced in the marrow of human bone. When mature, white blood cells actively seek out possible pathogens or unknown substances, they attack directly or provide for the removal of this substance. If a white blood cell is alerted to the presence of unwanted bacteria in the blood, it will find this bacteria and surround it. After a type of white blood cell, called a T cell, has the bacteria trapped, it releases a deadly toxin that destroys the bacteria by breaking its outer membrane.

Tissue Fluid, Lymph, and Lymph Nodes

Lymph is a clear fluid that travels through the body's arteries and circulates through the tissues in order to cleanse them and keep them firm. It then drains away through the lymphatic system. Lymph nodes are the filters along the lymphatic system. Their job is to filter out and trap bacteria, viruses, cancer cells, and other unwanted substances, and to make sure they are safely eliminated from the body. Also traveling through the arteries is fresh blood, which brings oxygen and other nutrients to all parts of the body (see Figure 25-16).

After lymph enters the lymphatic vessels, which contain valves that prevent its backflow, the lymph is pushed through the vessels by the movement of skeletal muscles. If lymph is not pushed through a lymphatic vessel, a leakage can occur, causing the surrounding tissue to swell and eventually leading to a condition called *edema.*

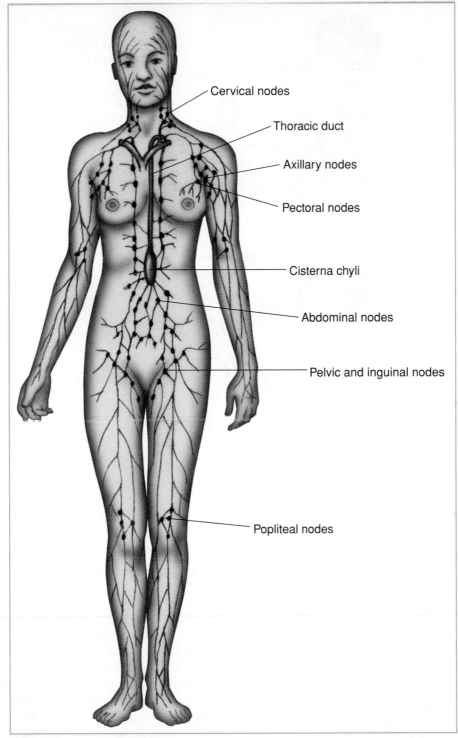

FIGURE 25-15 The lymphatic system.

Labels in figure:
- Cervical nodes
- Thoracic duct
- Axillary nodes
- Pectoral nodes
- Cisterna chyli
- Abdominal nodes
- Pelvic and inguinal nodes
- Popliteal nodes

Thymus and Spleen

The thymus, which lies just above the heart, and the spleen, located in the upper left portion of the abdominal cavity and considered the largest lymphatic organ, are both part of the lymphatic system. While the thymus carries out many of the same functions as the lymph nodes, it is also responsible for the production of lymphocytes and the hormone called thymosin, which stimulates the production of mature lymphocytes.

The spleen also plays an important part in a person's immune system and helps the body fight infection. Like the lymph nodes, the spleen contains antibody-producing lymphocytes. These antibodies weaken or kill bacteria, viruses, and other organisms that cause infection. Also, if the blood passing through the spleen carries damaged cells, white blood cells called macrophages in the spleen will destroy them and clear them from the bloodstream.

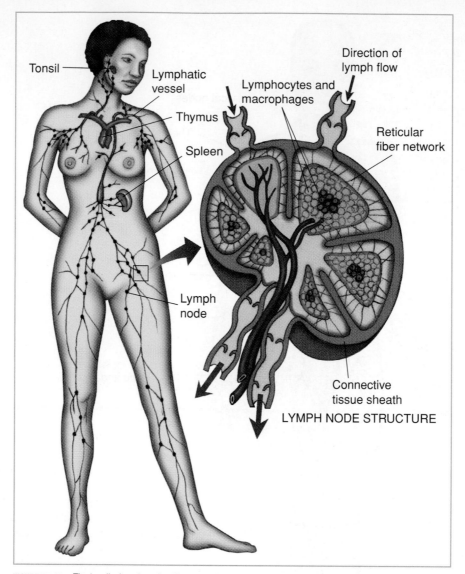

FIGURE 25-16 The tonsils, lymph nodes, thymus, spleen, and lymphatic vessels with an expanded view of a lymph node.

Common Disorders Associated with the Circulatory System

Disorders of the circulatory system are very common in the United States. Many are the result of a combination of lifestyle (lack of exercise, stress, obesity) and genetics.

Coronary Heart Disease

Coronary heart disease (CHD), also known as *coronary artery disease (CAD)*, is considered one of the most common forms of heart disease. This heart disease is due to a narrowing of the coronary arteries that supply blood to the heart. CHD is a more progressive disease that, if left untreated, can lead to a higher risk of myocardial infarction, or heart attack, and possibly sudden death.

Considered one of the leading causes of death in the United States for both men and women, according to the American Heart Association, at least two people per minute in the United States suffer from a CHD-related event, and someone dies about once a minute from cardiac events. During middle age, men have about a 40 to 49 percent risk of a cardiac event, and women have a 32 percent risk. After menopause, the risk increases for women to the same risk level as men.

CHD affects people of all races. It can be caused by lifestyle factors, including obesity, unhealthy diet choices, lack of exercise, and stress, as well as by genetic factors. High levels of lipoproteins or LDL cholesterol are associated with increased deposits on the interior of the arteries, leading to increased CHD. Total cholesterol should be below 200 mg/dL, and the HDL cholesterol (good cholesterol) should be above 35 mg/dL. Steps people can take to increase the HDL cholesterol and decrease total cholesterol include daily aerobic exercise, a dietary increase of vegetables and grain products, weight loss, and smoking cessation.

Atherosclerosis

Atherosclerosis, or narrowing of the vessel lumen of the arteries, results from a buildup of fatty material and plaque within the vessel (see Figure 25-17). It is the leading cause of CHD. As the coronary arteries become narrower and constricted, the flow of blood within the coronary arteries can slow or stop. Blood clots can form as a result of restricted blood flow. The arteries of the heart can narrow to the point that it becomes totally blocked. Plaque that breaks loose forms an embolus that can move and occlude a narrow vessel, causing death to the area supplied by that vessel.

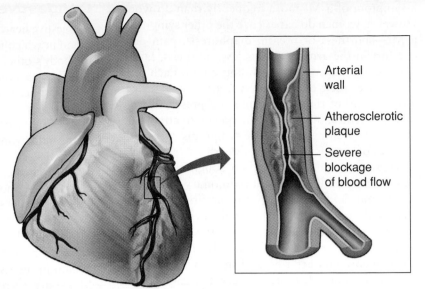

FIGURE 25-17 An atherosclerotic artery.

Small blockages may not always affect the heart's performance. When the heart needs more oxygen-rich blood than the vessels can supply, chest pain or other warning symptoms may occur. This commonly occurs during exercise or other activity. The pain that results is called angina. If the blockage is large, the anginal pain can occur with little or no activity. This pain is known as unstable angina. Sometimes, with unstable angina, the flow of blood to the heart is so limited that the person is restricted in his or her daily activities due to the chest pain. Typically, anginal pain decreases with rest and oxygen, but unrelieved angina is a common symptom of impending myocardial infarction.

Arteriosclerosis

Often referred to as "hardening of the arteries," **arteriosclerosis** is a term used to describe the thickening and loss of elasticity of the arteries. It is a condition that occurs over a period of many years during which the arteries of the circulatory system develop areas that become hard and brittle due to deposits of calcium on the walls. It can involve the arteries of the brain, kidneys, and upper and lower extremities.

A number of factors are causative for arteriosclerosis, including hypertension, diabetes mellitus, smoking, and obesity. Since this disease occurs within the body where it cannot be seen, it is not always recognized early or easily. There are, however, a series of signs and symptoms that should warn the individual and his or her physician. These include high blood pressure, recurrent kidney infections, and impaired circulation, particularly to the fingers and toes, due to peripheral vascular disease. Once recognized, arteriosclerosis can be treated through relieving symptoms and causes. And although several drugs for treating arteriosclerosis are on the

market, it is most important to prevent its occurrence by treating the causative factors.

Heart Attack (Myocardial Infarction)

A heart attack or **myocardial infarction** (MI) occurs when the blood supply to a part of the myocardium is severely reduced or stopped (see Figure 25-18). The blockage is usually due to atherosclerosis, preventing blood flow in the coronary arteries. The accumulated plaque can even tear loose or rupture and trigger a blood clot that blocks the artery. This event is called a coronary thrombosis or coronary occlusion. If the blood supply is cut off, then the muscle tissues fed by that artery suffer irreversible injury and die. Depending on the extent of the injury, disability or death can result.

The most common symptom of an MI is chest pain. Angina is often described as a crushing or squeezing pain, with a feeling of fullness, heaviness, or aching in the center of the chest that may radiate down the arm or into the neck or back. Men experience chest pain as

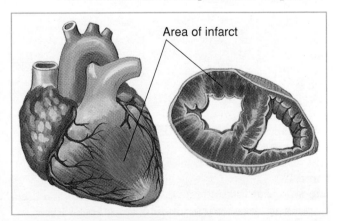

FIGURE 25-18 Cross-section of myocardial infarction.

a symptom of a MI more frequently than do women. However, women do experience the other symptoms of a MI—shortness of breath, diaphoresis, pain or discomfort in the arms, back or jaw, dizziness, fainting, nausea, and a sense of impending doom. Each person experiences their own set of symptoms with an MI—anytime any of these symptoms are present for more than 2 minutes, immediate emergency treatment must be started. Waiting to treat the symptoms increases the chances of serious disability or death.

Treatment for an MI, when sought quickly, can benefit most patients. Cardiopulmonary resuscitation (CPR) and defibrillation within the first few minutes increase the survival rate. Thrombolytics ("clot-busters") can stop some heart attacks in progress. **Angioplasty**, surgical vessel repair, is frequently used to reopen blocked coronary arteries, and stents are used to hold the arteries open. If more conservative measures fail, or if the heart attack is too severe, open heart surgery will be attempted to bypass the blocked artery using a vein from the leg or arm, called a coronary artery bypass graft (CABG).

The most important key for heart attack survival is immediate intervention. Patients need to be educated on the necessity of seeking medical assistance immediately when they have any symptoms of a heart attack. Delay because "it's just indigestion" only decreases the patient's chance of survival.

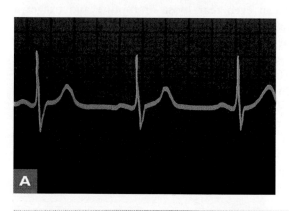

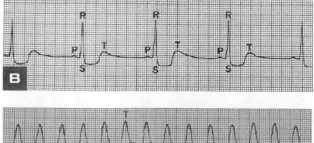

FIGURE 25-19 (A) Example of normal heart rhythm. (B) Example of sinus bradycardia. (C) Example of ventricular tachycardia.

Congestive Heart Failure

Congestive heart failure (CHF), or heart failure, is a condition in which the heart cannot pump enough blood to the body's other organs. This can result from any number of other conditions, including coronary artery disease, past heart attack, hypertension, heart valve disease due to past rheumatic fever or other causes, primary diseases of the heart muscle itself, heart defects present at birth, and any infection of the heart valves or heart muscle, such as endocarditis and myocarditis.

The "failing" heart keeps working but not as efficiently as it should. People with heart failure cannot exert themselves because they become extremely short of breath and tired.

As blood flowing out of the heart slows, blood returning to the heart through the veins backs up, causing congestion in the tissues. Often swelling, or edema, results. Most often there is edema in the legs and ankles, but it can also occur in other parts of the body, too. Sometimes fluid collects in the lungs and interferes with breathing, causing shortness of breath, which becomes more pronounced when a person is lying down. Heart failure also affects the kidneys' ability to dispose of sodium and water. The retained water increases the edema.

Congestive heart failure usually requires a treatment program consisting of rest, proper diet, modified daily activities, and medications such as angiotensin-converting enzyme (ACE) inhibitors, beta blockers, digitalis, diuretics, and vasodilators.

When a specific cause of CHF is discovered, it should be treated or, if possible, corrected. For example, some cases of congestive heart failure can be treated by treating high blood pressure. If the heart failure is caused by an abnormal heart valve, the valve can be surgically replaced.

Arrhythmia

An **arrhythmia** is an irregular heartbeat caused by a disturbance of normal electrical activity of the heart. There are two types of arrhythmias: tachycardias, or fast rhythms, and bradycardias, or slow heart rates. **Tachycardia** is an abnormally fast heartbeat of more than 100 beats per minute. The rhythm may be regular or irregular, but, if it is too fast, it may not allow the ventricles of the heart to fill properly, causing a lack of oxygen to the brain and body. Some tachycardias have such high rates that they can be fatal if not treated immediately. **Bradycardia** is an abnormally slow heart rate, less than 60 beats per minute, which may be regular or irregular. Figure 25-19 shows examples of normal heart rhythm and two examples of arrhythmias, sinus bradycardia and ventricular tachycardia.

While the causes of an arrhythmia may vary, both tachycardias and bradycardias produce similar symptoms, including dizziness, palpitations, shortness of breath, fatigue, weakness, angina, and fainting.

Arrhythmias can be life threatening, especially when they significantly impact the pumping function of the heart. If the oxygen supply to the brain and major organs is interrupted for more than a few minutes, death can occur. Most arrhythmias are caused by heart diseases, including CHD, heart valve disease, heart failure, or infections such as endocarditis.

Carditis (Endocarditis, Myocarditis, Pericarditis)

Carditis is an inflammation of the heart. It is more accurately referred to as endocarditis, myocarditis, or pericarditis, depending on the layer of the heart that is affected.

Endocarditis refers to an inflammation of the lining of the heart, including the heart valves. It is most commonly caused by a bacterial infection and frequently affects patients with existing abnormal conditions of their heart valves. Persons who suffer from this life-threatening condition may experience weakness, fever, diaphoresis or excessive sweating, **dyspnea** or difficulty breathing, and the formation of embolisms that lodge in other organs. Treatment generally consists of antibiotics given intravenously followed by the administration of oral antibiotics over a 6-week period.

When inflammation of the muscular layer of the heart occurs, the condition is referred to as *myocarditis*. Considered relatively uncommon, myocarditis is a very serious condition that, if left untreated, can also lead to death. The most common cause of myocarditis is a viral infection; however, exposure to bacteria and certain drugs, chemicals, and allergens may also lead to its development. Symptoms generally include palpitations or chest pains that closely resemble a heart attack, fever, dyspnea, general fatigue and malaise, and fainting. The person may also experience a decreased urine output. The best treatment for myocarditis includes reduction of the inflammation, bed rest, and a low-sodium diet.

When the inflammation affects the pericardium, that is, the membrane that surrounds the heart, the condition is known as *pericarditis*. It is most commonly seen as a complication of a viral or bacterial infection. Symptoms of this deadly condition frequently include sharp, stabbing chest pain, fatigue, fever, and dyspnea, especially while lying down. Treatment frequently includes analgesics, diuretics to help reduce the amount of fluid around the heart, and antibiotics to decrease the inflammation. Chronic cases of pericarditis may necessitate pericardiocentesis to remove fluid around the heart.

Thrombophlebitis

Thrombo means "clot"; *phlebitis* is the inflammation of a vein. Thrombophlebitis occurs when a blood clot causes inflammation in one or more veins, typically, those in the lower extremities (see Figure 25-20). On rare occasions, thrombophlebitis can also affect the veins in

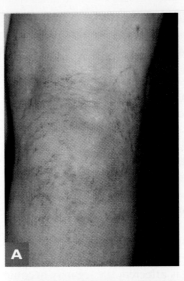

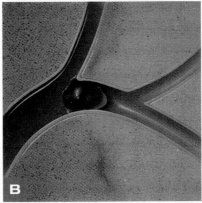

FIGURE 25-20 Example of thrombophlebitis: (A) superficial thrombophlebitis of the leg; (B) cross-section of vein where thrombophlebitis is present.

the upper extremities. The affected vein may be near the surface of the skin (superficial thrombophlebitis) or deep within a muscle (deep venous thrombosis). A clot in a deep vein increases the risk of serious health problems, including the possibility that a dislodged clot will travel to the lungs and block an artery (pulmonary embolism).

Thrombophlebitis is often caused by prolonged inactivity, such as sitting during a long period of travel in an airplane or automobile, by trauma, or from lengthy bed rest following surgery. Such inactivity decreases blood flow through the veins and may cause a clot to form. Paralysis and the use of oral contraceptives or hormone replacement therapy may also lead to thrombophlebitis. A history of varicose veins or an inherited tendency for blood clots can also place someone at higher risk for thrombophlebitis.

If thrombophlebitis occurs in a superficial vein, the physician generally recommends self-care steps that include the application of heat to the pain area, elevation of the affected limb, and the use of nonsteroidal anti-inflammatory drugs, such as aspirin. The condition usually subsides within a week or two. In more severe cases, as in deep venous thrombosis, an injection of a blood-thinning (anticoagulant) medication often prevents the clot from growing. Additional treatments may include the application of support stockings, in order to constrict the superficial veins and increase blood flow in the deep veins, and varicose vein ligation or stripping, in which the doctor surgically removes the varicose veins that causes pain or recurrent thrombophlebitis. In the most severe cases, a thrombectomy or bypass surgery may be required in order to remove an acute clot blocking a pelvic vein or an abdominal vein.

The most common signs and symptoms of thrombophlebitis include redness, swelling, warmth, tenderness, and a dull ache or pain in the affected area. When a superficial vein is affected, a red, hard and tender cord may also be present just under the surface of the skin. When a deep vein is affected, the leg may become swollen, tender, and painful, particularly when the person stands or walks.

Varicose Veins

Varicose veins are gnarled, enlarged veins. They are usually dilated and twisted, usually involving the superficial veins in the leg. These visible and bulging veins are often linked with symptoms such as tired, heavy, or aching limbs. This may be due to prolonged periods of standing, pregnancy or aging. In severe cases, varicose veins can rupture, or form open sores, called varicose ulcers, on the skin.

Varicose veins occur when the valves in the veins malfunction. As one gets older, the veins tend to lose elasticity, causing them to stretch. Blood pools in the veins, causing the veins to become engorged with deoxygenated blood.

Treatment for varicose veins falls into two categories: relief of the symptoms and ligation, or removal of the affected veins. Symptom relief includes such measures as moderate exercise, avoiding long periods of standing, elevating the legs, and wearing support stockings, which compress the veins and hold them in place. Cosmetic treatments may be used to decrease the size and visibility of the affected veins.

Anemia

Anemia is a condition in which there are abnormally low numbers of healthy red blood cells circulating in the body. More specifically, it is the result of low amounts of hemoglobin or abnormal hemoglobin in the red blood cells. Hemoglobin is the iron-containing pigment of the red blood cells that carries oxygen from the lungs to the tissues. Often considered the most common dysfunction of the red blood cells, it affects about 3.5 million Americans.

The three general causes of anemia are (1) decreased healthy red cell production by the bone marrow, (2) increased erythrocyte destruction, or hemolysis, and (3) blood loss from heavy menstrual periods or internal bleeding. A diet lacking in certain vitamins and minerals can also slow down the production of hemoglobin.

Some of the more common symptoms of anemia include fatigue, weakness, fainting, breathlessness, heart palpitations and tachycardia, dizziness, headache, ringing in the ears, difficulty sleeping, and trouble concentrating.

Types of Anemia

There are several types of anemia. Some forms of this condition may be inherited, while others are brought on by poor nutrition or toxins.

IRON DEFICIENCY ANEMIA   The body needs iron for hemoglobin production. Low hemoglobin results in pale red blood cells with a reduced capacity to transport oxygen. In general, most people need just 1 milligram of iron daily. Menstruating or pregnant women may require iron supplements.

VITAMIN DEFICIENCY ANEMIAS   Vitamin B_{12} is also essential for normal hemoglobin production. However, some people can't readily absorb B_{12}. The result is a vitamin B_{12} deficiency, or a condition known as *pernicious anemia.*

HEMOLYTIC ANEMIAS   Anemia caused by the premature destruction of red blood cells is known as hemolytic anemia. In this type of anemia, antibodies produced by the immune system damage red blood cells. This condition is sometimes associated with disorders such as lupus or lymphoma. Toxic materials, such as lead, copper, and benzene, can also lead to the destruction of red blood cells.

SICKLE CELL ANEMIA   Sickle cell anemia, which is characterized by a sickle-shaped red blood cell, is also known as hemoglobin S disease. This is a serious, life-threatening inherited form of anemia, and persons with the disease often suffer from pain in the joints and bones. Infections and heart failure can also occur. Sickle cell anemia occurs in about 0.6 percent of the population, and is highest among African Americans.

APLASTIC ANEMIA This is one of the deadliest and most rare forms of anemia, affecting only one to six people per million. The condition results from an unexplained failure of the bone marrow to produce certain types of blood cells. Instead, fat cells replace bone marrow.

Aplastic anemia is usually found in adolescents and young adults. Symptoms can include bleeding in the mucous membranes, infections with high fevers, pallor, and dyspnea. Injury to the bone marrow or chemicals, such as benzene and certain pesticides, can cause this type of anemia.

Treatments for Anemia

The treatment for anemia will depend on the type and cause. In some cases, injections of vitamin B_{12} may be necessary or specific medications that suppress the body's immune system may need to be eliminated. Blood transfusions, painkilling drugs, and antibiotics may also be required.

Leukemia

Leukemia is a malignant cancer of the bone marrow and blood and, like all cancers, it involves the uncontrolled growth of abnormal cells. In most cancers, these out-of-control cells form tumors, but in leukemia, the problem is with the white blood cells.

There are four major types of leukemia, and this cancer can be acute or chronic. Acute leukemias progress rapidly and cause a marked increase of cells that do not develop normally and never become functional. The leukemia cells crowd out the normal healthy blood cells, increasing the risk of anemia and infection. Patients with acute leukemia also lack platelets that help blood to clot, so they may bleed extensively. Chronic leukemias worsen gradually because the abnormal cells accumulate over time and affect other body tissues.

Leukemia is classified by the type of leukocyte affected. When it strikes the lymphoid cells, it is called lymphocytic leukemia. When it strikes the myeloid cells, it is called myeloid or myelogenous leukemia.

The symptoms of the disease are broad. These include excessive bruising, fatigue, weakness, dyspnea, bleeding of the mucous membranes, bone and joint pain, abdominal pain, weight loss, abdominal bleeding, and enlargement of the lymph nodes, spleen, and/or liver. Anemia and frequent infections are common.

Treatments for Leukemia

There are three major approaches to treating leukemia, depending on the severity and phase of the disease. These include chemotherapy to kill leukemia cells using strong anticancer drugs, radiation therapy to kill cancer cells by exposure to high-energy radiation, and bone marrow transplantation.

Aneurysm

An **aneurysm** is an abnormal widening or ballooning of a portion of an artery, related to weakness in the wall of the blood vessel. Some common locations for aneurysms include the aorta (major artery from the heart), brain (cerebral aneurysm), leg (popliteal artery aneurysm), and intestine (mesenteric artery aneurysm).

Aneurysms can be congenital or acquired. The cause of aneurysms is unknown; however, defects in some of the components of the artery wall may be responsible. High blood pressure and atherosclerotic disease may also contribute to the formation of certain types of aneurysms.

The symptoms of an aneurysm will vary depending on its location. Swelling with a throbbing mass at the site of an aneurysm is often seen if it occurs near the body's surface. Unfortunately, aneurysms within the body or brain often have no symptoms, and frequently go undetected until it is too late.

Surgical intervention may be indicated to repair the vessel and prevent rupturing. Some people may also be candidates for stent placement. This procedure involves the use of a tube placed inside the vessel with specialized catheters that are introduced through arteries at the groin.

Cerebrovascular Accident

A cerebrovascular accident (CVA), or stroke, occurs when the blood supply to part of the brain is suddenly interrupted by an occlusion of a blood vessel (ischemia or embolism) or a ruptured blood vessel (hemorrhage) in the brain. Brain cells die when they no longer receive oxygen and nutrients from the blood. The symptoms of a CVA include sudden numbness or weakness on one side of the body, sudden confusion or trouble speaking, sudden vision problems, severe dizziness, loss of balance or coordination, or sudden severe headaches.

Therapies to prevent a first or recurrent CVA are based on managing an individual's underlying risk factors, such as hypertension, atrial fibrillation, and diabetes. Permanent neurological damage may be avoided with prompt treatment of the underlying cause. Post-CVA rehabilitation helps individuals overcome speech, movement, and mobility disabilities resulting from damage to the affected side of the brain. Drug therapy includes the administration of antithrombotics and thrombolytics.

Hypertension

Hypertension (high blood pressure) is a term used to describe a blood pressure that is higher than 140/90. When the blood vessels can become rigid and constricted, the pressure within the vessels increases. When this force stays high for a period of time, the diagnosis of hypertension is made. Hypertension has few if any symptoms, thus is it called the "silent killer." If left untreated, hypertension can lead to kidney failure, stroke, heart attack, peripheral artery disease, and eye damage.

TABLE 25-2 Disorders of the Cardiovascular System

Disorder	Description
Anemia	A reduction in the number of circulating red blood cells per cubic millimeter of blood. It is not a disease but a symptom of disease.
Aneurysm	An abnormal dilation of a blood vessel, usually an artery, due to a congenital weakness or defect in the wall of the vessel.
Angina pectoris	Condition in which there is severe pain with a sensation of constriction around the heart. It is caused by a deficiency of oxygen to the heart muscle.
Angioma	Tumor, usually benign, consisting of blood vessels.
Angiospasm	Spasm of contraction of blood vessels.
Aortic aneurysm	Localized, abnormal dilation of the aorta, causing pressure on the trachea, esophagus, veins, or nerves. This is due to a weakness in the wall of the blood vessels.
Aortic insufficiency	A failure of the aortic valve to close completely, which results in leaking and inefficient heart action.
Aortic stenosis	Condition caused by a narrowing of the aorta.
Arrhythmia	An irregularity in the heartbeat or action.
Arterial embolism	Blood clot moving within an artery. This can occur as a result of arteriosclerosis.
Arteriosclerosis	Thickening, hardening, and loss of elasticity of the walls of arteries.
Atherosclerosis	This is the most common form of arteriosclerosis. It is caused by the formation of yellowish plaques of cholesterol building up on the inner walls of the arteries.
Bradycardia	An abnormally slow heart rate (under 60 beats per minute).
Congenital heart disease	Heart defects that are present at birth, such as patent ductus arteriosus, in which the opening between the pulmonary artery and the aorta fails to close at birth. This condition requires surgery.
Congestive heart failure	Pathological condition of the heart in which there is a reduced outflow of blood from the left side of the heart. This results in weakness, breathlessness, and edema.
Coronary artery disease	A narrowing of the coronary arteries that is sufficient enough to prevent adequate blood supply to the myocardium.
Coronary thrombosis	Blood clot in a coronary vessel of the heart causing the vessel to close completely or partially.
Embolus	Obstruction of a blood vessel by a blood clot that moves from another area.
Endocarditis	Inflammation of the membrane lining the heart. May be due to microorganisms or to an abnormal immunological response.
Fibrillation	Abnormal quivering or contractions of heart fibers. When this occurs within the fibers of the ventricle of the heart, arrest and death can occur. Emergency equipment to defibrillate, or convert the heart to a normal beat, will be necessary.

(continued)

TABLE 25-2 **Disorders of the Cardiovascular System** (*continued*)

Disorder	Description
Hypertensive heart disease	Heart disease as a result of persistently high blood pressure that damages the blood vessels and ultimately the heart.
Hypotension	A decrease in blood pressure. This can occur in shock, infection, anemia, cancer, or as death approaches.
Infarct	Area of tissue within an organ or part that undergoes necrosis (death) following the cessation of the blood supply.
Ischemia	A localized and temporary deficiency of blood supply due to an obstruction to the circulation.
Mitral stenosis	Narrowing of the opening (orifice) of the mitral valve, which causes an obstruction in the flow of blood from the atrium to the ventricle on the left side of the heart.
Mitral valve prolapse (MVP)	Common and serious condition in which the cusp of the mitral valve drops back (prolapses) into the left atrium during systole.
Murmur	A soft blowing or rasping sound heard upon auscultation of the heart.
Myocardial infarction	Condition caused by the partial or complete occlusion or closing of one or more of the coronary arteries. Symptoms include a squeezing pain or heavy pressure in the middle of the chest. A delay in treatment could result in death. This is also referred to as MI or heart attack.
Myocarditis	An inflammation of the myocardial lining of the heart resulting in an extremely weak and rapid beat, and irregular pulse.
Patent ducts arteriosus	Congenital presence of a connection between the pulmonary artery and the aorta that remains after birth. This condition is normal in the fetus.
Pericarditis	Inflammatory process or disease of the pericardium.
Phlebitis	Inflammation of a vein.
Reynaud's phenomenon	Intermittent attacks of pallor or cyanosis of the fingers and toes associated with the cold or emotional distress. There may also be numbness, pain, and burning during the attacks. It may be caused by decreased circulation due to smoking.
Rheumatic heart disease	Valvular heart disease as a result of having had rheumatic fever.
Tetralogy of Fallot	Combination of four symptoms (tetralogy), resulting in pulmonary stenosis, a septal defect, abnormal blood supply to the aorta, and the hypertrophy of the right ventricle. A congenital defect that is present at birth and needs immediate surgery to correct.
Thrombophlebitis	Inflammation and clotting of blood within a vein.
Thrombus	A blood clot.
Varicose veins	Swollen and distended veins, usually in the legs, resulting from pressure, such as occurs during a pregnancy.

Hypertension can be controlled by a variety of methods, including antihypertensive and diuretic medications, dietary changes, and exercise.

Prehypertension

A newer classification of hypertension is *prehypertension*. This diagnosis is used on individuals who are over 18 years old with a blood pressure that ranges from 120/80 to 139/89 mmHg. This diagnosis was deemed necessary for prevention and treatment of hypertension by the Joint National Committee of the National Institutes of Health National Heart, Lung, and Blood Institute (NHLBI) seventh report. According to the NIH/ NHLBI report, adults at the upper end of the prehypertension blood pressure range are twice as likely to progress to hypertension than those with lower blood pressures. The committee recommends lifestyle changes, including reducing dietary fat and sodium, increasing exercise, and limiting alcohol consumption.

Hypotension

Hypotension, or low blood pressure, is an abnormal condition in which a person's blood pressure is much lower than usual, generally below 90/60 mmHg. When blood pressure drops significantly, blood flow to the heart, brain, and other vital organs is inadequate.

Low blood pressure can also be a sign of a well-conditioned heart in those who get regular aerobic exercise, such as running. In these individuals, the myocardium is able to produce strong contractions to easily pump the blood through the body.

A sudden significant drop in blood pressure is a warning that the body is not receiving enough oxygen and is in danger of shutting down. Normal body functions like breathing, movement, and brain function can be impaired and damage can occur. Rapid drops in blood pressure that threaten life can occur due to loss of blood, shock, severe infections, or low body temperature due to cold exposure. Emergency treatment for these conditions raises blood pressure to a more normal level.

Other causes of hypotension include dehydration, heart failure, heart attack, changes in the heart's rhythm (arrhythmias), syncope (fainting), anaphylaxis, and drug overdose. Another common cause type of low blood pressure is orthostatic hypotension, which results from a sudden change in body position, usually moving from lying down to an upright position.

For more information on disorders, see Table 25-2.

SUMMARY

The circulatory system is concerned with the body's ability to circulate blood, oxygen, nutrients, and other substances. The structures that carry on these processes include the heart and the blood vessels. The heart is a pump used to move oxygen and nutrients to the body and waste and carbon dioxide back to the lungs for excretion from the body. Arteries carry blood away from the heart to the body; the exchange of oxygen and carbon dioxide and carbon dioxide and waste happens in the capillaries, then the veins carry the blood back to the heart and lungs. The lymphatic system acts as a defense system for the body, as well as a means of circulating blood, oxygen, and other fluids throughout the entire body.

- -

Chapter Review

COMPETENCY REVIEW

1. Define and spell the terms to learn for this chapter.
2. Name the components of the circulatory system.
3. Name the three layers of the heart.
4. Name the upper chambers of the heart.
5. Name the lower chambers of the heart.
6. What role do the arteries play in circulation?
7. What role do the veins play in circulation?
8. Name the heart's pacemaker.
9. Define blood pressure.
10. Define pulse pressure.

1. Another name for the mitral valve of the heart is the
   A. tricuspid
   B. pulmonary semilunar
   C. bicuspid
   D. aortic semilunar
   E. intraventricular septum

2. Blood enters the right atrium of the heart through the
   A. pulmonary artery
   B. superior and inferior venae cavae
   C. pulmonary veins
   D. descending aorta
   E. coronary artery

3. What are the two lower chambers of the heart called?
   A. superior and inferior venae cavae
   B. right and left pulmonary arteries
   C. right and left pulmonary veins
   D. right and left ventricles
   E. right and left atria

4. The inner layer of the heart is called the
   A. pericardium
   B. myocardium
   C. apex
   D. endocardium
   E. mediastinum

5. The largest artery in the body is the
   A. superior vena cava
   B. aorta
   C. pulmonary artery
   D. pulmonary vein
   E. jugular

6. The blood pressure that is considered hypertension is
   A. 90/60
   B. 120/40
   C. 120/80
   D. 130/85
   E. 160/90

7. Bradycardia means
   A. abnormally fast heartbeat
   B. abnormally slow heartbeat
   C. average heartbeat
   D. diseased heart
   E. throbbing pulse

8. The artery at the wrist where the pulse is taken is the
   A. radial artery
   B. temporal artery
   C. carotid artery
   D. facial artery
   E. femoral artery

9. What is another term for red blood cells?
   A. erythrocytes
   B. leukocytes
   C. platelets
   D. monocytes
   E. thrombocytes

10. What is a person with type AB blood often referred to as?
    A. universal donor
    B. universal recipient
    C. double antigen donor
    D. double antibody donor
    E. double antigen–antibody recipient

CRITICAL THINKING

1. What are signs and symptoms of angina?
2. Why was the patient given nitroglycerin?
3. If the patient does not get relief from his chest pain, what should he do next?

INTERNET ACTIVITY

Access one of the many "health heart" websites and see what type of education that they provide for their readers. What are some good points of the sites you access?

MediaLink   More on the Circulatory System, including interactive resources, can be found on the Student CD-Rom accompanying this textbook.

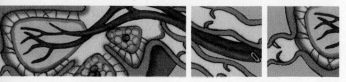

Medical Assistant Role Delineation Chart

HIGHLIGHT indicates material covered in this chapter.

ADMINISTRATIVE

Administrative Procedures

- Perform basic administrative medical assisting functions
- Schedule, coordinate and monitor appointments
- Schedule inpatient/outpatient admissions and procedures
- Understand and apply third-party guidelines
- Obtain reimbursement through accurate claims submission
- Monitor third-party reimbursement
- Understand and adhere to managed care policies and procedures
- *Negotiate managed care contracts*

Practice Finances

- Perform procedural and diagnostic coding
- Apply bookkeeping principles

- Manage accounts receivable
- *Manage accounts payable*
- *Process payroll*
- *Document and maintain accounting and banking records*
- *Develop and maintain fee schedules*
- *Manage renewals of business and professional insurance policies*
- *Manage personnel benefits and maintain records*
- *Perform marketing, financial, and strategic planning*

CLINICAL

Fundamental Principles

- Apply principles of aseptic technique and infection control
- Comply with quality assurance practices
- Screen and follow up patient test results

Diagnostic Orders

- Collect and process specimens
- Perform diagnostic tests

Patient Care

- Adhere to established patient screening procedures
- Obtain patient history and vital signs
- Prepare and maintain examination and treatment areas
- Prepare patient for examinations, procedures and treatments

- Assist with examinations, procedures and treatments
- Prepare and administer medications and immunizations
- Maintain medication and immunization records
- Recognize and respond to emergencies
- Coordinate patient care information with other health care providers
- Initiate IV and administer IV medications with appropriate training and as permitted by state law

GENERAL

Professionalism

- Display a professional manner and image
- Demonstrate initiative and responsibility
- Work as a member of the health care team
- Prioritize and perform multiple tasks
- Adapt to change
- Promote the CMA credential
- Enhance skills through continuing education
- Treat all patients with compassion and empathy
- Promote the practice through positive public relations

Communication Skills

- Recognize and respect cultural diversity
- Adapt communications to individual's ability to understand
- Use professional telephone technique

- Recognize and respond effectively to verbal, nonverbal, and written communications
- Use medical terminology appropriately
- Utilize electronic technology to receive, organize, prioritize and transmit information
- Serve as liaison

Legal Concepts

- Perform within legal and ethical boundaries
- Prepare and maintain medical records
- Document accurately
- Follow employer's established policies dealing with the health care contract
- Implement and maintain federal and state health care legislation and regulations
- Comply with established risk management and safety procedures
- Recognize professional credentialing criteria
- *Develop and maintain personnel, policy and procedure manuals*

Instruction

- Instruct individuals according to their needs
- Explain office policies and procedures
- Teach methods of health promotion and disease prevention
- Locate community resources and disseminate information
- *Develop educational materials*
- *Conduct continuing education activities*

Operational Functions

- Perform inventory of supplies and equipment
- Perform routine maintenance of administrative and clinical equipment
- Apply computer techniques to support office operations
- *Perform personnel management functions*
- *Negotiate leases and prices for equipment and supply contracts*

- *Denotes advanced skills.*

SOURCE: Reprinted by permission of the American Association of Medical Assistants from the AAMA Role Delineation Study: Occupational Analysis of the Medical Assisting Profession.

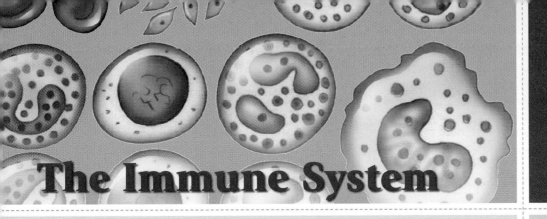

The Immune System

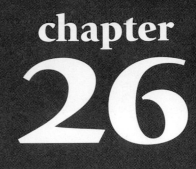

Learning Objectives

After completing this chapter, you should be able to:

- Explain the immune system and its response.
- Identify and discuss the anatomy of the immune system.
- Discuss the functions of the immune system.
- List and briefly discuss disorders of the immune system.

Terms to Learn

active immunity

antibodies

antigen

B lymphocytes

chemotherapy

chronic fatigue syndrome (CFS)

complement

cortex

germinal centers

immune response

immune system

infectious mononucleosis

leukocytes

lymphedema

lymphocytes

medulla

metastasis

neutrophils

oncogenes

phagocytes

radiation therapy

rheumatoid arthritis

systemic lupus erythematosus (SLC)

T lymphocytes

trabeculae

Case Study

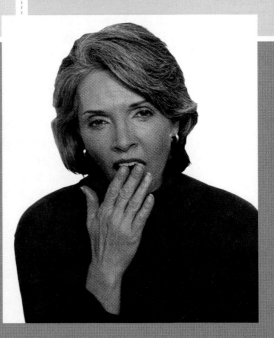

JULIE IS A 62-YEAR-OLD FEMALE SEEN BY THE PHYSICIAN. She has been suffering from what appears to be a multitude of individual problems, including low blood pressure, cold and flu-like symptoms, extreme fatigue, and what she describes as "hot" and "cold flashes." Upon a thorough physical exam, which includes a complete blood cell count and an evaluation of her entire treatment history, Julie is diagnosed with CFS. As part of her care, Julie's doctor has informed her that she must take an active role in her treatment. This includes getting plenty of rest and monitoring her for any additional viral infections.

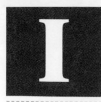

Inside the body there is an amazing protection mechanism called the **immune system**. The immune system consists of the tissues, organs, and physiological processes used by the body to identify abnormal cells, foreign substances, and foreign tissues, such as transplants, and defend against those substances that might be harmful to the body. It is a protective mechanism designed to defend the body against invaders. Those invaders can be bacteria, microbes, viruses, toxins, and parasites. To understand the power of the immune system, all one has to do is look at what happens to a living being once it dies. When a person dies, the immune system shuts down. In a matter of hours, the body is invaded by all sorts of bacteria, microbes, and parasites. None of these things are able to enter when the immune system is working properly; however, once this system shuts down, the door to many of the invading microorganisms is wide open. Once a person is deceased, it only takes a short time for these organisms to completely dismantle the body and carry it away, until all that is left is a skeleton.

Several structures are central to the immune system. These include the central lymphoid tissue, which is comprised of the bone marrow and thymus, and the peripheral lymphoid tissue, consisting of the lymph nodes, spleen, and mucosa-associated lymphoid tissue.

Anatomy of the Immune System

The immune system operates throughout the body. There are, however, certain sites where the cells of the immune system are organized into specific structures. These are classified as central lymphoid tissue and peripheral lymphoid tissue. All of these structures are also part of the lymphatic system (see Figure 26-1), which is a subsystem of the circulatory system. The primary responsibility of the lymphatic system is to defend the body from foreign invasion by disease-causing agents such as viruses, bacteria, or fungi. The lymphatic system consists macroscopically of the bone marrow, spleen, thymus gland, lymph nodes, tonsils, appendix, and a few other organs.

Central Lymphoid Tissue

The central lymphoid tissue consists of the bone marrow and the thymus. The bone marrow contains stem cells that create all the cells in the immune system. The bone marrow is also the origin of the red blood cells, the white blood cells, and the platelets. During a procedure called hematopoiesis, the bone marrow–derived cells either become mature cells of the immune system or precursors of cells that will mature in a place other than the bone marrow. The bone marrow produces B cells, natural killer cells, granulocyte and red blood cells, and platelets.

The thymus gland is located posterior to the sternum, in the anterior mediastinum. It enlarges during childhood, but begins to shrink again after maturity. It continues to function even though the size is small throughout life. It is arranged into an outer cortex and an internal medulla. Immature lymphoid cells enter the cortex and reproduce and mature, then move to the medulla where they reenter the circulation. The thymus manufactures infection fighting T cells and helps distinguish normal T cells from those that attack the body's own tissues.

Peripheral Lymphatic System

The peripheral lymphatic system consists of the lymph nodes, spleen, and other lymphoid tissue. (refer back to Figure 25-18 in the previous chapter). The lymphatic system is also composed of lymphatic capillaries, lymphatic vessels, and lymphatic ducts.

Lymph Nodes

Lymph nodes can take on many different sizes and shapes, but most are bean shaped and are about 1 inch in length. The node is covered thickly with a fibrous capsule and is subdivided into different compartments by inward-pointing **trabeculae**. As with many organs, the lymph node has two basic parts, the **cortex** and the **medulla**. The cortex is populated mainly with lymphocytes. The **germinal centers** are the primary resting place for B-cell lymphocytes, which are the cells responsible for production of circulating antibodies. In the event of an infecting antigen, these B lymphocytes will rapidly undergo mitosis and divide. Each unique kind of B cell produces only one type of antibody. Thus, by dividing, they can produce large quantities of a specific antibody to seek out and help destroy the antigen. The rest of the cortex contains T lymphocytes, that is, cells that circulate through the lymph nodes, bloodstream, and lymphatic ducts to seek out any infection. The medulla of the lymph nodes is primarily made up of macrophages attached to reticular fibers.

Lymph nodes have two functions. First, the phagocytic cells act as filters for particulate matter and microorganisms. The phagocytic cells are also called macrophages, and are one type of B cell. These cells destroy the invading cells.

The second function of lymph nodes has to do with the development of antigens. The antigens act as "invaders" to inhibit such substances as bacteria, viruses, or other toxic substances that may have breached the other protective mechanisms of the body, possibly causing infection or inflammation.

Spleen

Located in the upper left quadrant of the abdomen, the spleen is responsible for receiving blood from an artery off of the aorta. After passing through an intricate meshwork of tiny blood vessels, the blood continues to the liver. The blood vessels of the spleen are surrounded by nests of B lymphocytes, mainly of the memory type. As the blood slowly moves through the spleen, it is monitored by T cells for any non–self-invaders. If some suspicious cell or molecule is detected, it is presented to the B cells for a match to an appropriate memory B cell. Once a matching B cell is activated, the cell divides rapidly and begins producing antibodies directed against the invading antigen.

The spleen blood vessels are also lined with macrophages, which swallow and digest debris in the blood such as worn-out red blood cells and platelets. In a disease such as mononucleosis, the macrophages in the spleen become overactive and trap a higher number of

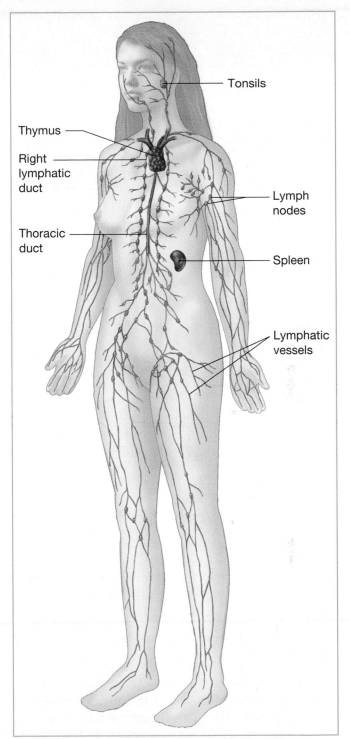

FIGURE 26-1 Components of the lymphatic system.

white blood cells. In the process, the spleen becomes swollen and may even rupture.

Tonsils

The tonsils are located in the depressions of the mucous membranes of the face and the pharynx (see Figure 26-2). There are three sets: the palatine, the pharyngeal, and the lingual. The function of the tonsils

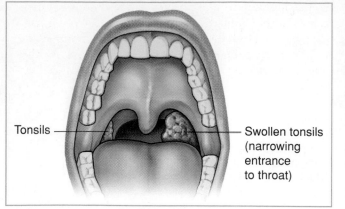

FIGURE 26-2 Tonsils—normal and enlarged.

is to filter bacteria and aid in the formation of white blood cells.

The Immune System and the Body's Defense

As previously noted, the immune system is the body's defense against infectious organisms and other pathogenic invaders. Through a series of steps called the **immune response**, the immune system attacks organisms and substances that invade body systems and cause disease. This occurs because the network of cells, tissues, and organs comprising the immune system works together to protect the body.

Leukocytes, or white blood cells (WBCs), combine to seek out and destroy harmful organisms. There are two types of WBCs: **phagocytes** and **lymphocytes**. The phagocytes attack the invading organism. A number of different cells are considered phagocytes; however, the most common are **neutrophils**, which primarily fight off bacteria. Lymphocytes allow the body to re-

Professionalism

As a medical assistant, you work under the license of the physician. You are a team member with the physician, but still subordinate to physicians and their levels of education. Always address physicians by their title and name, for example, "Dr. Morales." Even if the physician has invited you to call him or her by their first name, never do so in front of a patient. This can undermine the doctor–patient relationship. Physicians refer to each other as Doctor "so-and-so" when talking to their patients, and the staff should take their cue from the physician. They have earned the right to be called "Dr." and the medical assistant should honor that right.

member and recognize previous invading organisms. There are two kinds of lymphocytes: **B lymphocytes** and the **T lymphocytes**. Lymphocytes start out in the bone marrow and either stay there and mature into B cells, or they leave for the thymus gland, where they mature into T cells. B lymphocytes and T lymphocytes have separate responsibilities within the immune system. The B lymphocytes seek out the invading organisms and send defenses to attach onto them; the T cells destroy the organisms that the B lymphocytes identified.

How Immunity Works: Antigens versus Antibodies

When a foreign substance invades the body, it is called an **antigen**. When an antigen is detected, several types of cells work together to recognize and respond to it. These cells trigger the B lymphocytes to produce antibodies. This occurs through a process known as *humoral immunity*. **Antibodies** are specialized proteins that lock onto specific antigens. Immunoglobulins are glycoproteins that function as antibodies. The terms *antibody* and *immunoglobulin* are often used interchangeably. They are found in the blood and tissue fluids, as well as many secretions. Structurally they are globulins, which means they are synthesized and secreted by plasma cells that are derived from the B cells of the immune system. B cells are activated upon binding to their specific antigen and differentiate into plasma cells. In some cases the interaction of the B cell with a T cell is also necessary.

Once the B lymphocytes have produced antibodies, they continue to exist in a person's body. That means if the same antigen is presented to the immune system again, the antibodies are already there. That is why if a person becomes ill with a specific disease, such as chickenpox, that person typically will not get sick from it again. This is also why we use immunizations to prevent getting certain diseases. Immunizations, which are also called vaccinations, help protect a person from a specific disease. When an individual is given an immunization, that person is also receiving a vaccine that contains fragments of a disease organism or small amounts of a weakened disease organism. The vaccine causes the person's immune system to develop antibodies that can subsequently recognize and attack the organism if he or she is exposed to it. Sometimes an immunization does not completely prevent the disease, but it will significantly reduce its severity. More information on immunizations will be covered in Volume III, Chapter 49.

Although antibodies can recognize an antigen and lock onto it, they are not capable of destroying it without help. That is the job of the T cells. The T cells are part of the system that destroys antigens that have been tagged by antibodies or cells that have been infected or somehow changed. T cells are also involved in assisting other cells, such as phagocytes. Antibodies can also neutralize toxins produced by different organisms. Finally, antibodies can activate a group of proteins called **complement** that are also part of the immune system. Complement assists in destroying bacteria, viruses, or infected cells. All of these specialized cells and parts of the immune system offer the body protection against disease. This protection is called *immunity*. There are three types of immunity: innate, active, and passive.

Innate Immunity

Everyone is born with innate, or natural, immunity. Because of that fact, many of the viruses and bacteria that affect other species are not capable of harming human beings. For example, the viruses that cause leukemia in cats or distemper in dogs do not affect humans. The way in which innate immunity works to protect humans against illnesses that affects other species also works to protect nonhumans against human diseases. For example, the HIV/AIDS virus is not capable of making cats or dogs sick. Innate immunity also includes the external barriers of the body, including the skin and mucous membranes that line the nose, throat, and gastrointestinal tract, all of which are the body's first line of defense in preventing diseases from entering it. If this outer defensive wall is broken, such as when a person cuts himself or herself, the skin attempts to heal the break quickly, and special immune cells on the skin attack invading microorganisms.

Active Immunity

The introduction of immunity by infection or with a vaccine is called **active immunity**. Active immunity is permanent, meaning that the individual is protected from the disease all of his or her life. Acquired active immunity occurs when the person is exposed to a live pathogen, develops the disease, and becomes immune as a result of the primary immune response. Artificially acquired active immunity can be induced by a vaccine, a substance that contains the antigen. A vaccine stimulates a primary response against the antigen without causing symptoms of the disease.

Passive Immunity

Passive immunity is "borrowed" from another source and only lasts for a short time. For example, antibodies in a mother's breast milk provide an infant with temporary immunity to diseases to which the mother has been exposed. This can help protect the infant against infection during the early years of childhood.

It is important to remember that everyone's immune system is different. Some people never seem to get infections, whereas others seem to be sick all the time. As a person gets older, he or she usually becomes immune to more germs as the immune system comes into contact with more and more of them. That's why adults and teens tend to get fewer colds than children; their bodies have learned to recognize and immediately attack many of the viruses that cause colds.

Common Disorders Associated with the Immune System

Immune system disorders occur when the immune response is inappropriate, excessive, or lacking. And lack of one or more components of the immune system can result in any number of immunodeficiency disorders. Disorders may be inherited, acquired through infection or other illness, or produced as an inadvertent side effect of certain drug treatments. (See Table 26-1).

Allergies

Allergies are disorders of the immune system. Most allergic reactions are a result of an immune system that responds to a "false alarm." When a harmless substance such as dust, mold, or pollen is encountered by a person who is allergic to that substance, the immune system may react dramatically, by producing antibodies that "attack" the allergen (substances that produce allergic reactions). The result of an allergen entering a susceptible person's body may include wheezing, itching, runny nose, watery or itchy eyes, and other symptoms.

Cultural Considerations

Because some diseases of the immune system appear to have psychological implications associated with them, many cultures also see them as disorders that can be avoided. In fact, some physicians view some of these disorders, such as chronic fatigue syndrome, as more "psychosomatic" than physical. Providing emotional support and knowledge of resources may help patients with these illnesses to rebuild a support system and a new community for themselves. The most important help the medical assistant can give these individuals is the feeling that they can be self-sufficient and that they are not alone in the world, even though the medical assistant must be certain to maintain a professional relationship with the patient.

TABLE 26-1   Disorders of the Lymphatic System

Disorder	Description
Acquired immune deficiency syndrome (AIDS)	A disease that involves a defect in the cell-mediated immunity system. A syndrome of opportunistic infections occurs in the final stages of infection with the human immunodeficiency virus (HIV). This virus attacks T4 lymphocytes and destroys them, which reduces the person's ability to fight infection.
AIDS-related complex (ARC)	A complex of symptoms that appears in the early stages of AIDS. This is a positive test for the virus but only mild symptoms of weight loss, fatigue, skin rash, and anorexia.
Elephantiasis	Inflammation, obstruction, and destruction of the lymph vessels, which results in enlarged tissues due to edema.
Epstein-Barr virus	Virus believed to be the cause of infections mononucleosis.
Hodgkin's disease	Lymphatic system disease that can result in solid tumors in any lymphoid tissue.
Lymphadenitis	Inflammation of the lymph glands. Referred to as swollen glands.
Lymphangioma	A benign mass of lymphatic vessels.
Lymphoma	Malignant tumor of the lymph nodes and tissue.
Lymphosarcoma	Malignant disease of the lymphatic tissue.
Mononucleosis	Acute infections disease with a large number of atypical lymphocytes. Caused by the Epstein-Barr virus. There may be abnormal liver function and spleen enlargement.
Multiple sclerosis	Autoimmune disorder of the central nervous system in which the myelin sheath of nerves is attacked.
Non-Hodgkin's lymphoma	Malignant, solid tumors of lymphoid tissue.
Peritonsillar abscess	Infection of the tissues between the tonsils and the pharynx. Also called quinsy sore throat.
Sarcoidosis	Inflammatory disease of the lymph system in which lesions may appear in the liver, skin, lungs, lymph nodes, spleen, eyes, and small bones of the hands and feet.
Splenomegaly	Enlargement of the spleen.
Systemic lupus erythematosus (SLE)	A chronic autoimmune disorder of connective tissue that causes injury to the skin, joints, kidneys, mucous membranes, and nervous system.
Thymoma	Malignant tumor of the thymus gland.

Allergies are rarely cured, but many medications, supplements, and treatment options are available to help relieve allergy symptoms. The best way to treat an allergic reaction is for a person to stay away from the offending allergen. If that is not possible, treatment may include the use of antihistamines or decongestants to help combat allergy symptoms. Other forms of treatment for some types of airborne allergens may include the use of air filters and dehumidifiers. There are also various ways to cope with allergic symptoms other than traditional medical treatment and medications. Those methods often include the use of acupressure and chiropractic treatments. In severe cases, treatment may only be identified through specific allergy testing and desensitization. See Volume III, Chapter 35, for more information on allergies.

Cancer

Cancer is actually a group of many related diseases that all have to do with cells. Cells are the very small units that make up all living things, including the human body. Each person's body has billions of cells. Cancer cells are not normal; instead, they grow and spread very fast. Normal body cells grow and, through mitosis, divide and know to stop growing. Over time, they also die. Unlike these normal cells, cancer cells just continue to grow and divide out of control and do not die.

Cancer cells usually group or clump together to form tumors. A growing tumor becomes a lump of cancer cells that can destroy the normal cells around the tumor and damage the body's healthy tissues. Sometimes the cancer cells break away from the original tumor and travel to other areas of the body, where they keep growing and can go on to form new tumors. That occurs through a process known as **metastasis**.

Causes and Treatment of Cancer

While the causes of cancer are relatively unknown, there are certain risk factors that may make predisposed person to cancer. These include the presence of a suppressed immune system, radiation, tobacco, and some viruses.

Cancer may be treated with surgery, chemotherapy, radiation, or sometimes a combination of all of these treatments. The choice of treatment generally depends on the type of cancer someone has and the stage of the tumor, meaning how much and to where, if at all, the cancer has spread within the body. Surgery is the oldest form of treatment for cancer. Three out of every five people with cancer may require surgery to remove the cancer. During surgery some healthy cells or tissue may also be removed to make sure that all the cancer is removed.

Chemotherapy involves the use of anticancer drugs to treat the cancerous growth or tumor. These medicines are sometimes taken as a pill, but are usually given intravenously. Chemotherapy is usually given over a number of weeks to months. Often, a permanent IV catheter is placed under the skin into a larger blood vessel of the upper chest. This way, a person can easily get several courses of chemotherapy and other medicines through this catheter without having a new IV needle inserted. The catheter remains under the skin until the cancer treatment is completed. **Radiation therapy** may also be used to treat cancer. It uses high-energy waves, such as x-rays, to damage and destroy the cancer cells. This form of treatment may cause tumors to shrink and, in some cases, disappear completely. Radiation therapy is one of the most common treatments for cancer.

Cancer and the Immune System

When the immune system is at its peak, it recognizes, attacks, and destroys the cancerous cells before potentially deadly growth and multiplication of the cancer

can occur. However, when not destroyed immediately by the immune system, the new cancer cells avoid the usual controls on growth and multiplication in normal cells. The growth begins when the genes controlling cell growth and multiplication, called **oncogenes**, are transformed by cancer-causing agents, called carcinogens, into cancer cells.

Normal cells can undergo a malignant change to become cancer-infested cells. These small groups of abnormal cancer cells divide more rapidly than the normal surrounding cells. The fast multiplication results in invasion and destruction of normal body cells.

Cancerous cells act as uncontrollable parasites, consuming needed nutrients while contributing nothing except malnutrition. If not killed and removed, these cancerous cells can then metastasize via the bloodstream and lymphatic system to other parts of the body from their original site and potentially be fatal if they cause organs to fail.

The immune response is critical to beating or controlling cancer because cancerous tumors develop and multiply when the white immune cells fail to recognize, respond, and kill the cancerous cell invaders. If not at its peak, the immune response often fails to respond in a timely manner when overwhelmed due to the massive number of corrupted cancer cells that have multiplied rapidly when undetected and unchecked. When the immune response is in peak condition, it is better able to recognize the cancerous cells quickly and respond to kill the health invaders rapidly in most instances. A suppressed or impaired immune response exposes a body to both development and spread (metastasis) of too-often deadly cancer cells in the body.

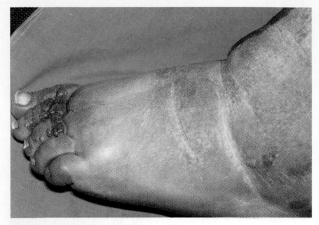

FIGURE 26-3 Chronic lymphedema.

Chronic Fatigue Syndrome

While there is no known single cause of chronic fatigue syndrome (CFS), some authorities believe it is a condition shared by many different underlying diseases rather than an entity unto itself. Others believe it is caused by a defect of the immune system. Hormonal deficits, low blood pressure, and viral infections have been studied as possible causes or contributors. There has also been some correlation between chronic single or multiple viral infections, but CFS has also been identified in the absence of any apparent viral infection. Food allergies are commonly associated with this disorder, as is candidiasis, intestinal parasites, and toxic chemical exposure.

The goal in any treatment regimen for CFS generally begins with the patient undergoing a thorough evaluation of his or her prior treatment history. And the treatment plan must also take into consideration the patient's ability to optimize sleep quality and quantity. Educating the patient with emphasis on becoming an active participant of his or her own treatment is extremely important in the treatment of CFS.

Infectious Mononucleosis

Infectious mononucleosis is a viral infection caused by the Epstein-Barr virus (EBV), which is part of the herpes family of diseases. It is characterized by an increase of white blood cells that are mononuclear, that is, containing a single nucleus. For that reason, this disease is frequently referred to as "mono." Because it often develops in young adults between the ages of 15 and 24 and is frequently spread through saliva, mono is also commonly referred to as the "kissing disease." The illness is less severe in young children and the incubation period for mono is generally between 4 and 8 weeks. Symptoms include fever, fatigue, sore throat, and swollen lymph glands. There is usually no treatment for this disorder except getting plenty of rest, gargling with saltwater or using throat lozenges to soothe a sore throat, taking aspirin or acetaminophen to reduce fever and relieve a sore throat and headache. If left untreated, mono can lead to liver inflammation or hepatitis and enlargement of the spleen; recovery from mono generally occurs within several weeks. However, for some people, it may take as long as several months before they regain their normal energy levels.

Lymphedema

Lymphedema is a condition that occurs from a damaged or dysfunctional lymphatic system (see Figure 26-3). There are two different types of lymphedema. The first, called primary lymphedema, can be hereditary. Each stage of the disease is called by a different name. It is known as Milroy's disease or syndrome when it expresses itself at birth or in the very early years. Meige lymphedema, also known as lymphedema praecox, generally begins sometime during puberty. Lymphedema tarda begins in or around middle age. Lymphedema that has not expressed itself as an active condition is referred to as latent lymphedema. Primary lymphedema can also be congenital. Secondary lymphedema is generally caused by an obstruction, or damage to, or injury to the lymph system that leads to an interruption of the normal lymphatic flow.

Causes of congenital primary lymphedema can be a developmental disorder of the lymphatics, *in utero* infection, injury, or delivery difficulties. The causes of secondary lymphedema are multiple. Infections from insect bites, serious wounds, or burns can cause lymphedema when they damage or destroy lymphatics as can any type of serious injury. Radiation for cancer treatments is also a cause. Outside the tropics the number one cause of secondary lymphedema is the removal of lymph nodes for cancer biopsies. Through improved techniques of small-needle biopsies, radiological diagnostic improvements, and site-specific node biopsies, there has been a marked decrease in secondary lymphedema.

The preferred treatment for lymphedema is decongestive therapy. The forms of therapy are complete decongestive therapy (CDT) or manual decongestive therapy (MDT). CDT is used primarily in the treatment of lymphedema and venous insufficiency edema. It is a combination of MDT, bandaging exercises, and skin care. CDT may also involve breathing exercises, compressive garments, and dietary measures. A frequent indication for CDT is lymphedema caused by irradiation or surgery due to cancer. It can relieve edema, fibrosis and the accompanying pain and discomfort. Other treatments include the use of compression pumps, surgery, and newer approaches such as the use of lasers, liposuction, and even acupuncture.

Rheumatoid Arthritis

Rheumatoid arthritis is a chronic disease that causes great suffering, reduced quality of life, major financial outlays, and loss of income due to functional impairment and the prospect of invalidity. One person out of every 100 suffers from chronic rheumatoid arthritis. It is a condition that occurs when the body's immune defenses attack tissue in the joints, leading to pain and degeneration of the articular cartilage. The disease or its treatment also increases mortality, and patients with rheumatoid arthritis often have a shorter life expectancy than their healthy peers. Drugs used to limit the symptoms have a limited effect and do not improve the long-term prognosis.

The treatment of rheumatoid arthritis is based on medical treatment and providing the patient with advice about how to facilitate daily activities. While preventive treatment of persons who may be genetically exposed to the disease is currently not an issue, persons with a family history of rheumatoid arthritis are four times more at risk of developing the disease than others. It is also important to note that treating the symptoms is only part of the regime for the rheumatoid arthritis patient. Maintenance of articular, or joint, function is equally important.

Systemic Lupus Erythematosus

Systemic lupus erythematosus or SLE is one of a group of illnesses called autoimmune diseases. One of the ways in which the immune system works is by producing antibodies that allow the cells of the immune system to destroy the invading organisms such as viruses and bacteria. Sometimes, the immune system starts to make antibodies that stick to the body's own cells. These antibodies are called *autoantibodies* and when they stick to the body's own cells they can cause an inflammatory reaction, which results in damage to the cells. This is what occurs with SLE. Patients suffering from SLE produce abnormal antibodies in their blood that target tissues within their own body rather than foreign infectious agents. SLE is called a "systemic" disorder because its effects can show in many parts of

the body, that is, it is systemwide. *Lupus* refers to a type of skin rash and *erythematosus* means "red." SLE can produce many different symptoms and can imitate many other diseases. Many patients with SLE have pain and swelling in the joints. They may also suffer from general fatigue, fever, chills, and headache.

About one-fifth of SLE patients have round (discoid) lesions that are raised and scaly. This condition is known as discoid lupus erythematosus. If left untreated, these lesions grow and can cause severe scarring.

A condition that may be present with lupus is vasculitis, or inflamed blood vessels. The inflammation may cause red marks in any area of the body. Sometimes deep red lumps appear, especially on the leg, where they may develop into ulcers. In some people, reddish-purple lesions appear on the tips of the fingers and toes.

Ninety percent of patients with SLE are women and it is more common before menopause. There is a genetic component to SLE because there is a higher risk of developing SLE if a close family member also has it.

Unfortunately, there is no cure for most autoimmune diseases and SLE is no different. Treatment is usually aimed at reducing the immune response using drugs such as steroids. It is important to note that SLE is a chronic, lifelong condition that is characterized by periods of remission and relapse. The course in any individual is difficult to predict but with immediate treatment, most patients have a normal life span.

Patient Education

Patients who take medication for a chronic or other disease must be educated that they need to be extremely compliant when taking their medications. They need to take all of the medications exactly as prescribed, every day, without exception. This requires dedication on the part of the patient. If the patient is not compliant with the regimen, the medications may not be effective in treating the disease and a relapse may occur.

SUMMARY

The immune system is the body's defense against infectious organisms and other pathogenic invaders, keeping the body healthy. There are three types of immunity: innate, active, and passive. Immune system disorders occur when the immune response is inappropriate, excessive, or lacking. Disorders may be inherited, acquired through infection or other illness, or produced as an inadvertent side effect of certain drug treatments.

Chapter Review

COMPETENCY REVIEW

1. Define and spell the terms to learn for this chapter.
2. What is the function of leukocytes?
3. What is the most common type of leukocyte?
4. What is the main function of the immune system?
5. Name the three accessory organs of the lymphatic system.
6. What is the difference between innate immunity and active immunity?
7. What does the central lymphoid tissue include?
8. What does the peripheral lymphoid tissue include?
9. What is the spleen responsible for?
10. What role do phagocytes perform?

PREPARING FOR THE CERTIFICATION EXAM

1. What structures are responsible for allowing the body to remember and recognize previous invaders?
   A. neutrophils
   B. lymphocytes
   C. phagocytes
   D. antigens
   E. antibodies

2. Accessory lymph organs include
   A. pharynx, larynx, trachea, and bronchi
   B. liver, gallbladder, and pancreas
   C. tonsils, spleen, and thymus gland
   D. lymphatic duct, thoracic duct, and lymph nodes
   E. ureters, urethra, and kidneys.

3. Humoral immunity refers to
   A. the binding of an antigen with an antibody
   B. the production of plasma lymphocytes or B cells
   C. the production of lymphocytes or T cells
   D. a severe reaction to an antigen
   E. a hypersensitivity to an allergen

4. An autoimmune viral disease characterized by an increase of white blood cells is
   A. allergies
   B. Epstein-Barr virus
   C. lymphedema
   D. rheumatoid arthritis
   E. Infectious mononucleosis

5. Which organ has a secondary purpose of the destruction of red blood cells?
   A. thymus
   B. bone marrow
   C. spleen
   D. tonsils
   E. liver

6. What condition of the immune system creates autoantibodies that stick to the body's own cells, causing an inflammatory reaction that eventually causes damage to the cells?
   A. chronic fatigue syndrome
   B. systemic lupus erythematosus
   C. cancer
   D. lymphedema
   E. infectious mononucleosis

continued on next page

7. What disorder do some authorities believe is a condition shared by many different underlying diseases, rather than an entity onto itself?
   A. cancer
   B. chronic fatigue syndrome
   C. rheumatoid arthritis
   D. SLE
   E. lymphedema

8. What disorder can produce all sorts of symptoms and can initiate many other diseases?
   A. cancer
   B. systemic lupus erythematosis
   C. CFS
   D. Infectious mononucleosis
   E. lymphedema

9. What organ manufactures infection-fighting T cells and helps distinguish normal T cells from those that attack the body's own tissues?
   A. spleen
   B. thyroid
   C. thymus
   D. pancreas
   E. large intestine

10. When expressing itself at birth or in the very early years, lymphedema is known as
    A. Milroy's disease
    B. Meige lymphedema
    C. lymphedema praecox
    D. lymphedema tarda
    E. latent lymphedema

CRITICAL THINKING

1. Why was it important to note that Julie was having many cold and flu-like symptoms?

2. Why did the physician order a complete blood cell count?

3. Why did the physician tell Julie to get plenty of rest and decide to monitor her for any other viral infections?

INTERNET ACTIVITY

Do an Internet search for chronic fatigue syndrome services in your hometown. What resources are available in your area?

 MediaLink More on the immune system, including interactive resources, can be found on the Student CD-Rom accompanying this textbook.

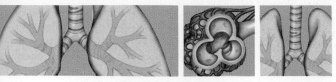

Medical Assistant Role Delineation Chart

HIGHLIGHT indicates material covered in this chapter.

ADMINISTRATIVE

Administrative Procedures

- Perform basic administrative medical assisting functions
- Schedule, coordinate and monitor appointments
- Schedule inpatient/outpatient admissions and procedures
- Understand and apply third-party guidelines
- Obtain reimbursement through accurate claims submission
- Monitor third-party reimbursement
- Understand and adhere to managed care policies and procedures
- *Negotiate managed care contracts*

Practice Finances

- Perform procedural and diagnostic coding
- Apply bookkeeping principles

- Manage accounts receivable
- *Manage accounts payable*
- *Process payroll*
- *Document and maintain accounting and banking records*
- *Develop and maintain fee schedules*
- *Manage renewals of business and professional insurance policies*
- *Manage personnel benefits and maintain records*
- *Perform marketing, financial, and strategic planning*

CLINICAL

Fundamental Principles

- Apply principles of aseptic technique and infection control
- Comply with quality assurance practices
- Screen and follow up patient test results

Diagnostic Orders

- Collect and process specimens
- Perform diagnostic tests

Patient Care

- Adhere to established patient screening procedures
- Obtain patient history and vital signs
- Prepare and maintain examination and treatment areas
- Prepare patient for examinations, procedures and treatments

- Assist with examinations, procedures and treatments
- Prepare and administer medications and immunizations
- Maintain medication and immunization records
- Recognize and respond to emergencies
- Coordinate patient care information with other health care providers
- Initiate IV and administer IV medications with appropriate training and as permitted by state law

GENERAL

Professionalism

- Display a professional manner and image
- Demonstrate initiative and responsibility
- Work as a member of the health care team
- Prioritize and perform multiple tasks
- Adapt to change
- Promote the CMA credential
- Enhance skills through continuing education
- Treat all patients with compassion and empathy
- Promote the practice through positive public relations

Communication Skills

- Recognize and respect cultural diversity
- Adapt communications to individual's ability to understand
- Use professional telephone technique

- Recognize and respond effectively to verbal, nonverbal, and written communications
- Use medical terminology appropriately
- Utilize electronic technology to receive, organize, prioritize and transmit information
- Serve as liaison

Legal Concepts

- Perform within legal and ethical boundaries
- Prepare and maintain medical records
- Document accurately
- Follow employer's established policies dealing with the health care contract
- Implement and maintain federal and state health care legislation and regulations
- Comply with established risk management and safety procedures
- Recognize professional credentialing criteria
- *Develop and maintain personnel, policy and procedure manuals*

Instruction

- Instruct individuals according to their needs
- Explain office policies and procedures
- Teach methods of health promotion and disease prevention
- Locate community resources and disseminate information
- *Develop educational materials*
- *Conduct continuing education activities*

Operational Functions

- Perform inventory of supplies and equipment
- Perform routine maintenance of administrative and clinical equipment
- Apply computer techniques to support office operations
- *Perform personnel management functions*
- *Negotiate leases and prices for equipment and supply contracts*

- *Denotes advanced skills.*

SOURCE: Reprinted by permission of the American Association of Medical Assistants from the AAMA Role Delineation Study: Occupational Analysis of the Medical Assisting Profession.

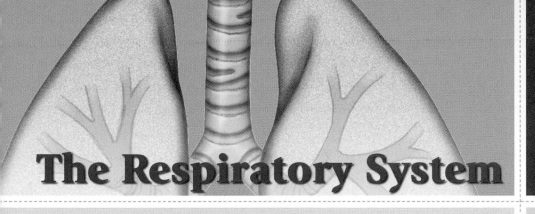

chapter 27

The Respiratory System

Learning Objectives

After completing this chapter, you should be able to:

- Define and spell the terms to learn for this chapter.
- Explain the purpose and function of the respiratory system.
- List and explain the structures and functions of the organs of the respiratory system.
- Explain the different respiratory volumes and capacities.
- Identify and discuss common disorders associated with the respiratory system.

Terms to Learn

asthma

atmospheric pressure

bronchitis

chronic obstructive pulmonary disease (COPD)

cilia

common cold

cyanosis

cystic fibrosis (CF)

emphysema

hay fever

hemoptysis

influenza

Legionnaire's disease

lung cancer

pleurisy

pneumonia

pulmonary edema

pulmonary embolism (PE)

severe acute respiratory syndrome (SARS)

sinusitis

tuberculosis (TB)

Case Study

JOE F. IS A 65-YEAR-OLD MALE being seen in your clinic for minor shortness of breath. Upon taking his medical history, it is learned that he has a distant history of "some asthma" and has been a two-pack-a-day smoker for 40 years. He has recently been coughing up greenish-tinted sputum. He denies any exposure to tuberculosis or other infectious diseases. Sputum cultures, chest x-rays, and pulmonary function tests indicate a bacterial infection, no masses or infiltrates in the lungs, and decreased forced expiratory volumes and a low FEV_1/FEC ratio. The physician diagnoses COPD with an overlying bacterial bronchial infection. The patient is started on Levaquin, 500 mg a day, as an antibiotic; albuterol, two puffs every 4 hours or as needed; Tessalon for his cough; and guaifenesin, 600 mg twice a day. In 2 weeks, the patient reports back, stating he feels better, is breathing much better, and rarely coughs. He is beginning to cut back on his tobacco usage.

he primary function of the respiratory system is to supply the blood with oxygen so the blood can deliver oxygen to all parts of the body. It does this through breathing. When we breathe, we inhale oxygen and exhale carbon dioxide. This exchange of gases is the respiratory system's means of getting oxygen to the blood.

Respiration is achieved through the mouth, nose, trachea, lungs, and diaphragm. Oxygen enters the respiratory system through the mouth and the nose. The oxygen then passes through the larynx (where speech sounds are produced) and the trachea, which is a tube that enters the chest cavity. In the chest cavity, the trachea splits into two smaller tubes called the bronchi. Each bronchus then divides again, forming the bronchial tubes. The bronchial tubes lead directly into the lungs where they divide into many smaller tubes, which connect to tiny sacs called alveoli. The average adult's lungs contain about 600 million of these spongy, air-filled sacs that are surrounded by capillaries. The alveoli are the final branchings of the respiratory tree and perform gas exchange for the lungs. The inhaled oxygen passes into the alveoli and then diffuses through the capillaries into the arterial blood. Meanwhile, the waste-rich blood from the veins releases its carbon dioxide into the alveoli. The carbon dioxide follows the same path out of the lungs when you exhale.

The diaphragm's job is to help pump the carbon dioxide out of the lungs and pull the oxygen into the lungs. The diaphragm is a sheet of muscles that lie across the bottom of the chest cavity.

Organs of the Respiratory System

The organs of the respiratory system extend from the nose to the lungs and are divided into the upper and lower respiratory tracts (see Figure 27-1). The upper respiratory tract consists of the nose and the pharynx, or throat. The lower respiratory tract includes the larynx, or voice box; the trachea, or windpipe, which splits into two main branches called bronchi;

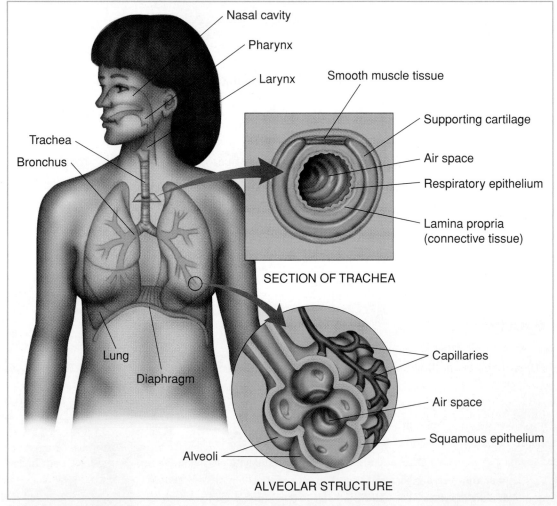

FIGURE 27-1 The respiratory system: nasal cavity, pharynx, larynx, trachea, bronchus, and lung with expanded views of the trachea and alveolar structure.

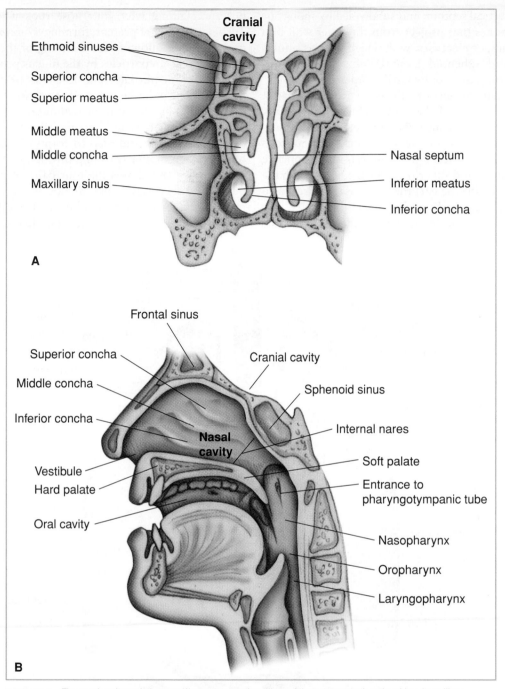

FIGURE 27-2 The nasal cavity and pharynx: (A) meatuses and positions of the entrance to the ethmoid and maxillary sinuses; (B) sagittal section of the nasal cavity and pharynx.

tiny branches of the bronchi called bronchioles; and the lungs, a pair of sac-like, spongy organs. The nose, pharynx, larynx, trachea, bronchi, and bronchioles conduct air to and from the lungs. The lungs interact with the circulatory system to deliver oxygen and remove carbon dioxide.

Nose

The nose is the organ of smell, and also part of the apparatus of respiration and voice (see Figure 27-2). In addition to being our organ of smell, it is also respon-

sible for performing several other functions, including being a passageway for air to move; warming and moistening inhaled air; using hair-like projections, called cilia, to trap and prevent dust, pollens, and other foreign matter from entering the nasal cavity; and assisting in the making of sounds that occur during speaking and singing. Considered anatomically, the nose is divided into an external portion—the visible projection portion, to which the term *nose* is popularly restricted—and an internal portion, consisting of two principal cavities, or nasal fossae, separated from each other by a vertical septum, and subdivided by spongy or turbinated bones that project from the outer wall into three passages, or meatuses, with which various sinuses in the ethmoid, sphenoid, frontal, and superior maxillary bones communicate by narrow apertures.

The external entrances of the nose are called nares. The inside structure of the nose includes the septum, which divides the nose into right and left sides. The septum is a cartilaginous wall. It is also lined with mucous membranes. Each side of the nose has three conchae (inferior, middle, and superior), which connect with the eustachian tube (to the ear) the paranasal sinuses (also known as "the sinuses") and nasolacrimal ducts. The nasolacrimal ducts drain fluid from the eyes into the

nose, explaining why your nose runs when you cry. Turbinates also are present, forming a "maze" for air to move around, allowing for warming of the air and removal of foreign particles by the mucus produced from the mucous membranes. The nose is separated from the mouth by the palatine bones of the skull.

The nasal mucosa produces about one quart per day of mucus, which is used to moisten the air moving through the nose and also to trap pollens, dust, and other foreign matter traveling through the nose.

The nose also drains the four pairs of paranasal sinuses. The maxillary sinuses are located over the medial portion on the cheekbones, while the frontal sinuses are found over the eyebrows. The ethmoidal sinuses reside

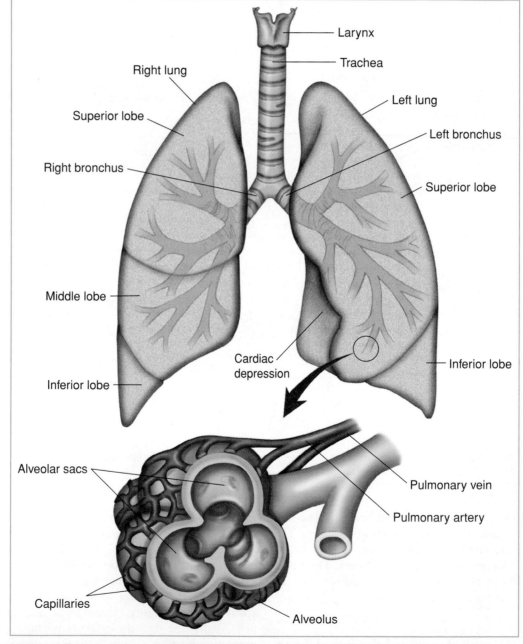

FIGURE 27-3 The larynx, trachea, bronchi, and lungs with an expanded view showing the structures of an alveolus and the pulmonary blood vessels.

in the area between and behind the eyes and the sphenoidal sinuses are located behind the ethmoidal sinuses. The sinuses decrease the weight of the skull with the creation of "air pockets" and also aid in phonation.

Pharynx

The pharynx is the musculo-membranous tube approximately 5 inches long that stretches from the base of the skull to the cervical spine and connects to the trachea and esophagus. The major functions of the pharynx include being a passageway for air and food and assisting in the production and sound of speech.

The pharynx has three parts: the nasopharynx, connects with the nose; the oropharynx, which connects with the back of the mouth; and the laryngopharynx, which is where the pharynx is located. Three paired sets of tonsils reside in the pharynx. The adenoids are located behind the nose and are often blamed for snoring, especially in children. The palatine tonsils are in the oropharynx and are often referred to as "the tonsils," and are located on either side of the throat on the anterior portion of the oropharynx. The lingual tonsils are located at the base of the tongue. The tonsils are part of the immune system and help in infection control.

Larynx

The larynx is also known as the voice box (see Figure 27-3). It is a muscular, cartilaginous structure lined with mucous membrane and connected to the inferior (lower) end of the pharynx. The larynx has several cartilaginous structures to help protect it from trauma. The thyroid cartilage is the largest of the cartilage structures, and is also known as the "Adam's apple." The epiglottic cartilage is also known as the epiglottis. Its function is to cover the trachea (windpipe) during swallowing so that food is all directed down the esophagus to the stomach rather than down the trachea and into the lungs. The cricoid cartilage is the lowest cartilage in the larynx. It is C shaped and wraps around the larynx to protect it from pressure. The "opening" in the "C" allows for large boluses of food to be swallowed down the esophagus. The inside of the larynx contains the false and true vocal folds and the entrance of the glottis—the opening between the vocal folds through which air passes.

The larynx functions in the production of vocal sounds. If the larynx is relaxed, then low sounds are produced. If it is tense, then higher pitched notes occur. The nose, mouth, pharynx, and bony sinuses impact the other aspects of speaking and singing.

Trachea

The trachea is also known as the windpipe (Figure 27-3). It is a cartilaginous tube that extends between the larynx to the main bronchi, and is about 1 inch wide and 4.5 inches long. Like the larynx, it has C-rings of cartilage that protect its structure and shape.

Lifespan
Considerations

THE CHILD

- Infants born before the age of 24 weeks gestation are frequently administered a product called surfactant, which the body produces in more mature lungs to help increase the surface tension of the fluid lining in the alveoli, making oxygen exchange more efficient. By administering this fluid to more immature lungs, there is a decrease in the occurrence of respiratory distress syndrome and lung damage in these infants.
- A newborn has a respiratory rate of 30 to 80 breaths per minute. As the infant matures, the respiratory rate drops to 20 to 40 by the first birthday. A 5-year-old has a respiratory rate of approximately 20 to 25 breaths per minute, while a 15-year-old usually demonstrates a rate of 15 to 20 breaths per minute. Healthy adults also breathe in the range of 15 to 20 breath per minute.

THE OLDER ADULT

- Older adults may increase their respiratory rates as the cumulative effects of pollution, smoking, and disease begin to wear on the integrity of the tissues. Mucous membranes produce less mucus, and the cilia decrease in their function. As a result, less foreign matter is trapped prior to entering the lungs and an increase in infections results.
- With skeletal changes of aging, oftentimes breathing in the elderly is diaphragm based rather than rib based, decreasing the tidal volume of external respiration. The lungs also lose their flexibility and become stiffer, so the volume of air that can be moved decreases. As a result, older adults are less able to move out foreign and disease-causing materials, and are more susceptible to bronchitis and pneumonia.

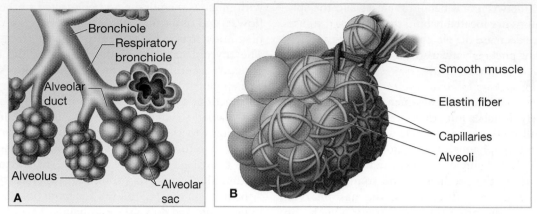

FIGURE 27-4 (A) Alveolar sac; (B) alveoli with capillaries.

The interior is lined with mucous membrane and cilia to trap foreign matter. One of the most important functions of the trachea is to transfer oxygen to the lungs and carbon dioxide from the lungs; in other words, breathing.

Bronchi

The bronchi are the two main branches of the trachea that stretch between the trachea and the lungs (Figure 27-3). These structures are responsible for providing a passageway for air between the trachea and the lungs. The right bronchus is the longer, larger branch moving down the right side of the heart. The left bronchus is shorter and more vertical, as it makes room for the heart in the chest cavity. After entering the lungs at the hilum, the lungs subdivide into the bronchial tree, which continues to branch into smaller and small branches called bronchioles. Eventually, those bronchioles terminate at the alveoli. The alveoli are small air sacs that support a network of capillaries used for oxygen and carbon dioxide transfer (see Figure 27-4). In healthy individuals, the alveoli resemble small balloons that inflate and deflate as air moves in and out. The bronchial tubes are lined with a mucous membranes and cilia to assist in removing foreign matter prior to its entry into the lungs.

Lungs

The lungs are large, conical-shaped, lobed organs in the chest (Figure 27-3). At birth the lungs are pinkish in color, but as adulthood approaches, the lungs turn a dark, slate gray color. The lungs are porous and spongy in texture and highly elastic. The right lung is made up of three lobes, called the upper, middle, and lower lobes, and weighs about 625 grams, whereas the left lung weighs 567 grams and only has two lobes: upper and lower. Each lung is between 10 and 12 inches in length, and they are separated by the mediastinum. The mediastinum contains the heart, trachea, esophagus, and blood vessels.

Pleura, thin sheets of epithelium sometimes referred to as pleural membranes, cover the outer surface of the lungs and the inside of the thoracic cavity. The gap between the pleura is called the pleural space. The pleura produce a lubricating fluid called surfactant that fills the pleural space. Surfactant helps the lungs glide smoothly in the chest cavity during inhalation and exhalation.

The lungs have three important roles: to supply oxygen, remove wastes and toxins, and defend against hostile intruders.

The lungs have three dozen distinct types of cells. Some of these cells scavenge foreign matter. Others have cilia that sweep the mucous membranes lining the smallest air passages. Some cells act on blood pressure control, while others spot infection invaders.

Mechanism of Breathing

Ventilation is the term used for movement to and from the alveoli. The two aspects of ventilation are inhalation and exhalation, which are brought about by the nervous system and the respiratory muscles. The respiratory centers are located in the brainstem, specifically, in the medulla oblongata and the pons. The respiratory muscles are the diaphragm and the internal and external intercostal muscles. The diaphragm is a dome-shaped muscle below the lungs. When it contracts, the diaphragm flattens and moves downward. The intercostal muscles are found between the ribs. The external intercostal muscles pull the ribs upward and outward, and the internal intercostal muscles pull the ribs downward and inward. Ventilation is the result of the respiratory muscles producing changes in the pressure within the alveoli and bronchial tree. Breathing involves three important pressure measurements:

- **Atmospheric pressure**—the pressure of the air around us. At sea level the atmospheric pressure is 760 mmHg; at higher altitudes the pressure is lower.

- Intrapleural pressure—the pressure within the potential pleural space between the parietal and visceral pleura. This space is a potential rather than a real space. Intrapleural pressure is always slightly below atmospheric pressure. This is called negative pressure because the elastic lungs are always tending to collapse and pull the visceral pleura away from the parietal pleura. The serous fluid, however, prevents separation of the pleural membranes.
- Intrapulmonic pressure—the pressure within the bronchial tree and alveoli. This pressure fluctuates below and above atmospheric pressure during each cycle of breathing.

Inhalation

Inhalation, which is also called *inspiration,* involves a precise sequence of events. The nervous system sends an impulse to the diaphragm and external intercostal muscles. The diaphragm flattens, which increases the top-to-bottom length of the thorax. Contraction elevates the ribs and increases the size of the thorax from the front to the back and from side to side. This increase in the size of the chest cavity reduces pressure within it, and what follows is an active process through which air moves into the lungs.

Expiration

Quiet *expiration* is ordinarily a passive process. During expiration the thorax returns to its resting size and shape. Elastic recoil of lung tissues aids in expiration. However, expiratory muscles used in forceful expiration are the internal intercostals and abdominal muscles. Reduction of the size of the thoracic cavity builds pressure and air leaves the lungs. Figure 27-5 shows how the actual mechanism of breathing takes place.

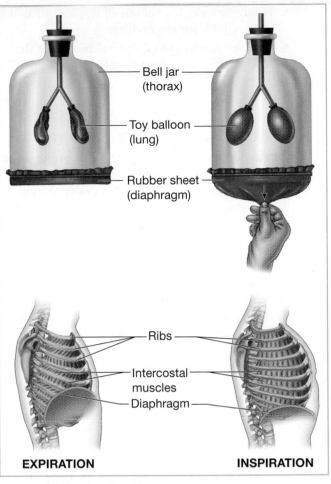

FIGURE 27-5 Mechanism of breathing.

Respiratory Volumes and Capacities

During the act of breathing, different volumes of air are moving in and out at different capacities, and these capacities can be calculated by adding specific respiratory volumes together. For example, when measuring lung volume, the following volumes would be used:

- Tidal volume (V_T) = volume of air entering or leaving the lungs during a single breath.
- Inspiratory reserve volume (IRV) = volume of air that can be inspired over and above the resting tidal volume
- Expiratory reserve volume (ERV) = volume of air that can be expired after a normal expiration

- Residual volume (RV) = volume of air remaining in the lungs after a maximal expiration, which can be estimated as 25 percent of the vital capacity

When measuring lung capacities, the following measurements would be used:

- Inspiratory capacity (IC) = maximum volume that can be inspired after a normal expiration = VT + IRV
- Vital capacity (VC) = maximum volume that can be expired after a maximal inspiration = VT + IRV + ERV
- Functional residual capacity (FRC) = volume of air left in the lungs after a normal expiration = ERV + RV
- Total lung capacity (TLC) = volume of the lungs when fully inflated = VC + RV (or 1.25 × VC)

When measuring a person's respiratory volume and capacity, other measurements may be used including the following:

- Respiratory rate (f) = number of breaths per minute
- Minute ventilation (V_E) = total volume of air expired per minute = $V_T \times f$

- Dead space (V_D) = volume of inspired air that is not available for gas exchange
- Alveolar ventilation (V_A) = volume of air that reaches the alveoli per minute = $(V_T - V_D) \times f$

Common Disorders Associated with the Respiratory System

Pulmonary diseases have a wide range of presentation, from life-threatening to mildly irritating. Many are present in childhood, while others develop during the aging process.

Asthma

Asthma is a chronic, inflammatory disease. It is typically caused when allergens or other irritating substances cause swelling in the lining of the trachea and bronchial tubes, aggravating sensitive tissues. The tissues create mucus in an attempt to trap the offending intruder, which can cause coughing or a sense of struggling to breathe. This, in turn, causes more swelling, which causes more mucous production. It becomes a vicious cycle. Most individuals with asthma carry an inhaler of a beta-2 medication called albuterol or pirbuterol. This medication is a rescue medicine used during an asthma episode. Long-term, preventive medications are also used, including long-acting beta-2 medications (such as Serevent [salmeterol]), leukotrienes (Singulair), and inhaled corticosteroids (Flovent, Intal, beclomethasone). These medications do not stop an already occurring asthma episode, but must be used on a daily basis to keep medication levels in the tissues at an effective level for preventing the asthma episodes. In an asthma exacerbation, prescribers will give the patient steroids, such as prednisone, to help reduce the inflammation and allow the patient to heal faster with fewer complications.

Asthma is related to the same process that causes allergic reactions, so the two disorders are usually related. Asthma can have its onset during childhood, but adult-onset asthma is also common.

Chronic Obstructive Pulmonary Disease

Chronic obstructive pulmonary disease (COPD) is comprised primarily of two related diseases: chronic bronchitis and emphysema. In both diseases, there is chronic obstruction of the flow of air through the airways and out of the lungs, and the obstruction generally is permanent and progressive over time. Smoking is responsible for 90 percent of COPD in United States. Although not all cigarette smokers will develop COPD, it is estimated that 15 percent will. Smokers with COPD have higher death rates than nonsmokers with COPD. They also have more frequent respiratory symptoms (coughing, shortness of breath, etc.) and more deterioration in lung function than nonsmokers. Air pollution and some occupational pollutants such as cadmium and silica may increase the risk of COPD.

COPD usually is first diagnosed on the basis of a medical history that discloses many of the symptoms of COPD and a physical examination that discloses signs of COPD. Other tests to diagnose COPD include chest x-ray, computerized tomography (CT or CAT scan) of the chest, tests of lung function (pulmonary function tests), and the measurement of oxygen and carbon dioxide levels in the blood.

The goals of COPD treatment include prevention of further deterioration in lung function, alleviation of symptoms, and improvement in the performance of daily activities and quality of life. The treatment strategies include quitting smoking, taking medications to dilate airways (bronchodilators) and decrease airway inflammation, vaccinating against influenza and pneumonia, regular oxygen supplementation, and pulmonary rehabilitation.

Bronchitis

Bronchitis is a respiratory disease in which the mucous membrane in the lungs' bronchial passages becomes inflamed. As the irritated membrane swells and grows thicker, it narrows or shuts off the tiny airways in the lungs, resulting in coughing spells accompanied by thick phlegm and breathlessness. The disease comes in two forms: acute (lasting less than 6 weeks) and chronic (reoccurring frequently for more than 2 years). In addition, people with asthma also experience an inflammation of the lining of the bronchial tubes called asthmatic bronchitis.

Acute bronchitis is generally caused by lung infections. In most cases the infection is viral in origin, but sometimes it is caused by bacteria. Chronic bronchitis may be caused by repeated attacks of acute bronchitis, which weaken and irritate bronchial airways over time, and by industrial pollution. Chronic bronchitis is found in higher than normal rates among coal miners, grain handlers, metal molders, and other people who are continually exposed to dust. But the chief cause is heavy, long-term smoking, which irritates the bronchial tubes and causes them to produce excess mucus. The symptoms of chronic bronchitis are also worsened by air pollution.

Symptoms of acute bronchitis include a hacking cough; appearance of yellow, white, or green phlegm, usually appearing 24 to 48 hours after a cough; fever and chills; soreness and tightness in the chest; some pain below the breastbone during deep breathing; and some shortness of breath. Symptoms of chronic bronchitis generally include a persistent cough that produces yellow, white, or green phlegm (for at least 3 months of the year, and for more than two consecutive years) and sometimes wheezing, and breathlessness.

Conventional treatment for acute bronchitis may consist of simple measures such as getting plenty of rest, drinking lots of fluids, avoiding smoke and fumes, and possibly getting a prescription for an inhaled bronchodilator and/or cough syrup. In severe cases of chronic bronchitis, inhaled or oral steroids to reduce inflammation or supplemental oxygen may be necessary. In severe cases of chronic bronchitis with COPD, a physician may prescribe oxygen therapy, either on a continuous or as-needed basis.

Emphysema

Emphysema is a long-term, progressive disease of the lung that primarily causes shortness of breath. In people with emphysema, the lung tissues necessary to support the physical shape and function of the lung are destroyed. It is considered an obstructive lung disease because the destruction of lung tissue around smaller airways, called bronchioles, makes these airways unable to hold their shape properly when you exhale.

Tobacco smoking is by far the most dangerous reason why people develop emphysema, and it is also the most preventable cause. Other risk factors include a deficiency of an enzyme called alpha-$_1$-antitrypsin, air pollution, airway reactivity, heredity, gender (male), and age.

Shortness of breath is the most common symptom of emphysema. Cough, sometimes caused by the production of mucus, and wheezing may also be symptoms of emphysema. A tolerance for exercise may also decrease over time. Emphysema usually develops slowly. There may not be any acute episodes of shortness of breath. Slow deterioration is the rule, and it may go unnoticed.

Treatment for emphysema can take many forms and different approaches to treatment are available. Generally, a doctor will prescribe these treatments in

a stepwise approach, depending on the severity of the condition. Smoking cessation is a treatment that most doctors require of people with emphysema. Quitting smoking may halt the progression of the disease and should improve the function of the lungs to some extent. Bronchodilating medications, which cause the air passages to open more fully and allow better air exchange, are usually the first medications that a physician will prescribe. Other medications that may be prescribed include steroids and antibiotics. In cases where there is shortness of breath, oxygen may also be a prescribed treatment, and in very severe cases, surgery may be required. This may involve the actual removal of a lung.

Common Cold

A **common cold** is an infection of the upper respiratory tract. Because any one of more than 200 viruses

Patient Education

Patients with pulmonary diseases must be educated on the need to be aware of their respiratory status and to alter their daily activities accordingly. Environmental irritants such as smoke, pollution, and allergens will irritate respiratory symptoms and should be avoided. Compliance with medication instructions is another way in which patients can avoid exacerbations of their disease. If prescribed medications do not relieve their symptoms, then the patient should contact the office for further instructions.

Patients who have pulmonary diseases are also at higher risk for developing bronchitis and pneumonia. Because they may be unable to clear their secretions, and because of inflammation blocking the bronchial tubes, an increased amount of bacteria can collect in the bases of the lungs and thrive in the dark, stagnant environment. As a result, these patients should avoid other individuals who are sick.

In the current American culture, tobacco smoking has become less acceptable, especially as the medical profession continues to discover more links to chronic, life-threatening diseases. However, not every patient (or medical assistant) is part of a culture that accepts these tenets. Be sure that all information is presented in a nonjudgmental, factual, accepting manner. There are cultures that consider habits such as cigarette smoking as not only acceptable, but expected. These choices are the patient's own, and, although medical professionals will present factual information, they should never force this information on patients.

can cause a common cold, symptoms tend to vary greatly. The symptoms of a common cold usually appear about 1 to 3 days after exposure to a cold virus. Signs and symptoms may include a runny or stuffy nose, itchy or sore throat, cough, congestion, slight body aches or a mild headache, sneezing, watery eyes, low-grade fever of less than 102°F, and mild fatigue. Discharge from the nose may become thicker and yellow or green in color as a common cold runs its course. What makes a cold different from other viral infections is that generally a high fever does not accompany a cold. A person is also unlikely to experience significant fatigue from a common cold.

Although more than 200 viruses can cause a common cold, the rhinovirus is the most common culprit. Many cold viruses are highly contagious. Although a common cold can spread through sneezing and coughing, it often spreads by hand-to-hand contact with someone who has a cold or by using shared objects, such as utensils, towels, toys, or telephones.

There is no cure for the common cold. Antibiotics are of no use against cold viruses, and over-the-counter cold preparations will not cure a common cold or make it go away any sooner. However, over-the-counter medications can relieve some symptoms. For fever, sore throat, and headache, mild pain relievers may help. For runny nose and nasal congestion, antihistamines or decongestants may be useful. Because so many different viruses can cause a common cold, no effective vaccine has been developed. However, there are some common-sense precautions a person can follow that will help to slow the spread of cold viruses. These in-

clude washing their hands; scrubbing countertops clean, especially when someone in the household has a common cold; using tissues to sneeze and cough into and then discarding them right away; and not sharing drinking glasses or other utensils with family members who may be sick.

Cystic Fibrosis

Cystic fibrosis (CF) is a chronic and progressive disease usually diagnosed in childhood that causes mucus to become thick, dry, and sticky. The mucus builds up and clogs passages in many of the body's organs, but primarily the lungs and the pancreas. In the lungs, the mucus can lead to serious breathing problems and lung disease. In the pancreas, the mucus can lead to malnutrition and problems with growth and development. People with CF have an average life expectancy of about 32 years, although new treatments offer hope for longer and healthier lives. It is an incurable genetic disorder that occurs when a child inherits a specific defect in the cystic fibrosis transmembrane regulator (CFTR) gene from both parents. If the gene defect is inherited from only one parent, the child will not have the disease but is considered a carrier. Symptoms of cystic fibrosis are usually caused by the production of thick, sticky mucus. Symptoms vary from person to person and are not always present at birth; in some people, symptoms may be very mild and not be noticed or develop until later in childhood or early adulthood. The goal of treatment for CF is to manage symptoms and prevent complications.

Hay Fever

Hay fever, which is also called seasonal allergic rhinitis or pollinosis, is a seasonal allergy causing inflammation of the mucous membranes of the nose and eyes. About 26.1 million Americans experience hay fever symptoms each year. During the seasons when plants are pollinating, people breathe in the pollen and have an allergic reaction to it. Some of the symptoms of hay fever include repeated and prolonged sneezing; a stuffy and watery nose; redness, swelling, and itching of the eyes; itching of the nose, throat, and mouth; and itching of the ears or other ear problems. Sometimes breathing difficulties occur at night. Coughing is sometimes a symptom and is a result of postnasal dripping of clear mucus. Loss of smell is common and sometimes loss of taste occurs. In severe conditions, nose bleeding occurs.

Hay fever is best controlled by avoiding the substance that causes a reaction, and using medications that counteract the histamine that is released during the reaction. In more severe cases, corticosteroids may be also be used. The best way to control hay fever is by removing pollen from the air by means of air conditioners and filters.

Influenza

Influenza, commonly called the flu, is an illness caused by viruses that infect the respiratory tract. Compared with most other viral respiratory infections, such as the common cold, influenza (flu) infection often causes a more severe illness.

Influenza viruses continually change over time, usually by mutation. This constant changing enables the virus to evade the immune system of its host, so that people are susceptible to influenza virus infection throughout life.

Typical symptoms of influenza include fever (usually 100°F to 103°F in adults and often even higher in children), respiratory symptoms such as cough, sore throat, and runny or stuffy nose, headache, muscle aches, and extreme fatigue. Although nausea, vomiting and diarrhea can sometimes accompany influenza infection, especially in children, gastrointestinal symptoms are rarely prominent. The term "stomach flu" is a misnomer that is sometimes used to describe gastrointestinal illnesses caused by other microorganisms.

Most people who get the flu recover completely in 1 to 2 weeks, but some people develop serious and potentially life-threatening medical complications, such as pneumonia.

Legionnaire's Disease

Legionnaire's disease is a type of pneumonia or lung infection. It causes 2 percent of pneumonia cases that need hospital treatment. The disease came to be known as Legionnaire's disease, or legionellosis, in 1976. More than 40 different strains of the Legionella germ have now been discovered. Outbreaks of the disease tend to occur in healthy people staying in hotels or other buildings in which the cooling systems or showers have become contaminated by Legionella germs. They may also occur as single cases in which the source of the germs is uncertain. About three-quarters of all cases in the United States occur as isolated instances rather than as epidemics. It usually affects middle-aged or elderly people and it more commonly affects smokers or people with other respiratory problems.

The symptoms of the disease generally start 2 to 10 days after a person has been infected. They include high fever with sweating, severe headache, shortness of breath, a worsening cough, with greenish thick mucus (can be bloodstained), and muscle aches and pains. In severe cases, other systems of the body may be affected, leading to diarrhea, vomiting, mental confusion, and kidney and liver damage. The most serious effects are on the lungs. The mortality rate in previously fit and well people is about 10 percent. Many people experience fatigue, lack of energy,

and difficulty concentrating for some time after recovering from the disease. Joint pain and muscle weakness are also fairly common. These symptoms may last for some months or less commonly for a year or two.

Treatment normally includes antibiotics. In some cases, where the patient experiences difficulty breathing, intensive care with ventilation may be necessary, especially if the pneumonia is severe.

Lung Cancer

Lung cancer is the leading cause of cancer deaths in both women and men in the United States and throughout the world.

Smoking is the most significant cause of lung cancer. About 85 percent of lung cancers occur in a smoker or former smoker. The risk of developing lung cancer is related to the number of cigarettes smoked, the age at which a person started smoking, and how long a person has smoked (or had smoked before quitting). Other causes of lung cancer include passive smoking. Air pollution from motor vehicles, factories, asbestos exposure, and the presence of other lung diseases may increase the risk for lung cancer.

The most widely used therapies for lung cancer are surgery, chemotherapy, and radiation therapy.

Pleurisy

Pleurisy is an inflammation of the membrane that surrounds and protects the lungs (the pleura). The condition, which is also called *pleuritis*, is a disorder that generally stems from an existing respiratory infection, disease, or injury. In people who have otherwise good health, respiratory infections or pneumonia are the main causes of pleurisy.

A variety of conditions can give rise to pleurisy. These include infections, such as pneumonia, tuberculosis, and other bacterial or viral respiratory infections; immune disorders, including systemic lupus erythematosus, rheumatoid arthritis, and sarcoidosis; and other diseases, including pancreatitis, liver cirrhosis,

Professionalism

and heart or kidney failure. Pleurisy may also result from an injury.

The chief symptom of pleurisy is sudden, intense chest pain that is usually located over the area of inflammation. Although the pain can be constant, it is usually most severe when the lungs move during breathing, coughing, sneezing, or even talking. In some cases the pain may be felt in other areas such as the neck, shoulder, or abdomen (referred pain). Another indication of pleurisy is that holding one's breath or exerting pressure against the chest causes pain relief.

Pleurisy is also characterized by certain respiratory symptoms. In response to the pain, pleurisy patients commonly have a rapid, shallow breathing pattern. If severe breathing difficulties persist, patients may experience a blue-colored complexion (**cyanosis**).

The pain of pleurisy is usually treated with analgesic and anti-inflammatory drugs, such as acetaminophen. People with pleurisy may also receive relief from lying on the painful side. Sometimes, a painful cough will be controlled with codeine-based cough syrups. However, as the pain eases, a person with pleurisy should try to breathe deeply and cough to clear any congestion, otherwise pneumonia may occur.

Pneumonia

Pneumonia is an inflammation of the lung or lungs, caused by bacteria, viruses, fungi, or chemical irritants. The most common bacterial cause of pneumonia in the United States is *Streptococcus pneumoniae* (pneumococcus). Oftentimes, pneumonia follows influenza in the elderly and debilitated. Symptoms include a productive cough with greenish mucus or pus-like sputum, fever, chills, fatigue, chest pain, and muscle aches. Diagnostic indicators include chest auscultation with a stethoscope, sputum cultures, and chest x-rays. Treatment of pneumonia includes drinking fluids, rest, antibiotics, and nonprescription drugs for pain relief. Supportive care includes oxygen therapy and respiratory treatments to thin out and remove secretions as necessary.

Pulmonary Edema

Pulmonary edema is a condition in which fluid accumulates in the lungs, usually because the heart's left ventricle does not pump adequately. Pulmonary edema can be a chronic condition, or it can develop suddenly and quickly become life threatening.

Most cases of pulmonary edema are caused by failure of the heart's main chamber, the left ventricle. It can be brought on by an acute heart attack, severe ischemia, volume overload of the heart's left ventricle, and mitral stenosis. Non-heart-related pulmonary edema is caused by lung problems such as pneumonia, an excess of intravenous fluids, some types of kidney disease, bad burns, liver disease, nutritional problems, and Hodgkin's disease.

Early symptoms of pulmonary edema include shortness of breath upon exertion, sudden respiratory distress after sleep, difficulty breathing, except when sitting upright, and coughing. In cases of severe pulmonary edema, the symptoms may worsen and will frequently include labored and rapid breathing; frothy, bloody fluid containing pus coughed from the lungs (sputum); a fast pulse and possibly serious disturbances in the heart's rhythm; cold, clammy, sweaty, and bluish skin; and a drop in blood pressure resulting in a thready pulse.

Pulmonary edema requires immediate emergency treatment. Treatment includes placing the patient in a sitting position and, in some cases, oxygen, assisted or mechanical ventilation, and drug therapy. The goal of treatment is to reduce the amount of fluid in the lungs, to improve gas exchange and heart function, and, where possible, to correct the underlying disease.

Pulmonary Embolism

A **pulmonary embolism** (PE) is a blood clot in the lung. It usually comes from smaller vessels in the leg, pelvis, arms, or heart. The clot travels through the vessels of the lung continuing to reach smaller vessels until it becomes wedged in a vessel that is too small to allow it to continue farther. The clot gets wedged and prevents any further blood from traveling to that section of the lung. When no blood reaches a section of the lung, that portion of the lung suffers an infarct, meaning it dies because no blood or oxygen is reaching it. This is referred to as a pulmonary (or lung) infarct.

Several factors can make someone more susceptible to developing a blood clot that can eventually break loose and travel to the lung. These factors may include immobilization due to illness or injury, or prolonged sitting, such as on an airplane or a long car trip, which allows the blood to sit in the legs and increases the risk of clot formation. Other factors are recent surgery, trauma or injury (especially to the legs), obesity, heart disease, burns, and a previous history of blood clot in the legs.

There are specific symptoms that may indicate that a PE has occurred. These include chest pain that is very sharp and stabbing in nature, has a sudden onset, and is worse when taking a deep breath; shortness of breath; anxiety or apprehension; dry cough; sweating; and passing out.

For someone who is critically ill and may have severe shortness of breath, low blood pressure, and low oxygen concentrations, the treatment may be much more aggressive, and often includes medications to elevate the blood pressure and increase the oxygen in the blood. Additional treatment might also include the use of "clot-buster" medications to help dissolve the emboli, and blood pressure elevators to raise the blood pressure. In cases where the PE is not as severe, oxygen therapy and the administration of blood-thinning medications are generally all that are needed.

Severe Acute Respiratory Syndrome

Severe acute respiratory syndrome (SARS) is a newly identified respiratory illness that first infected people in parts of Asia, North America, and Europe in early 2003. SARS is caused by a previously unknown type of coronavirus, a family of viruses that often cause mild to moderate upper respiratory illness, such as the common cold. This new virus is known as SARS-CoV. It is possible that outbreaks of SARS may be seasonal, appearing during winter months. Experts believe SARS may have first developed in animals, since the virus has been found in civets—a cat-like wild animal that is eaten as a delicacy in China.

The World Health Organization (WHO) reported that 8,096 people became sick with SARS, 774 of whom died, in the first outbreak. In 2004, China reported five confirmed and four possible cases of SARS by April 30. By May 18, 2004, WHO reported that the outbreak had been contained.

Like most respiratory illnesses, SARS is spread mainly through contact with infected saliva or droplets from coughing. You cannot get SARS from brief, casual exposure to an infected person, such as passing someone on the street. Close proximity, that is, less than 3 feet, or contact is probably necessary to become infected. Close contact includes living with or caring for a person who has SARS or having direct contact with saliva or respiratory droplets from an infected person. Treatment of SARS usually consists of antibiotics, antiviral medications, and steroids.

Sinusitis

Sinusitis is an infection or inflammation of the mucous membranes that line the inside of the nose and sinuses. Sinuses are hollow spaces, or cavities, located around your eyes, cheeks, and nose. When a mucous membrane becomes inflamed, it swells, blocking the drainage of fluid from the sinuses into the nose and throat, which causes pressure and pain in the sinuses. Bacteria and fungus are more likely to grow in sinuses that are unable to drain properly.

Sinuses can become blocked during a viral infection such as a cold, and sinus inflammation and infection can develop as a result. One key distinction between a cold and sinusitis is that cold symptoms, including a stuffy nose, begin to improve within 5 to 7 days. Sinusitis symptoms last longer and get worse after 7 days. There are two types of sinusitis: acute (sudden) and chronic (long term). With chronic sinusitis, a person is never really free from symptoms and always has a low level of sinusitis symptoms.

Pain and pressure in the face along with a stuffy or runny nose are the main symptoms of sinusitis. You also may have a yellow or greenish discharge from your nose. Leaning forward or moving your head often increases facial pain and pressure. The location of pain and tenderness may depend on which sinus is affected. Pain over the cheeks and upper teeth is often caused by maxillary sinus inflammation. Pain in the forehead, above the eyebrow, may be caused by frontal sinus inflammation. Pain behind the eyes, on top of the head, or in both temples may be caused by sphenoid sinus inflammation. And pain around or behind the eyes is caused by ethmoid sinus inflammation.

Sinusitis is generally treated with medications and home treatment measures, such as applying moist heat to the face. The goals of treatment for sinusitis are to improve drainage of mucus and reduce swelling in the sinuses, relieve pain and pressure, clear up any infection, prevent the formation of scar tissue, and avoid permanent damage to the tissues lining the nose and sinuses. Medications may also be used to treat sinusitis, especially when it is caused by a bacterial infection. There are varying lengths of treatment with medications—as short as 3 days or lasting as long as several weeks or more. The medications most often used to treat the condition include a combination of antibiotics, decongestants, analgesics, corticosteroids, and mucolytics.

Tuberculosis

Tuberculosis (TB) is a contagious disease caused by the bacillus *Mycobacterium tuberculosis*. The bacteria are spread from person to person by inhaling droplets infected with the bacteria. This often happens when an individual with this bacteria coughs, sneezes, or laughs, spreading those bacteria for others to breathe.

TB bacteria can grow anywhere in the body, but are most commonly found in the lungs. They produce granulomas (granular tumors) in the infected tissues. Symptoms for lung infections include coughing, hemoptysis (coughing up blood), white/gray frothy sputum, and night sweats. Other symptoms can include fatigue, chills, weakness, and anorexia.

Diagnosis is done by chest x-ray and sputum culture. The PPD skin test is done to see if an individual has ever been exposed to the bacteria, but is not indicative of whether the person actually has the disease.

Treatment of this disease is long term, usually taking 9 to 12 months to eradicate the bacteria. The first period requires that individuals take respiratory precautions to prevent the spread of the bacteria. Antibiotics are used to begin eradication of the bacteria, usually rifampin, isoniazid, and ethambutol HCl. After the patient shows negative sputum cultures, they will still need to continue antibiotic treatment for another 6 to 9 months to prevent multi-drug-resistant TB that is more difficult to treat.

Individuals who are immunocompromised, such as the homeless, those with AIDS, infants, the elderly, and individuals on chemotherapy, are the most at risk for developing TB.

SUMMARY

The respiratory system is made of a system of tubes lined with mucous membranes and cilia, which serve a protective function. The function of the system is external, internal, and cellular respiration. Multiple disease processes can result from infection and inflammation within the system.

Chapter Review

COMPETENCY REVIEW

1. Define and spell the terms to learn for this chapter.
2. List the organs of the respiratory system.
3. What is the primary function of the respiratory system?
4. What does atmospheric pressure represent?
5. What are the five functions of the nose?
6. What are the three functions of the pharynx?
7. What is the function of the epiglottis?
8. Describe the bronchi. What are the differences between the left and right bronchus?
9. What are the alveoli?
10. What does tidal volume represent?

PREPARING FOR THE CERTIFICATION EXAM

1. What organ is responsible for being a passageway for air and food and also assists in the production and sound of speech?
   A. pharynx
   B. nares
   C. trachea
   D. bronchi
   E. epiglottis

2. The sac that encases the lungs is called the
   A. thorax
   B. pleura
   C. bronchiole
   D. pneumoderma
   E. pneumocardium

3. Another name for the windpipe is the
   A. bronchial tube
   B. trachea
   C. larynx
   D. pharynx
   E. epiglottis

4. The function of the epiglottis is to
   A. aid in swallowing
   B. aid in speaking
   C. prevent swallowing
   D. prevent aspiration
   E. aid in aspiration

continued on next page

5. A genetic condition characterized by the production of thick sticky mucus is called
   A. asthma
   B. pneumonia
   C. cystic fibrosis
   D. COPD
   E. tuberculosis

6. The volume of air remaining in the lungs after a maximal expiration is called the
   A. tidal volume
   B. inspiratory reserve volume
   C. expiratory reserve volume
   D. residual volume
   E. vital capacity

7. What term is used to describe the number of breaths per minute?
   A. ventilation rate
   B. respiratory rate
   C. alveolar ventilation rate
   D. minute ventilation
   E. respiratory ventilation

8. Bronchitis is
   A. inflammation of the bronchial tubes
   B. constriction of the bronchial tubes
   C. destruction of the bronchial tubes
   D. seen only in the elderly
   E. seen only in infants

9. What disease is smoking most responsible for causing in the United States?
   A. asthma
   B. COPD
   C. cystic fibrosis
   D. pneumonia
   E. tuberculosis

10. Tuberculosis is spread by
    A. touching the infected person
    B. breathing an allergen
    C. breathing infected droplets
    D. the casual handshake
    E. smoking

CRITICAL THINKING

1. What could Joe have done early on to reduce his chances of getting COPD?
2. Why did the physician prescribe an antibiotic for Joe?
3. Why did the physician prescribe two puffs of albuterol every 4 hours?

INTERNET ACTIVITY

Do an Internet search for COPD services in your hometown and see what resources are available in your area.

MediaLink More on the respiratory system, including interactive resources, can be found on the Student CD-ROM accompanying this textbook.

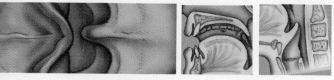

Medical Assistant Role Delineation Chart

HIGHLIGHT indicates material covered in this chapter.

ADMINISTRATIVE

Administrative Procedures

- Perform basic administrative medical assisting functions
- Schedule, coordinate and monitor appointments
- Schedule inpatient/outpatient admissions and procedures
- Understand and apply third-party guidelines
- Obtain reimbursement through accurate claims submission
- Monitor third-party reimbursement
- Understand and adhere to managed care policies and procedures
- *Negotiate managed care contracts*

Practice Finances

- Perform procedural and diagnostic coding
- Apply bookkeeping principles

- Manage accounts receivable
- *Manage accounts payable*
- *Process payroll*
- *Document and maintain accounting and banking records*
- *Develop and maintain fee schedules*
- *Manage renewals of business and professional insurance policies*
- *Manage personnel benefits and maintain records*
- *Perform marketing, financial, and strategic planning*

CLINICAL

Fundamental Principles

- Apply principles of aseptic technique and infection control
- Comply with quality assurance practices
- Screen and follow up patient test results

Diagnostic Orders

- Collect and process specimens
- Perform diagnostic tests

Patient Care

- Adhere to established patient screening procedures
- Obtain patient history and vital signs
- Prepare and maintain examination and treatment areas
- Prepare patient for examinations, procedures and treatments

- Assist with examinations, procedures and treatments
- Prepare and administer medications and immunizations
- Maintain medication and immunization records
- Recognize and respond to emergencies
- Coordinate patient care information with other health care providers
- Initiate IV and administer IV medications with appropriate training and as permitted by state law

GENERAL

Professionalism

- Display a professional manner and image
- Demonstrate initiative and responsibility
- Work as a member of the health care team
- Prioritize and perform multiple tasks
- Adapt to change
- Promote the CMA credential
- Enhance skills through continuing education
- Treat all patients with compassion and empathy
- Promote the practice through positive public relations

Communication Skills

- Recognize and respect cultural diversity
- Adapt communications to individual's ability to understand
- Use professional telephone technique

- Recognize and respond effectively to verbal, nonverbal, and written communications
- Use medical terminology appropriately
- Utilize electronic technology to receive, organize, prioritize and transmit information
- Serve as liaison

Legal Concepts

- Perform within legal and ethical boundaries
- Prepare and maintain medical records
- Document accurately
- Follow employer's established policies dealing with the health care contract
- Implement and maintain federal and state health care legislation and regulations
- Comply with established risk management and safety procedures
- Recognize professional credentialing criteria
- *Develop and maintain personnel, policy and procedure manuals*

Instruction

- Instruct individuals according to their needs
- Explain office policies and procedures
- Teach methods of health promotion and disease prevention
- Locate community resources and disseminate information
- *Develop educational materials*
- *Conduct continuing education activities*

Operational Functions

- Perform inventory of supplies and equipment
- Perform routine maintenance of administrative and clinical equipment
- Apply computer techniques to support office operations
- *Perform personnel management functions*
- *Negotiate leases and prices for equipment and supply contracts*

- *Denotes advanced skills.*

SOURCE: Reprinted by permission of the American Association of Medical Assistants from the AAMA Role Delineation Study: Occupational Analysis of the Medical Assisting Profession.

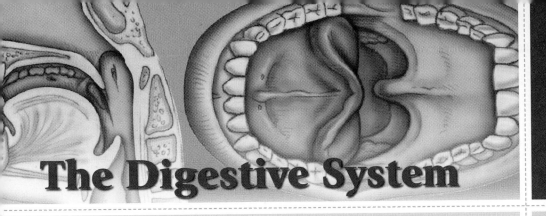

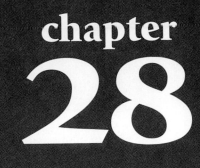

chapter 28

The Digestive System

Learning Objectives

After completing this chapter, you should be able to:

- Define and spell the terms to learn for this chapter.
- Describe the purpose and function of the digestive system.
- Identify the primary organs of the digestive system and briefly explain the function of each.
- Name the two sets of teeth with which a person is born.
- Discuss the three main portions of a tooth.
- Identify the accessory organs of the digestive system and state the function of each.
- Briefly explain common disorders associated with the digestive system.

Terms to Learn

appendicitis
cirrhosis
colitis
colorectal cancer
constipation
Crohn's disease
diarrhea
diverticulitis

diverticulosis
gastroesophageal reflux disease (GERD)
hemorrhoid
hernia
hiatal hernia
inguinal hernia

irritable bowel syndrome (IBS)
oral cancer
pancreatic cancer
peptic ulcer disease (PUD)
pyloric stenosis
stomach ulcers

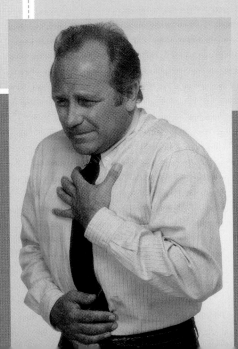

Case Study

NATE SYLVANS IS A 38-YEAR-OLD MALE seen by Dr. Sammons. He is complaining of "a lot of heartburn" and frequent "belching." He admits to being under a lot of pressure at work lately, and has a frequent dull aching pain in his stomach and back. Pain is localized in the midepigastrium. Mr. Sylvans is diagnosed with an acute gastric ulcer after receiving an upper GI series, gastric analysis and histology with culture, indicating no presence of *H. pylori* bacteria.

he digestive system contains those organs that are responsible for getting food into and out of the body and for making use of it. These organs include the salivary glands, the mouth, esophagus, stomach, small intestine, liver, gallbladder, pancreas, colon, rectum, and anus. The main part of the digestive system is the digestive tract. This is like a long tube, some 30 feet long in adults, through the middle of the body. It starts at the mouth, where food and drink enter the body, and finishes at the anus, where leftover food and wastes leave the body. The three main functions of the digestive system include digestion, absorption, and elimination (by means of urine or feces). Each of the various organs commonly associated with digestion is described in this chapter, and the organs of digestion are shown in Figure 28-1.

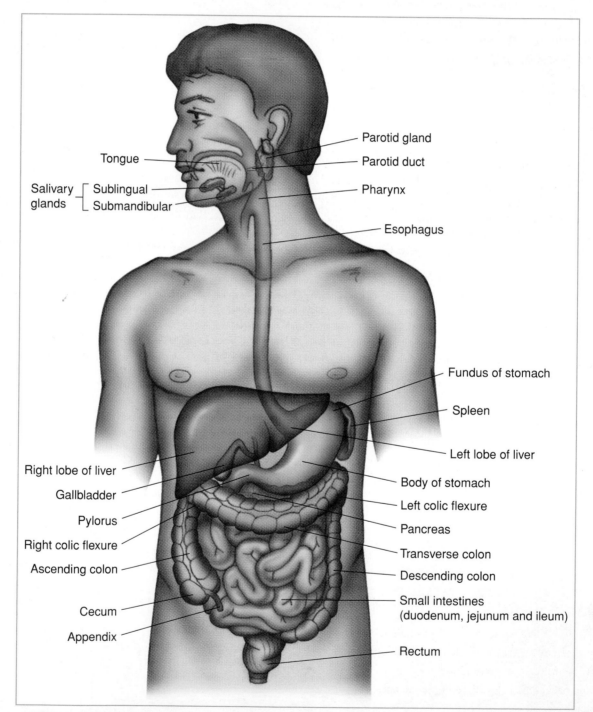

FIGURE 28-1 The digestive system.

Organs of the Digestive System

The digestive system is a series of hollow organs joined in a long, twisting tube from the mouth to the anus. Inside this tube is a lining called the mucosa. In the mouth, stomach, and small intestine, the mucosa contains tiny glands that produce juices to help digest food.

Mouth

The mouth is the cavity formed by the palate (roof), the lips and cheeks on the sides, and the tongue on the floor (see Figure 28-2). The oral cavity (the mouth) contains the teeth and the salivary glands. The cheeks form the lateral walls and are continuous with the lips. The vestibule includes the space between the cheeks and the teeth. The gingivae (gums) surround the neck of the teeth, helping to hold the teeth in place. The hard and soft palates form a roof for the oral cavity, and the tongue is connected to the floor of the mouth by the lingual frenulum. The tongue is made of skeletal muscle and is covered with mucous membrane. The tongue can be divided into the rear portion called the root, the central body, and the pointed tip. Papillae (elevations) and taste buds are located on the surface of the tongue. There are four types of taste buds—sweet, salt, sour, and bitter. Three pairs of salivary glands secrete saliva into the oral cavity. They are called the parotid, sublingual, and submandibular glands. The posterior margins of the soft palate support the muscular pharyngeal arches, which function in swallowing and phonation, and the uvula—the dangling tissue hanging down from the center of the pharyngeal arches. The line formed by the pharyngeal arches and the uvula separates the oral cavity from the pharynx. Digestion begins in the mouth with the process of mastication (chewing) and the secretion of saliva, which moistens the food and starts the chemical breakdown of food. The combination of the chewing action and the saliva helps to form the food into a bolus (ball) for swallowing.

Teeth

Humans have two sets of teeth: 28 deciduous teeth (the baby teeth) and 32 permanent teeth (see Figure 28-3). The 28 deciduous teeth include 8 incisors, 4 canines (cuspids), and 8 molars. The permanent teeth include 8 incisors, 4 canines, 8 premolars, and 12 molars. The incisors are so named because of their sharp, cutting edge used for biting food. The incisors are the four front teeth of the dental arch. The upper incisors are larger and stronger than the lower ones.

The canine teeth are also known as the cuspids. These teeth have their roots stuck deeply into the bones of the jaw. The upper canines are also known as the "eye teeth" and are larger than the lower canines. The lower canines are also known as the "stomach teeth."

The premolar teeth are situated lateral to, and behind, the canine teeth. They are also known as the bicuspid teeth and are smaller and shorter than the canine teeth. There are four premolars in each arch. The molar teeth are the largest teeth in the permanent set and are adapted to grinding and pounding food. An adult has 12 molars, six in each arch, placed posterior to the premolars.

The deciduous teeth are smaller than the permanent teeth, but generally resemble the permanent teeth on a smaller scale.

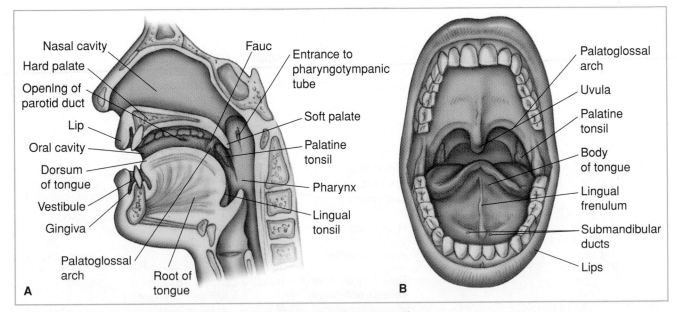

FIGURE 28-2   The oral cavity: (A) sagittal section; (B) anterior view as seen through the open mouth.

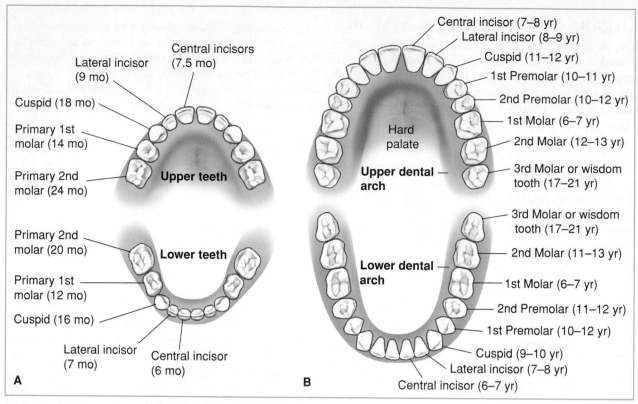

FIGURE 28-3 Deciduous and permanent teeth: (A) deciduous teeth, with the age at eruption given in months; (B) permanent teeth, with the age at eruption given in years.

Each tooth consists of three main portions: the crown (the part above the gum); the root (embedded in the gums); and the neck, the part between the root and the crown (see Figure 28-4). The root of each tooth sits in a bony socket called the alveolus. Collagen fibers of the periodontal ligament extend from the dentin of the root to the bone of the alveolus, creating a strong articulation known as a gomphosis (that binds the teeth to the bony sockets in the maxillary bone and mandible). A layer of cementum covers the dentin of the root, providing protection and firmly anchoring the periodontal ligament. The solid portion of the tooth consists of the dentin, which forms the bulk of the tooth, and the enamel, which covers the exposed

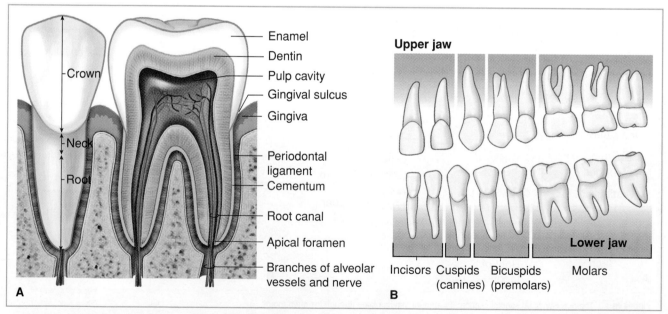

FIGURE 28-4 Teeth: (A) a diagrammatic section through a typical adult tooth; (B) the adult teeth.

part of the crown. The enamel is the hardest and most compact part of the tooth. The cementum is a think layer of bone, deposited on the surface of the root. The neck of the tooth is the part between the crown and the root. The gingiva is the soft tissue of the gum that surrounds the neck. A shallow groove called the gingival sulcus surrounds the neck of each tooth.

Teeth erupt from the gums when there is sufficient calcification for the tooth to be able to tolerate the stress that it will be subjected to later on. Deciduous teeth erupt from the gums starting at about 7 months and finishing at about age 2½. The permanent teeth erupt at about the following ages:

First molars	6th to 7th year
Two central incisors	7th to 8th year
Two lateral incisors	8th to 9th year
First premolars	10th to 11th year
Second premolars	10th to 12th year
Canines	11th to 12th year
Second molars	12th to 13th year
Third molars	17th to 21st year

Pharynx

The pharynx lies posterior to the mouth and is the beginning of the tube leading to the stomach. The pharynx is used by both the respiratory system and the digestive system. Both the larynx and the esophagus begin in the pharynx. Anything that is swallowed passes through the pharynx into the esophagus reflexively. Muscular constructions move the ball of food into the esophagus while closing the trachea to prevent food from entering the trachea.

Esophagus

The esophagus is a collapsible tube, about 10 inches long, that starts at the pharynx and ends at the stomach. Food is carried down the esophagus by a series of muscular contractions called peristalsis. These wave-like contractions will move the bolus of food along through the entire digestive system.

Stomach

The stomach is a large sac-like organ that holds food for the beginning of the digestive process (see Figure 28-5). The stomach holds about 1 to 1.5 liters of food and fluid at a time. The stomach secretes hydrochloric acid and gastric juices to convert food into a semiliquid state to be passed into the small intestine for further digestion.

Small Intestine

The small intestine is 21 feet long, and about 1 inch in diameter (see Figure 28-6). The opening of the small

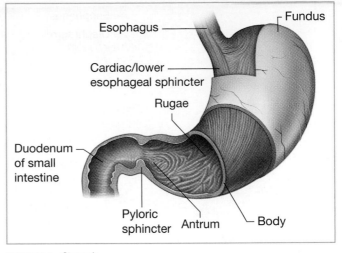

FIGURE 28-5 Stomach.

intestine, the pyloric sphincter, is at the base of the stomach. The first 12 inches of the small intestine is the duodenum, the second 8 feet is called the jejunum, and the ileum consists of the last 12 feet of intestine. Semi-liquid food (now called *chime*) is received from the stomach through the pylorus and mixed with bile from the liver and gallbladder along with pancreatic juice from the pancreas. Digestion and absorption of nutrients occur in the small intestine. Nutrients are absorbed into tiny capillaries and lymph vessels located in the walls of the small intestine and transmitted to the body cells via the circulatory system.

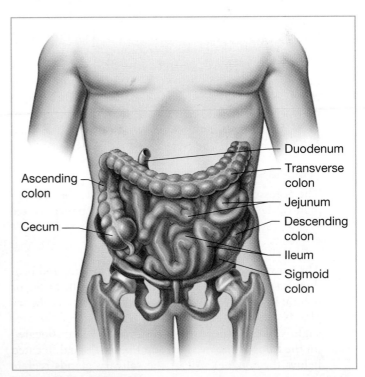

FIGURE 28-6 Small intestine.

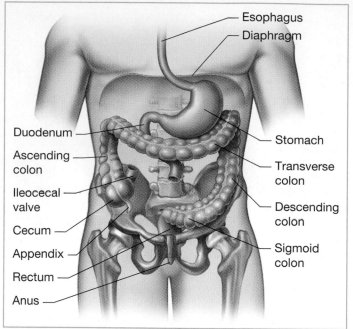

FIGURE 28-7 Large intestine (colon).

Large Intestine

The small intestine terminates at the ileocecal orifice at the large intestine. The large intestine starts at this terminus, and continues through the cecum (a small pouch about 3 inches long), the colon, the rectum, and the anal canal (see Figure 28-7). The large intestine is 5 feet long and about 2.5 inches in diameter. The appendix is a small appendage attached to the cecum that has no known function in humans. The colon makes up the bulk of the large intestine and is divided into several parts: the ascending colon (on the right side of the abdomen), the transverse colon (moves across the body transversely from right to left), the descending colon (on the right side of the abdomen), and the sigmoid colon, which leads to the rectum. The function of the large intestine is to complete digestion and absorption. The waste products of digestion are eliminated from the body via the rectum and the anus.

Accessory Organs

The accessory organs of digestion include the salivary glands, the gallbladder, the liver, and the pancreas (see Figure 28-8).

Salivary Glands

The salivary glands are located in the mouth, and produce saliva in response to the sight, smell, taste, or mental images of food. There are three pairs of salivary glands: the parotid (located on either side of the face slightly below the ear), the submandibular (located on the floor of the mouth), and the sublingual (located below the tongue). All of the salivary glands secrete saliva through openings into the mouth. Saliva con-

tains amylase—an enzyme that helps to start the break down of carbohydrates.

Gallbladder

The gallbladder is a membranous sac where bile is stored and concentrated. Any bile stored in the gallbladder is 10 times more concentrated than bile not stored in the gallbladder. Because of the function of concentrating bile, gallstones can occur, as can inflammation of the gallbladder. This condition is called cholelithiasis.

Liver

The liver is located on the upper right quadrant of the abdomen. It is the largest glandular organ and weight about 3.5 pounds. The liver plays an essential role in the metabolism of carbohydrates, fats, and proteins. The liver changes glucose to glycogen, and stores that glycogen as a product of carbohydrate metabolism.

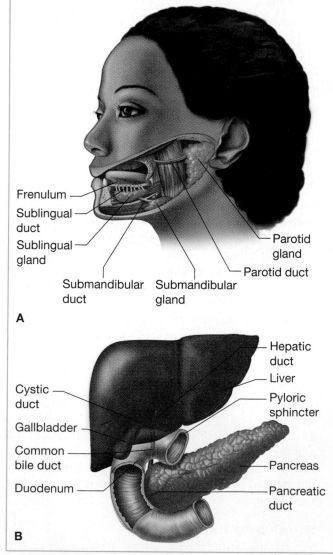

FIGURE 28-8 (A) Salivary glands; (B) gallbladder, liver, and pancreas.

The liver produces bile, which emulsifies fats for fat metabolism before releasing the products into the bloodstream. For protein metabolism, the liver acts as a storage place for the components of proteins, so the body can break down or build up proteins as it requires.

The liver manufactures four important substances for the function of the body:

- Bile—emulsifies fats
- Fibrinogen and prothrombin—essential for blood clotting
- Heparin—prevents the clotting of blood
- Blood proteins—albumin, gamma globulin

The liver also stores iron and the vitamins B_{12}, A, D, E, and K. The liver produces body heat and detoxifies the body from substances such as drugs and alcohol.

Pancreas

The pancreas is a long, elongated gland situated behind the stomach that secretes pancreatic juice into the small intestine. The pancreas is 6 to 9 inches long and contains cells that produce digestive enzymes. Other cells in the pancreas secrete the hormones insulin and glucagon, which lower and raise glucose levels in the blood.

Common Disorders Associated with the Digestive System

Digestive disorders range from the occasional upset stomach, heartburn, and nausea to the more serious and life-threatening colorectal cancer. These disorders encompass the gastrointestinal tract as well as the liver, gallbladder, and pancreas. Most digestive disorders and diseases are complex, with subtle symptoms, and the causes of many remain unknown (see Table 28-1). Some may be genetic or develop from multiple factors such as stress, fatigue, diet, or smoking. Alcohol abuse also poses a risk for digestive disorders. Diagnosis of a digestive disorder requires a thorough and accurate medical history and physical examination. Some may need to undergo more extensive diagnostic evaluations including laboratory tests, endoscopic procedures, and imaging techniques.

Appendicitis

The appendix is a small, tube-like structure attached to the first part of the large intestine, also called the colon. The appendix is located in the lower right portion of the abdomen. It has no known function, and removal of this structure appears to cause no change in digestive function. Appendicitis is an inflammation of the appendix.

Lifespan
Considerations

THE CHILD

- A child's digestive system continues to develop throughout the first year of life. Many environmental factors can stress a child's digestive system. Aside from the dietary factors, children are exposed to heavy metals, pollutants, solvents, and carcinogens found in food, water, air, medicine, and plastics that can injure the digestive system.

- Digestive disorders affecting infants and children range from simple problems that most children experience from time to time, such as vomiting or diarrhea, to more serious (and possibly life-threatening) birth defects such as tracheoesophageal fistula, or illnesses such as appendicitis.

- Digestive and liver disorders can have significant effects on the health of a child. A healthy digestive system processes the foods and liquids that we eat, replenishing vitamins, minerals, proteins, carbohydrates, and fats that are vital for the body to function properly. Occasional vomiting or diarrhea may lead to dehydration; however, long-term problems with the digestive system and/or liver can deplete these important nutrients, causing malnutrition that affects a child's physical and mental growth and development.

THE OLDER ADULT

- The digestive system becomes less motile with aging, as muscle contractions become weaker. Glandular secretions decrease, causing a drier mouth and a lower volume of gastric juices. Nutrient absorption decreases due to the atrophy of the mucosal lining. Because of age and continued use, the gums recede and the tooth surfaces wear down. There may be a loss of taste, and food preferences may change.

- Gastric motor activity slows, causing delayed gastric emptying and decrease in hunger contractions. Although there are no significant changes in the small intestine, the muscle layer and the blood flow through the large intestine begin to decline. Constipation can be a frequent problem, especially because of a decrease in dietary and fluid intake.

TABLE 28-1   Disorders and Pathology of the Digestive System

Disorder/Pathology	Description
Anorexia	Loss of appetite that can accompany other conditions such as a gastrointestinal (GI) upset.
Ascites	Collection or accumulation of fluid in the peritoneal cavity.
Bulimia	Eating disorder that is characterized by recurrent binge eating and then purging of the food with laxatives and vomiting.
Cholecystitis	Inflammation of the gallbladder.
Cholelithiasis	Formation or presence of stones or calculi in the gallbladder or common bile duct.
Cirrhosis	Chronic disease of the liver.
Cleft lip	Congenital condition in which the upper lip fails to come together. This is often seen along with cleft palate and is corrected with surgery.
Cleft plate	Congenital condition in which the roof of the mouth has a split or fissure. It is corrected with surgery.
Constipation	Experiencing difficulty in defecation or infrequent defecation.
Crohn's disease	Form of chronic inflammatory bowel disease affecting the ileum or colon. Also called regional ileitis.
Diarrhea	Passing of frequent, watery bowel movements. Usually accompanies gastrointestinal (GI) disorders.
Diverticulitis	Inflammation of a diverticulum or sac in the intestinal tract, especially in the colon.
Dyspepsia	Indigestion.
Emesis	Vomiting usually with some force.
Enteritis	Inflammation of only the small intestine.
Esophageal stricture	Narrowing of the esophagus, which makes the flow of foods and fluids difficult.
Fissure	Crack-like split in the rectum or anal canal or roof of mouth.
Fistula	Abnormal tube-like passage from one body cavity to another.
Gastritis	Inflammation of the stomach, which can result in pain, tenderness, nausea, and vomiting.
Gastroenteritis	Inflammation of the stomach and small intestine.
Halitosis	Bad or offensive breath, which is often a sign of disease.
Hepatitis	Inflammation of the liver.
Ileitis	Inflammation of the ileum of the small intestine.
Inflammatory bowel syndrome	Ulceration of the mucous membranes of the colon of unknown origin. Also known as ulcerative colitis.

(continued)

TABLE 28-1 **Disorders and Pathology of the Digestive System** (*continued*)

Disorder/Pathology	Description
Inguinal hernia	Hernia or outpouching of intestines into the inguinal region of the body. May require surgical correction.
Intussusception	Result of the intestine slipping or telescoping into another section of intestine just below it. More common in children.
Irritable bowel syndrome	Disturbance in the functions of the intestine from unknown causes. Symptoms generally include abdominal discomfort and an alteration in bowel activity.
Malabsorption syndrome	Inadequate absorption of nutrients from the intestinal tract. May be caused by a variety of diseases and disorders, such as infections and pancreatic deficiency.
Peptic ulcer	Ulcer occurring in the lower portion of the esophagus, stomach, and duodenum thought to be caused by the acid of gastric juices. Some peptic ulcers are now successfully treated with antibiotics.
Pilonidal cyst	Cyst in the sacrococcygeal region due to tissue being trapped below the skin.
Polyphagia	To eat excessively.
Polyps	Small tumors that contain a pedicle or foot-like attachment in the mucous membranes of the large intestine (colon).
Reflux esophagitis	Acid from the stomach backs up into the esophagus causing inflammation and pain. Also called GERD (gastroesophageal reflux disease).
Regurgitation	Return of fluids and solids from the stomach into the mouth. Similar to emesis but without the force.
Ulcerative colitis	Ulceration of the mucous membranes of the colon of unknown source. Also known as inflammatory bowel disease.
Volvulus	Condition in which the bowel twists upon itself and causes an obstruction. Painful and requires immediate surgery.

Once it starts, there is no effective medical therapy, so appendicitis is considered a medical emergency. When treated promptly, most patients recover without difficulty. If treatment is delayed, however, the appendix can burst, causing infection and even death. Anyone can get appendicitis, but it occurs most often between the ages of 10 and 30. The cause of appendicitis relates to blockage of the inside of the appendix, known as the lumen. This blockage leads to increased pressure, impaired blood flow, and inflammation.

Appendicitis is the most common acute surgical emergency of the abdomen. The appendix is almost always removed, even if it is found to be normal. With complete removal, any later episodes of pain will not be attributed to appendicitis. If the diagnosis is uncertain, people may be watched and sometimes treated with antibiotics. This approach is taken when the doctor suspects that the patient's symptoms may have a nonsurgical or treatable cause. If the cause of the pain is infectious, symptoms resolve with intravenous antibiotics and intravenous fluids.

Cirrhosis

Cirrhosis is a potentially life-threatening condition that occurs when scarring damages the liver. This scarring (also called *fibrosis*) replaces healthy tissue and prevents the liver from working normally. Cirrhosis usually develops after years of liver inflammation.

Cirrhosis can have many causes. Some people have cirrhosis without an obvious cause (cryptogenic cirrhosis). In the United States, the major causes of cirrhosis are drinking excessive amounts of alcohol over many years or having certain forms of viral hepatitis (mainly hepatitis B or C). Cirrhosis may be caused by a condition in which too much fat is stored in the liver, or when the ducts that carry bile out of the liver become inflamed and blocked. The latter may be related to a problem with the immune system. Another type of cirrhosis can be caused as a result of the immune system attacking the liver, a condition known as autoimmune hepatitis. Sometimes cirrhosis can be caused by an inherited disease, such as cystic fibrosis.

In many cases, symptoms develop only after the disease progresses. They may include fluid buildup in the legs (edema) and abdomen (ascites), fatigue, yellowing of the skin (jaundice), itching, nosebleeds, redness of the palms, bleeding from enlarged veins in the digestive tract, easy bruising, weight loss and muscle loss, abdominal pain, frequent infections, and confusion.

Treatment focuses on avoiding substances that can further damage the liver, especially alcohol and nonsteroidal anti-inflammatory drugs; making dietary changes; and using medications, surgery, and other treatment to prevent and treat complications. A liver transplant may be considered when liver damage is severe.

Colitis

Colitis is an inflammation of the large intestine that may be caused by many different disease processes, including acute and chronic infections, primary inflammatory disorders (ulcerative colitis, Crohn's colitis, lymphocytic and collagenous colitis), lack of blood flow (ischemic colitis), and history of radiation to the large bowel. Symptoms can include abdominal pain, diarrhea, dehydration, abdominal bloating, increased intestinal gas, and bloody stools. The disorder may be identified by flexible sigmoidoscopy or colonoscopy. In both of these tests, a flexible tube is inserted in the rectum, and specific areas of the colon are evaluated. Biopsies taken during these tests may show changes related to inflammation. Other studies that can identify colitis include barium enema, abdominal CT scan, abdominal MRI, and abdominal x-ray. Treatment is directed at the underlying cause of disease, whether it is infection, inflammation, lack of blood flow, or another cause.

Colorectal Cancer

Colon cancer is cancer of the large intestine (colon), the lower part of the digestive system. Rectal cancer is cancer of the last 8 to 10 inches of the colon. Together, they are often referred to as colorectal cancers, and they make up the second-leading cause of cancer-related deaths in the United States. Only lung cancer claims more lives.

Most cases of colon cancer begin as small, noncancerous (benign) clumps of cells called adenomatous polyps. Over time some of these polyps become cancerous. The polyps may be small and produce few, if any, symptoms; therefore, regular screening tests are important to help prevent colon cancer. If signs and symptoms of cancer do appear, they may include a change in bowel habits, blood in the stool, persistent cramping, gas, or abdominal pain.

Screening tests, along with a few simple changes in your diet and lifestyle, can dramatically reduce a person's overall risk of developing colon cancer. The type of treatment the physician recommends will depend largely on the stage of the cancer. The three primary treatment options are surgery, chemotherapy, and radiation. Surgery is the main treatment for colorectal cancer. How much of the colon is removed and whether other therapies, such as radiation or chemotherapy, are an option will be determined depending on how far the cancer has penetrated into the wall of the bowel and whether it has spread to the lymph nodes or other parts of the body.

Constipation

Constipation occurs when stools are difficult to pass. Constipation is said to be present if a person has two or fewer bowel movements each week or has two or more of the following problems at least 25% of the time: straining, a feeling of not completely emptying the bowels, and hard or pellet-like stools. Lack of fiber and dehydration are common causes of constipation. Other causes may include irritable bowel syndrome, travel or other changes in one's daily routine, lack of exercise, immobility caused by illness or aging, medication use, overuse of laxatives, and pregnancy. Constipation may occur with cramping and pain in the rectum caused by the strain of trying to pass hard, dry stools. There may also be some bloating and nausea. Sometimes there may be small amounts of bright red blood on the stool or on the toilet tissue, caused by bleeding hemorrhoids or a slight tearing of the anus (anal fissure) as the stool

Preparing for
Externship

Communicating with patients can be challenging, especially with those individuals who may have difficulties hearing or understanding. Communicating can be extra difficult for individuals who are not native to the area in which they live. Be sure to speak slowly and very clearly, and encourage patients and families to repeat your instructions to be sure that they understand.

is pushed through the anus. This should stop when the constipation is controlled.

Constipation can usually be treated effectively at home, often through exercise, good nutritional habits, and a change of lifestyle that provides for a scheduled time each day for bowel movements. Laxatives may also be used.

Crohn's Disease

Crohn's disease is a chronic inflammatory disease of the intestines. It primarily causes ulcerations, or breaks in the lining of the small and large intestines, but can affect the digestive system anywhere from the mouth to the anus. Crohn's disease is related closely to another chronic inflammatory condition that involves only the colon called ulcerative colitis. Together, Crohn's disease and ulcerative colitis are frequently referred to as inflammatory bowel disease (IBD). They affect approximately 500,000 to 2 million people in the United States. Crohn's disease also tends to be more common in relatives of patients with Crohn's disease or ulcerative colitis.

The cause of Crohn's disease is unknown. Some scientists suspect that infection by certain bacteria, such as strains of mycobacterium, may be the cause of Crohn's disease. Crohn's disease is not contagious. Although diet may affect the symptoms in patients with Crohn's disease, it is unlikely that diet is responsible for the disease.

Common symptoms of Crohn's disease include abdominal pain, diarrhea, and weight loss. Less common symptoms include poor appetite, fever, night sweats, rectal pain, and rectal bleeding. Patients with mild or no symptoms may not need treatment. Patients whose disease is in remission (where symptoms are absent) also may not need treatment. There is no medication that can cure Crohn's disease. Patients with Crohn's disease typically will experience periods of relapse (worsening of inflammation) followed by periods of remission (reduced inflammation) lasting months to years.

Because there is no cure for Crohn's disease, the goals of treatment are to induce remissions, maintain remissions, minimize side effects of treatment, and improve the quality of life. Treatment of Crohn's disease and ulcerative colitis with medications is similar though not always identical. These medications may include anti-inflammatory agents such as 5-ASA compounds, corticosteroids, topical antibiotics, or immunomodulators.

Diarrhea

Diarrhea is an increase in the frequency of bowel movements or a decrease in the form of stool (greater looseness of stool). Although changes in frequency of bowel movements and looseness of stools can vary in-

Professionalism

Ensuring that patients and their families understand instructions and explanations can present difficulties. Never address any patient with nicknames such as "sweetie" or "honey." Many individuals consider these terms derisive and unprofessional. Instead, address all adults as Mr. or Ms. or Mrs. unless otherwise instructed. If you are working in an office where English is the primary language and your first language is not English, or if you have a heavy regional accent not native to your office, practice speaking very clearly so that those who have hearing difficulties can still understand your instructions. Supplement verbal instructions with clearly written instructions to help increase understanding. Be sure all explanations are not in medical terminology, but do not oversimplify so that the patients feel "talked down to."

dependently of each other, changes usually occur in both.

Diarrhea generally is divided into two types, acute and chronic. Acute diarrhea lasts a few days or up to a week. Chronic diarrhea can be defined in several ways but almost always lasts more than 3 weeks. It is important to distinguish between acute and chronic diarrhea because they usually have different causes, require different diagnostic tests, and require different treatment.

The most common cause of acute diarrhea is infection—viral, bacterial, and parasitic. Bacteria can also cause acute food poisoning. A third important cause of acute diarrhea is medications.

Diarrhea is usually treated through the use of absorbents and antimotility medications. Absorbents are compounds that absorb water. When they are taken orally, they bind water in the small intestine and colon and make diarrheal stools less watery. They also may bind toxic chemicals produced by bacteria that cause the small intestine to secrete fluid; however, the importance of toxin binding in reducing diarrhea is unclear. Antimotility medications are drugs that relax the muscles of the small intestine or the colon. Relaxation results in slower flow of intestinal contents. Slower flow allows more time for water to be absorbed from the intestine and colon and reduces the water content of stool. Cramps, due to spasm of the intestinal muscles, also are relieved by the muscular relaxation.

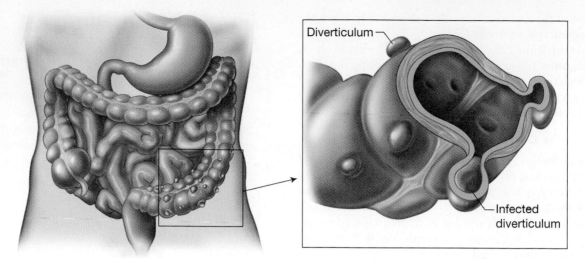

FIGURE 28-9 Colon with diverticulosis. An infected diverticulum is called diverticulitis.

Diverticulitis

Diverticulitis is an inflammation of a small pouch or sac of the walls called a diverticulum that may occur in the wall of the colon (see Figure 28-9). The exact cause of diverticulitis is not known, but generally begins when stool lodges in the diverticula. Infection can lead to complications, including swelling or rupture. Symptoms include pain, fever, chills, cramping, bloating, constipation, or diarrhea. The treatment will depend on the severity of the condition.

Diverticulosis

Diverticulosis is the condition of having diverticula, or small outpouchings, from the large intestine, the colon (see Figure 28-9). It can occur anywhere in the colon

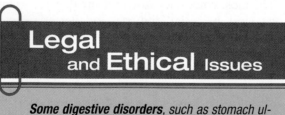

Legal
and Ethical Issues

Some digestive disorders, such as stomach ulcers, IBS, and GERD, may be associated with a person's lifestyle. Your role, as a member of the health care profession, is to provide care and assist with the treatment of your patients, and it is never acceptable, nor appropriate, to judge or make reference to how a person chooses to live his or her life. You are, however, when required, expected to provide patients with information and education regarding how they can best manage their conditions and, at the same time, live a long and productive life.

but it is most typical in the sigmoid colon, the S-shaped segment of the colon located in the left lower part of the abdomen. The incidence of diverticulosis increases with age. This is because age causes a weakening of the walls of the colon and this weakening permits the formation of diverticula. By age 80, most people have diverticulosis.

A key factor promoting the formation of diverticulosis is elevated pressure within the colon. The pressure within the colon is raised when a person is constipated and has to push down to pass small, hard bits of stool.

Most patients with diverticulosis have few or no symptoms although some have mild symptoms including abdominal cramping and bloating. This condition does, however, set the stage for inflammation and infection of the outpouching, a condition called diverticulitis.

The best way to avoid developing diverticulosis is to eat a healthy diet with plenty of fiber. A diet high in fiber keeps the bowels moving, keeps the pressure within the colon within normal limits, and slows or stops the formation of diverticula.

Gastroesophageal Reflux Disease

Gastroesophageal reflux disease (GERD) occurs when the muscle at the superior portion of the stomach (the cardiac sphincter) does not close tightly, or relaxes inappropriately, allowing for a "backwash" of gastric fluids and stomach contents back up the esophagus and into the throat. Individuals with GERD may have symptoms, but there are also quite a few incidences where the patient is symptom free. Symptoms may include heartburn, sore throat, hoarse voice, bad taste in the patient's mouth, belching, and regurgitation of food. If not treated, the patient may begin to suffer from reflux esophagitis, a potentially serious disease resulting from damage to the tissues of the esophagus

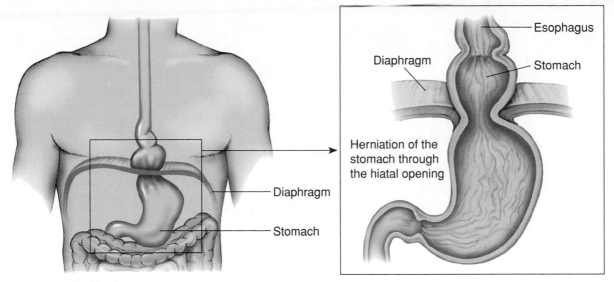

FIGURE 28-10 Hiatal hernia.

by the acidic fluids from the stomach. Barrett's esophagitis, a precancerous condition can also be a result of GERD, and must be treated. Other possible results of long-term, untreated GERD include perforation of the esophagus, esophageal cancer, esophageal stricture (abnormal narrowing of the esophagus), and esophageal ulcers.

Treatment of GERD relies on medications that block the production of hydrochloric acid (the chief digestive acid) and that protect the mucosa of the esophagus. Other simple treatments taught to patients include not lying down until at least 3 hours after eating, weight loss, sleeping on a bed that has the head raised 6 inches, and sleeping on the left side. If medications and basic treatments do not work, surgery called a fundoplication, which tightens the cardiac sphincter and its surrounding tissues, can be performed. Strictures are treated with dilation, or expansion, of the narrowed area.

Hemorrhoids

A hemorrhoid is a dilated, or enlarged, vein in the walls of the anus and sometimes around the rectum, usually caused by untreated constipation but occasionally associated with chronic diarrhea. Symptoms start with bleeding after defecation. If untreated, hemorrhoids can worsen, protruding from the anus. In their worst stage, they must be returned to the anal cavity manually. Fissures can develop, and these may cause intense discomfort. Treatment is by changing the diet to prevent constipation and avoid further irritation, the use of topical medication, and sometimes surgery or sclerotherapy.

Hernia

A hernia is an abnormal protrusion of an organ, or part of an organ through the wall of the body cavity where

it is located. The most common types of abdominal hernias are hiatal hernias and inguinal hernias.

Hiatal Hernia

Hiatal hernia is a condition in which the upper portion of the stomach protrudes into the chest cavity through an opening of the diaphragm called the esophageal hiatus (see Figure 28-10). This opening usually is large enough to accommodate the esophagus alone. With weakening and enlargement, however, the opening (or herniation) can allow upward passage or even entrapment of the upper stomach above the diaphragm. Hiatal hernia is a common condition. By age 60, up to 60 percent of people have it to some degree.

Suspected causes or contributing factors of hiatal hernia include obesity, poor seated posture (such as slouching), frequent coughing, straining with constipation, frequent bending over or heavy lifting, heredity, smoking, and congenital defects.

Some of the symptoms that may be present include chest pain or pressure, heartburn, difficulty swallowing, coughing, belching, and hiccups. Hiatal hernia also causes symptoms of discomfort when it is associated with gastroesophageal reflux disease. GERD is characterized by the upwelling of stomach acids and digestive enzymes into the esophagus through a weakened sphincter that is supposed to act as a one-way valve between the esophagus and stomach. Hiatal hernia is thought to contribute to the weakening of this sphincter muscle.

Inguinal Hernia

An inguinal hernia occurs when tissue or part of the intestine pushes through a weak spot in the abdominal wall in the groin area, causing a bulge in the groin or scrotum (see Figure 28-11).

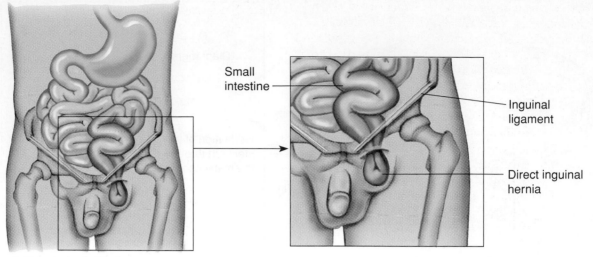

FIGURE 28-11   Inguinal hernia.

The bulge may appear gradually over a period of several weeks or months, or it may form suddenly after you have been lifting heavy weights, coughing, bending, straining, or laughing. Many hernias flatten when you lie down. Pain and discomfort may also be present and is usually worse when a person bends or lifts an object. While men may have pain or discomfort in the scrotum, many hernias do not cause any pain. Nausea and vomiting may also be present if part of the intestine bulges outside the abdomen and becomes trapped (incarcerated) in the hernia.

Other symptoms of a hernia may include heaviness, swelling, and a tugging or burning sensation in the area of the hernia, scrotum, or inner thigh. Males may have a swollen scrotum, and females may have a bulge in the large fold of skin (labia) surrounding the vagina. Discomfort and aching are relieved only when the person lies down. This is often the case as the hernia grows larger.

Surgery is the only treatment and cure for inguinal hernia. Hernia repair is one of the most common surgeries done in the United States. About 750,000 people have hernia repairs each year. However, if an inguinal hernia does not cause any symptoms, it may not need treatment.

Irritable Bowel Syndrome

Irritable bowel syndrome (IBS) is a common intestinal condition characterized by abdominal pain and cramps, changes in bowel movements (diarrhea, constipation, or both), gassiness, bloating, and nausea. Other symptoms—which vary from person to person—include cramps, a powerful and uncontrollable urge to defecate (urgency), passage of a sticky fluid (mucus) during bowel movements, or the feeling after finishing a bowel movement that the bowels are still not com-

pletely empty. There is no cure for IBS. Much about the condition remains unknown or poorly understood; however, dietary changes, drugs, and psychological treatment are often able to eliminate or substantially reduce its symptoms. The symptoms of IBS tend to rise and fall in intensity rather than growing steadily worse over time.

Researchers remain unsure about the cause or causes of IBS. It is called a functional disorder because it is thought to result from changes in the activity of the major part of the large intestine (the colon). Stress is an important factor in IBS because of the close nervous system connections between the brain and the intestines. Although researchers do not yet understand all of the links between changes in the nervous system and IBS, they point out the similarities between mild digestive upsets and IBS. Just as healthy people can feel nauseated or have an upset stomach when under stress, people with IBS react the same way, but to a greater degree. Finally, IBS symptoms sometimes intensify during menstruation, which suggests that female reproductive hormones are another trigger.

Dietary changes, sometimes supplemented by drugs or psychotherapy, are considered keys to the successful treatment of IBS.

Oral Cancer

Oral cancer starts in the cells of the mouth (oral cavity). Almost all cases of oral cancer start in the flat squamous cells that line the mouth. Squamous cell carcinoma can start on the lips, inside the lips and cheeks (buccal mucosa), the gums (gingiva), the front two-thirds of the tongue, the tissue under the tongue (the floor of the mouth), the tissue behind the wisdom teeth, and the bony roof of the mouth (hard palate).

There is no single cause of oral cancer, but several factors appear to increase the risk of developing it. These include age, particularly after 50; gender— more men develop oral cancer; smoking, particularly if combined with heavy alcohol consumption; chewing tobacco or using snuff; heavy alcohol consumption, particularly if combined with smoking; excessive sun exposure to the lips; some medical problems in the mouth tissues; and chewing betel nut.

The signs and symptoms of oral cancer can be seen and felt quite early. Pain is very rare in early oral cancer, but any sore, irritation, or swelling in the mouth or lump on the neck that lasts longer than 2 weeks should be checked by a doctor or dentist. Velvety red or white patches in the mouth may also indicate a precancerous condition. Sores or wart-like patches on the lip, a persistent sore throat, sores under dentures, a lump in the lip, tongue, or neck, and trouble chewing, swallowing, or speaking are all symptoms.

Treatment of oral cancer will depend on the extent of the condition. Surgery to remove part or all of the tumor and some surrounding tissue may be required. Radiation and chemotherapy, that is, the use of drugs or medications that interfere with the cancer cell's ability to grow and spread, may also be used in the treatment of oral cancer.

Pancreatic Cancer

The most common type of **pancreatic cancer** arises from the exocrine glands and is called adenocarcinoma of the pancreas. The endocrine glands of the pancreas can give rise to a completely different type of cancer, referred to as pancreatic neuroendocrine carcinoma or islet cell tumor, which is considered very rare. In 2004, approximately 31,800 people in the United States were diagnosed with pancreatic cancer, and approximately 31,200 people died of this disease. These numbers reflect the challenge in treating pancreatic cancer and the relative lack of curative options.

The symptoms of pancreatic cancer are generally vague and can easily be attributed to other less serious and more common conditions. This lack of specific symptoms explains the high number of people

Cultural Considerations

Culture seems to play a major role in how people eat and view disorders of their digestive system. Hindus, for example, believe in fasting and in eating a specific way. While Americans may believe such a lifestyle could lead to digestive problems, the Hindu religion believes their dietary experiences are part of what makes them at one with God. Other cultures, such as those in the Far East, believe that alternative medicine therapies, such as acupuncture, homeopathy, meditation, and biofeedback, are frequently more useful than western medicine in treating disorders of the digestive system. While there may appear to be many cultural stereotypes regarding specific diseases of the digestive system, as a member of the health care team, it is important to remember to always respect a person's beliefs and focus on supporting and treating the patient. When asking questions or assisting in a treatment, make sure that the questions are not disrespectful and your care is directed at the "total" patient, and not just the disease.

who have a more advanced stage of the disease when pancreatic cancer is eventually discovered. The main symptoms include pain in the abdomen, the back, or both; weight loss, often associated with loss of appetite; bloating; diarrhea or fatty bowel movements that float in water; and jaundice or yellowing of the skin.

Complete surgical removal of the cancer is the only known cure for pancreatic cancer. Only 15 to 20 percent of people with pancreatic cancer have disease that

Patient Education

When teaching patients about a bland diet, it is important to take their cultural preferences into consideration. Be sure patients understand which foods in their diet are appropriate and which should be temporarily avoided. This may require asking patients or their families for more information regarding their dietary preferences. It is also important to be sure that all patients understand the need to avoid alcohol and tobacco until their conditions have healed.

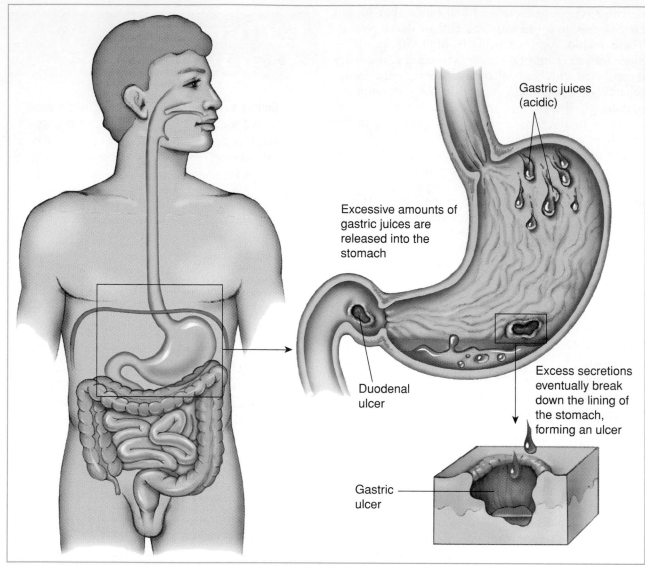

FIGURE 28-12   Peptic ulcer disease (PUD).

can be surgically removed at the time of diagnosis. Depending on how advanced the cancer is, chemotherapy and radiation therapy may also be included in the treatment of pancreatic cancer.

Peptic Ulcer Disease

Peptic ulcer disease (PUD) occurs when there is a disruption in the lining of the esophagus, stomach, or duodenum (see Figure 28-12). The most frequent location for PUD is in the duodenum (the upper part of the small intestine). Peptic ulcers (ones that occur in the stomach) are also common.

Peptic ulcers are most likely caused by an imbalance between acid and pepsin (a stomach acid) secretion and the defenses of the mucosal lining. Inflammation results, causing some of the discomfort. This inflammation may be caused or aggravated by aspirin or nonsteroidal anti-inflammatories (NSAIDs) such as ibuprofen. Because of the resulting erosion of the stomach mucosa, a bacteria

called *Helicobacter pylori* can cause infection, further aggravating the situation.

The most common symptoms of PUD are abdominal pain, nausea, vomiting, and weight loss. Esophageal ulcers often include heartburn and chest pain. Other symptoms that may occur include black, tar-like or maroon stools (indicating old blood), fresh blood in the stool, and a burning or gnawing pain in the stomach or the back.

Prevention of ulcers includes avoiding alcohol and tobacco, and limiting the use of NSAIDs and aspirin. Spicy foods do not cause ulcers, but can aggravate the condition.

Treatment of PUD depends on the cause. Any medications that may be causing or aggravating the condition need to be changed. Tobacco use and alcohol should be avoided because they delay healing. Medications that speed healing will be prescribed to protect the stomach from the stomach acid by either decreasing or stopping the secretion of stomach acids. Severe cases might require surgery.

Pyloric Stenosis

Pyloric stenosis is a condition in which a baby's pylorus gradually swells and thickens, which interferes with food entering the intestine. The pylorus is the connection between the stomach and the first part of the small intestine (duodenum). It can occur any time between birth and 5 months of age. However, it most commonly develops about 3 weeks after birth.

Vomiting all or most of feedings on a repeated basis is the main symptom of pyloric stenosis. The vomiting usually starts gradually and gets worse over time. As the pylorus becomes tighter, the vomiting becomes more frequent and more forceful. As the vomiting continues, the baby will lose weight, develop symptoms of not getting enough fluids (dehydration), be sleepier than normal, and be very fussy when awake.

Pyloric stenosis is always treated with surgery (pyloromyotomy). Once the baby has the surgery, the disorder usually will not develop again.

Stomach Ulcers

The stomach produces acid to break down food during the digestive process. The stomach and upper part of the small intestine (duodenum) are protected from the acid by a lining of sticky fluid (mucus). If this lining is damaged, the sensitive tissue underneath is exposed to acid. Irritation of the wall tissue in the stomach and duodenum may cause a stomach ulcer to form. Bacteria may also cause *stomach ulcers*.

Stomach or gastric ulcers are more common in people over the age of 50. Mild symptoms may be mistaken for indigestion or heartburn. Symptoms of a stomach ulcer that may occur include any or all of the following:

- Pain, or a burning sensation (similar to indigestion) in the upper abdomen and sometimes the lower chest. The pain from a duodenal ulcer can be worse when the stomach is empty and is relieved by eating, but then recurs a few hours afterward
- Pain that is often made worse by eating
- Difficulty swallowing or regurgitation (bringing up swallowed food into the mouth)
- Bloating, retching, and feeling sick, particularly after eating
- Vomiting and nausea
- Loss of appetite and weight loss

Severe ulcers may be very painful and bleed. Bleeding can indicate a serious problem—the ulcer may have burrowed through the stomach or duodenal wall, or it may be blocking the path of food trying to leave the stomach. Sometimes the stomach acid or the ulcer itself breaks a blood vessel in the lining of the stomach or duodenum.

If long-term treatment with aspirin or another (NSAID) is the cause, ulcer-healing drugs and additional drugs to protect the lining of the stomach and duodenum are advised. Antibiotics may be given to treat *H. pyloric* infections. Occasionally surgery is recommended if the ulcer does not respond to medication. This may include one of the following options:

- Vagotomy: cutting the vagus nerve that links the stomach to the brain. This reduces acid production
- Antrectomy: removal of the lower part of the stomach that produces the hormone that causes the stomach to produce digestive juices
- Pyloroplasty: enlarging the opening into the duodenum and small intestine to allow the contents of the stomach to move more freely

SUMMARY

The digestive system consists of a single tube starting at the mouth and ending at the rectum. Its function is to process food and other nutritional sources for energy for the body. The primary digestive system consists of the mouth, the pharynx, the esophagus, the stomach, the small intestine, the large intestine, and the rectum. The accessory organs of digestion include the salivary glands, pancreas, liver, and gallbladder.

- -

Chapter Review

COMPETENCY REVIEW

1. Define and spell the terms to learn for this chapter.
2. Name the primary organs associated with digestion.
3. What are the four accessory organs of digestion?

4. What are the three main functions of the digestive system?
5. What is the first portion of the intestine called?
6. The large intestine can be divided into four distinct sections. Name them.
7. What is the function of the gallbladder?
8. What sac-like organ holds food for the beginning of the digestive process?
9. How many deciduous teeth is a person born with?
10. What essential role does the liver play?

PREPARING FOR THE CERTIFICATION EXAM

1. The medical term for gallstones is:
   A. cholecystectomy
   B. cholecystotomy
   C. choledochal
   D. cholelithiasis
   E. choledochectomy

2. The muscle at the superior portion of the stomach is the
   A. pyloric sphincter
   B. esophageal sphincter
   C. cardiac sphincter
   D. gallbladder
   E. fundus

3. Which substance is not produced by the liver?
   A. heparin
   B. bile
   C. hydrochloric acid
   D. fibrogen and prothrombin
   E. blood proteins

4. Which is not a component of the small intestine?
   A. jejunum
   B. ileum
   C. duodenum
   D. cecum
   E. pyloric sphincter

5. What is the function of the gallbladder?
   A. production of bile
   B. storage of bile
   C. production of pepsin
   D. production of insulin
   E. storage of insulin

6. How many permanent teeth does the body produce?
   A. 20
   B. 24
   C. 28
   D. 32
   E. 36

7. A potentially life-threatening condition that occurs when scarring damages the liver is
   A. pancreatitis
   B. cirrhosis
   C. cholecystitis
   D. colitis
   E. stomatitis

8. An inflammation of the large intestine that may be caused by many different disease processes is
   A. pancreatitis
   B. cirrhosis
   C. cholecystitis
   D. colitis
   E. stomatitis

9. Symptoms of Crohn's disease include all of the following EXCEPT
   A. abdominal pain
   B. diarrhea
   C. weight loss
   D. night sweats
   E. constipation

10. GERD occurs when the muscle of what organ does not close tightly?
   A. stomach
   B. liver
   C. gallbladder
   D. pancreas
   E. large intestine

CRITICAL THINKING

1. Why did the physician order a gastric analysis and histology with culture?

2. What type of diet will the physician prescribe for Mr. Sylvans? Why?

3. What steps can Mr. Sylvans take to lower his risk of any future episodes of pain and discomfort from his condition?

INTERNET ACTIVITY

Do an Internet search on peptic ulcer disease.

MediaLink More on the digestive system, including interactive resources, can be found on the Student CD-ROM accompanying this textbook.

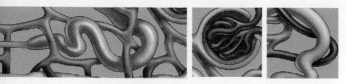

Medical Assistant Role Delineation Chart

HIGHLIGHT indicates material covered in this chapter.

ADMINISTRATIVE

Administrative Procedures

- Perform basic administrative medical assisting functions
- Schedule, coordinate and monitor appointments
- Schedule inpatient/outpatient admissions and procedures
- Understand and apply third-party guidelines
- Obtain reimbursement through accurate claims submission
- Monitor third-party reimbursement
- Understand and adhere to managed care policies and procedures
- *Negotiate managed care contracts*

Practice Finances

- Perform procedural and diagnostic coding
- Apply bookkeeping principles

- Manage accounts receivable
- *Manage accounts payable*
- *Process payroll*
- *Document and maintain accounting and banking records*
- *Develop and maintain fee schedules*
- *Manage renewals of business and professional insurance policies*
- *Manage personnel benefits and maintain records*
- *Perform marketing, financial, and strategic planning*

CLINICAL

Fundamental Principles

- Apply principles of aseptic technique and infection control
- Comply with quality assurance practices
- Screen and follow up patient test results

Diagnostic Orders

- Collect and process specimens
- Perform diagnostic tests

Patient Care

- Adhere to established patient screening procedures
- Obtain patient history and vital signs
- Prepare and maintain examination and treatment areas
- Prepare patient for examinations, procedures and treatments

- Assist with examinations, procedures and treatments
- Prepare and administer medications and immunizations
- Maintain medication and immunization records
- Recognize and respond to emergencies
- Coordinate patient care information with other health care providers
- Initiate IV and administer IV medications with appropriate training and as permitted by state law

GENERAL

Professionalism

- Display a professional manner and image
- Demonstrate initiative and responsibility
- Work as a member of the health care team
- Prioritize and perform multiple tasks
- Adapt to change
- Promote the CMA credential
- Enhance skills through continuing education
- Treat all patients with compassion and empathy
- Promote the practice through positive public relations

Communication Skills

- Recognize and respect cultural diversity
- Adapt communications to individual's ability to understand
- Use professional telephone technique

- Recognize and respond effectively to verbal, nonverbal, and written communications
- Use medical terminology appropriately
- Utilize electronic technology to receive, organize, prioritize and transmit information
- Serve as liaison

Legal Concepts

- Perform within legal and ethical boundaries
- Prepare and maintain medical records
- Document accurately
- Follow employer's established policies dealing with the health care contract
- Implement and maintain federal and state health care legislation and regulations
- Comply with established risk management and safety procedures
- Recognize professional credentialing criteria
- *Develop and maintain personnel, policy and procedure manuals*

Instruction

- Instruct individuals according to their needs
- Explain office policies and procedures
- Teach methods of health promotion and disease prevention
- Locate community resources and disseminate information
- *Develop educational materials*
- *Conduct continuing education activities*

Operational Functions

- Perform inventory of supplies and equipment
- Perform routine maintenance of administrative and clinical equipment
- Apply computer techniques to support office operations
- *Perform personnel management functions*
- *Negotiate leases and prices for equipment and supply contracts*

- *Denotes advanced skills.*

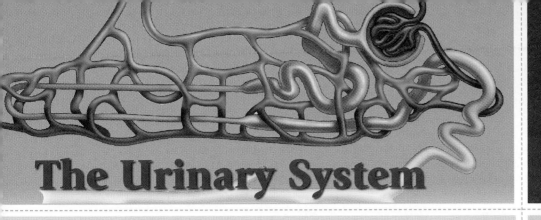

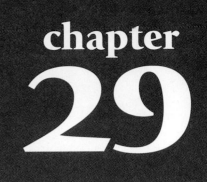

chapter
29

The Urinary System

Learning Objectives

After completing this chapter, you should be able to:

- Define and spell the terms to learn for this chapter.
- Describe the purpose and function of the urinary system.
- Identify the individual organs of the urinary system and briefly explain the function of each.

- List and discuss the three processes involved in the formation of urine.
- Explain the normal constituents of urine.
- List and briefly explain common disorders associated with the urinary system.

Terms to Learn

acute renal failure

ascites

chronic renal failure

cortex

cystitis

dialysis

glomerulonephritis

hilum

incontinence

interstitial cystitis (IC)

kidney stones

kidneys

lithotripsy

medulla

nephrons

polycystic kidney disease
(PKD)

pyelonephritis

renal calculi

renal pelvis

ureters

urethra

urinary bladder

urinary meatus

Case Study

MARTIN TEVIA ARRIVED AT THE EMERGENCY ROOM with severe right-sided flank pain and visible blood in his urine. He states that he has no previous history of kidney problems and no pelvic pain or difficulty urinating. He is sweating, nauseated and continues to complain of extreme pain. Mr. Tevia was diagnosed with a kidney stone (renal calculi) located in the right renal ureter. He receives IV fluids and pain medication. He eventually passes the stone and is discharged to home with instructions to follow up with a urologist in 1 week.

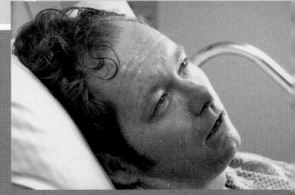

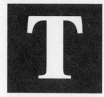

The urinary system consists of organs that produce and excrete urine from the body (see Figure 29-1). Urine is a transparent yellow fluid containing unwanted wastes, mostly excess water, salts, and nitrogen compounds. The primary organs of the system are the kidneys, which continuously filter substances from the blood and produce urine. Urine flows from the kidneys through two long, thin tubes called ureters. With the aid of gravity and wave-like contractions, the ureters transport the urine to the bladder, a muscular vessel. The normal adult bladder can store up to about 0.5 liter (1 pint) of urine, which it excretes through the tube-like urethra.

In addition to producing and excreting urine from the body, the urinary system is also responsible for regulating blood volume and blood pressure by adjusting the volume of water lost in the urine and releasing the

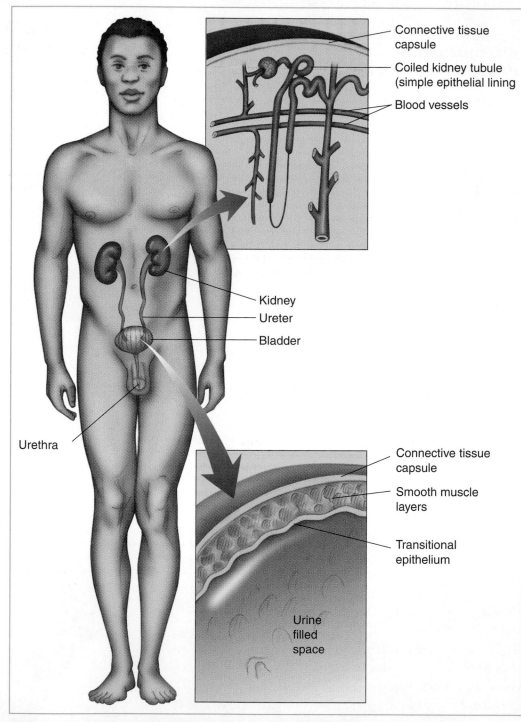

FIGURE 29-1 The urinary system: kidneys, ureters, bladder, and urethra with expanded view of a nephron and the urine-filled space within a bladder.

hormones erythropoietin and rennin. It is also responsible for regulating blood concentrations of sodium, potassium, chloride, and other ions by controlling the quantities lost in the urine. By doing this, the urinary system is able to conserve valuable nutrients by selectively preventing losses while eliminating waste products.

Organs of the Urinary System

The components of the urinary system include the kidneys, which are the primary organs of the system; the ureters, which transport urine from the kidney to the urinary bladder; the urinary bladder, which is a temporary storage reservoir for urine; and the urethra, which is the final passageway for the flow of urine. The flow of urine through the urethra is controlled by an involuntary internal urethral sphincter and voluntary external urethral sphincter.

Kidneys

The **kidneys** are paired, bean-shaped organs located at the back of the abdominal cavity, retroperitoneal between the 12th thoracic and 3rd lumbar vertebrae (see Figure 29-2). They lie on either side of the spinal column in the flank area, against the muscles of the back. Each kidney has three capsules surrounding it: the true capsule, the perirenal fat, and the renal fascia. The true capsule is a smooth, fibrous connective membrane that loosely adheres to the surface of the kidney. Surrounding that is the adipose capsule (the perirenal fat) that embeds the kidney in fatty tissue, providing a layer of protection. The renal fascia is a sheath of fibrous tissue that anchors the kidney to the surrounding structures and ensures that the normal position is maintained.

External Structure of the Kidney

The concave border of each kidney has a notch called the **hilum**. The hilum is the entrance for the renal artery and vein, nerves, and the lymphatic vessels. The hilum also houses the opening for the ureters, where it connects with the **renal pelvis**, which is a sac-like collecting area for urine.

Internal Structure of the Kidney

Two distinct parts of the kidney are visible on a cross section, the **cortex** (the outer layer) and the **medulla** (the middle portion). The arteries, veins, convoluted tubules, and glomerular capsules are found in the cortex, and the renal pyramids are found in the medulla.

Nephrons

Microscopic examination of the kidney reveals about 1 million **nephrons**, which is the functional unit of the kidney (see Figure 29-3). Each nephron contains a renal corpuscle and a tubule. The nephron removes the waste products of metabolism from the blood plasma. The waste products are urea, uric acid, and creatinine, along with sodium, chloride, and potassium ions and ketone bodies. Nephrons help the body to maintain fluid balance by helping regulate the amount of fluid and electrolytes reabsorbed into the blood and how much is excreted. Approximately 1,000 to 1,200 mL of blood passes through the kidney per minute; at that rate, about 1.5 million millileters of blood passes through the kidneys each day. The renal corpuscle consists of the glomerulus and the Bowman's capsule. The Bowman's capsule has a tubule extending from it called the proximal convoluted tubule, which becomes the loop of Henle and then the distal convoluted tubule, which opens into a collecting tubule.

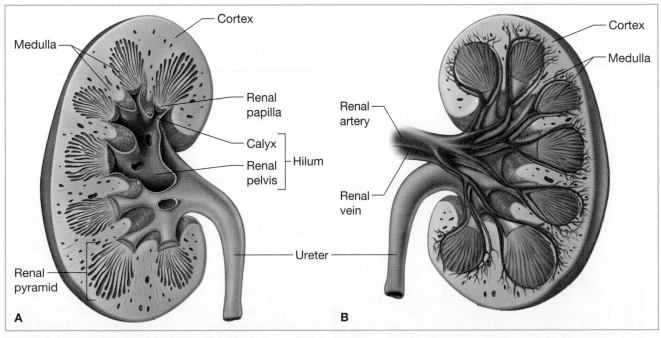

FIGURE 29-2 (A) Sectioned kidney; (B) renal artery and vein.

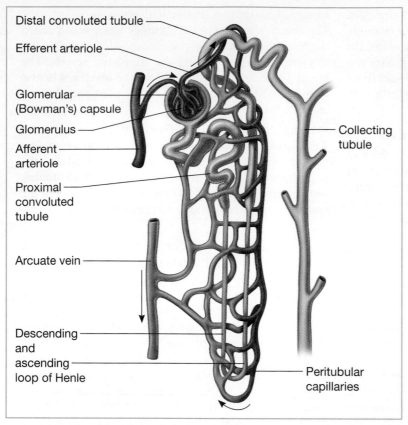

Distal convoluted tubule

Efferent arteriole

Glomerular (Bowman's) capsule

Glomerulus

Afferent arteriole

Proximal convoluted tubule

Arcuate vein

Descending and ascending loop of Henle

Collecting tubule

Peritubular capillaries

FIGURE 29-3 The structure of a nephron.

Ureters

The **ureters** are tubes that carry the newly formed urine from each kidney down to the bladder. There is one ureter from each kidney to the bladder. Each ureter is 28 to 34 cm long and has a diameter of 1 mm to 1 cm. There are three layers to the ureter wall: an inner coat of mucous membrane, a middle coat of smooth muscle, and an outer layer of fibrous tissue.

Legal and Ethical Issues

Patient privacy is always of utmost concern in any part of the medical field. Never leave a telephone message stating the results of any test, or even stating the type of test a patient had. All messages should simply request that the patient call you back during office hours. Never leave any more information, even on a cell phone. By following this procedure, you will avoid violating HIPAA regulations.

Urinary Bladder

The **urinary bladder** is the muscular sac that serves as a reservoir for urine. It is located in the pelvic cavity. The wall of the bladder consists of four layers: an inner layer of epithelium, a muscular coat of smooth muscle, an outer layer made of longitudinal muscle, and a fibrous layer. When the bladder is empty, the wall of the bladder feels firm because the walls of the bladder are thick. As the bladder becomes more full, it stretches so it can hold the urine present, and the walls become thinner.

Urethra

The **urethra** is the musculomembranous tube extending from the bladder to the **urinary meatus**, the external opening of the urinary system. The male urethra is approximately 20 cm long and has three sections, the prostatic, membranous, and penile sections. In males, the urethra transports both urine and semen. In females, the urethra is approximately 3 cm long, and its external opening is situated between the clitoris and the opening of the vagina. In females, the urethra transports only urine.

Urine

The formation of urine has three processes: filtration, reabsorption, and tubular secretion (see Figure 29-4). During filtration, or glomerular excretion, blood pressure forces all the small molecules in the blood into the lumen of the nephron through the pores both in the walls of the glomerular capillaries and in the wall of the Bowman's capsule. The filtrate has the same concentration of dissolved substances as the blood minus the formed elements and the plasma proteins that are too large to fit through the pores of the capillaries and the Bowman's capsule. As the filtrate passes through the tubules of the nephron, water and many dissolved materials are reabsorbed by the blood. In fact, during the filtrate's passage through the tubules up to 99 percent of the water is reabsorbed. In addition, the tubules also remove substances from the blood. This process, called tubular secretion, supplements the initial glomerular filtration. Water and some selected substances are reabsorbed from the filtrate by the capillaries surrounding the nephrons. Other substances, such as hydrogen ions and uric acid, will be transported into the filtrate, now known as urine.

Urine consists of 95 percent water and 5 percent solid substances. The average normal adult feels a need to void, or urinate, when the bladder contains 300 to 350 mL of urine. Typically, about 1,000 to 1,500 mL of urine is voided daily, depending on fluid intake. Normal urine is clear (not cloudy), straw colored, and has a faintly aromatic odor, with a specific gravity of 1.003 to 1.030 and a slightly acidic pH of about 6. Specific gravity measures the kidney's ability to concentrate or dilute urine in relation to plasma. Because urine is a solution of minerals, salts, and compounds dissolved in water, the specific gravity is greater than 1.000. The more concentrated the urine, the higher the urine specific gravity. An adult's kidneys have a remarkable ability to concentrate or dilute urine. In infants, the range for specific gravity is less because immature kidneys are not able to concentrate urine as effectively as mature kidneys.

Common Disorders Associated with the Urinary System

Compromised kidneys, and even healthy kidneys, can suffer from a variety of conditions that can affect an individual's lifestyle and activities of daily living (see Table 29-1)

Cystitis

Cystitis is an inflammation of the bladder, usually occurring as a result of ascending urinary tract infections. Cystitis occurs when bacteria, causing irritation and inflammation, infect the lower urinary tract. Most cases of urinary tract infection are caused by *Escherichia coli* (*E. coli*), a bacterium found in the lower gastrointestinal system.

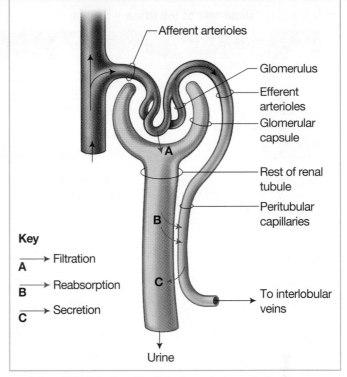

FIGURE 29-4 Schematic view of the three stages of urine production: (A) filtration; (B) reabsorption; (C) secretion.

Urinary tract infections are common, especially in sexually active women ages 20 to 50, but they can happen in anyone. Women are more frequently affected, secondary to the anatomy of the perineum, improper personal hygiene, and the short length of the urethra.

Lifespan Considerations

THE CHILD
- At about 10 weeks gestation, the kidneys begin forming urine. By 3 months gestation, the fetus actually begins to secrete small quantities of urine. Quantities continue to increase during the rest of fetal development. However, a newborn's kidneys are not able to concentrate urine. Because of this, newborns and even older infants are more prone to fluid volume excess or dehydration. Extreme changes in temperature and fluid intake must be avoided until their kidneys are better able to adjust for fluid needs. Because of the lack of fat pads in the flank, the kidneys of small children are more susceptible to trauma.
- Small children, especially those wearing diapers,

are susceptible to urinary tract infections. It is especially important that the diaper area be cleaned regularly and appropriately to prevent urinary tract infections.

THE OLDER ADULT
- As people age, the kidneys begin to lose mass as the blood vessels degenerate. The kidneys lose their ability to filter as well, and their ability to conserve water and sodium decreases. This means that dehydration can happen more quickly. In addition, the tubules' ability to balance the pH of the body decreases, as well as the ability to balance electrolytes. As a result, acid–base imbalances can happen much more easily. There is also a loss of muscle tone in the ureters, bladder, and urethra. Bladder capacity is reduced by as much as 50 percent, causing more frequent trips to the bathroom. In some adults, urge incontinence (the inability to voluntarily retain urine) is a big concern.

TABLE 29-1 Disorders of the Urinary System

Disorder	Description
Anuria	No urine formed by the kidneys and a complete lack of urine excretion.
Bladder neck obstruction	Blockage of the bladder outlet.
Dysuria	Painful or difficult urination.
Enuresis	Involuntary discharge of urine after the age by which bladder control should have been established. This usually occurs by the age of 5. Also called bed-wetting at night.
Glomerulonephritis	Inflammation of the kidney (primarily of the glomerulus). Since the glomerular membrane is inflamed, it becomes more permeable and this results in protein (proteinuria) and blood (hematuria) in the urine.
Hematuria	A condition of blood in the urine. This is a symptom of a disease process.
Hypospadius	A congenital opening of the male urethra on the underside of the penis.
Interstitial cystitis	Disease of an unknown cause in which there is inflammation and irritation of the bladder. It is most commonly seen in middle-aged women.
Nocturia	Excessive urination during the night. This may or may not be abnormal.
Pyelitis	Inflammation of the renal pelvis.
Pyelonephritis	Inflammation of the renal pelvis and the kidney. This is one of the most common types of kidney disease. It may be the result of a lower urinary tract infection that moved up to the kidney via the ureters. There may be large quantities of white blood cells and bacteria in the urine. Hematuria may also be present. This condition can occur whenever there is an untreated or persistent case of cystitis.
Pyuria	Presence of pus in the urine.
Renal colic	Pain caused by a kidney stone. This type of pain can be excruciating and generally requires medical treatment.

Sexual activity can introduce bacteria into the urethra. Bacteria in the bladder are often removed through urination, but occasionally, the bacteria reproduce more quickly than they are washed away, causing an infection. In men, cystitis is usually secondary to another infection, such as epididymitis, prostatitis, gonorrhea, syphilis, or kidney stones.

Frequently, the most common symptoms of cystitis are urgency and frequency. Urgency is a need to void immediately. Frequency is the need to void frequently. Another common symptom of cystitis is painful urination. Occasionally, the patient may suffer from chills and fever. If the cystitis is chronic, then dysuria (burning urination) may be the only symptom. Urinary tract infections are treated with antibiotics and antispasmodics.

Interstitial cystitis (IC) is a painful inflammation of the bladder wall. Ninety percent of the 450,000 people who suffer from this condition are women. The cause is unknown. The symptoms can be mild to severe, but IC does not respond to typical antibiotic therapy.

Glomerulonephritis

Glomerulonephritis is a type of kidney disease that hampers the kidneys' ability to remove waste and excess fluids. Also called glomerular disease, glomerulonephritis can be acute, referring to a sudden attack of inflammation, or chronic, which comes on gradually. Glomerular disease can be part of a systemic disease, such as lupus or diabetes, or it can be a disease by itself, called primary glomerulonephritis. Glomerulonephritis can lead to kidney failure.

There are many causes of glomerulonephritis. They include those related to infections, immune diseases, inflammation of the blood vessels (vasculitis) and conditions that scar the glomeruli. Chronic glomerulonephritis sometimes develops after a bout of acute glomerulonephritis. Infrequently, chronic glomerulonephritis runs in families. In many cases, the specific cause is unknown.

Signs and symptoms of glomerulonephritis may depend on whether the patient has the acute or chronic form, and the cause. The first indication that something is wrong may come from symptoms or from the results of a routine urinalysis. Signs and symptoms may include cola-colored or diluted iced-tea-colored urine from red blood cells in the urine (hematuria), foam in the toilet water from protein in the urine (proteinuria), high blood pressure (hypertension), fluid retention (edema) with swelling evident in the face, hands, feet, and abdomen, fatigue from anemia or kidney failure, and less frequent urination than usual.

Some cases of acute glomerulonephritis, especially those that follow a strep infection, often improve on their own and require no specific treatment. Other treatments may include the use of diuretics, angiotensin-converting enzyme (ACE) inhibitors, calcium channel blockers, and beta blockers.

Incontinence

More common in women who have had children, incontinence is the involuntary and unpredictable flow of urine. Stress incontinence is the most common, and happens when sneezing, laughing, or other causes of intra-abdominal pressure cause the involuntary release of urine. Urge incontinence occurs when the bladder contracts without warning. Leakage will occur if the patient is not able to respond to that need immediately. Overflow incontinence happens when a blockage prohibits normal emptying. The bladder simply overflows. Incontinence is diagnosed by a urologist, and treatment may include medications, surgery, and pelvic floor exercises.

Kidney Stones

Kidney stones, or renal calculi, are caused by deposits of mineral salts in the kidney (see Figure 29-5). The stones are usually benign when still in the kidney, but can pass into the ureter, slowing down or blocking urine flow. Because the stones have a rough surface, they irritate and scratch the ureters, causing bleeding. The kidney becomes irritated due to the bleeding and

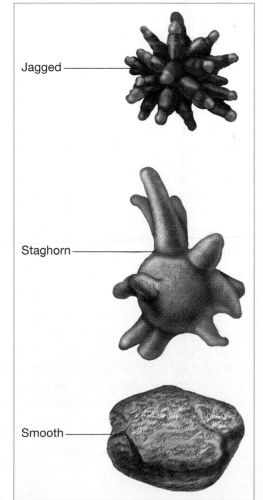

Jagged

Staghorn

Smooth

FIGURE 29-5 Types of kidney stones found in an adult.

the decreased urine flow, causing pain and spasms. Kidney stones are painful, and a person suffering from one presents with flank pain along with possible nausea and vomiting. On urinalysis, hematuria is usually present.

Kidney stones afflict about 10 percent of the people in the United States, and men are more often afflicted than women. A person with a family history of kidney stones is more likely to have stones that someone with no family history. Urinary tract infections, kidney disorders, and metabolic disorders, such as hyperparathyroidism are linked to kidney stones.

Most kidney stones are made of calcium oxalate. Calcium from food is absorbed in excess, and then excreted into the urine. There, it combines with oxalates, and creates the stones. Individuals with this type of stone are advised to control their intake of foods containing calcium and oxalate. Foods containing oxalate include beets, chocolate, tea, coffee, cola, nuts, rhubarb, strawberries, tea, wheat bran, and spinach. To prevent stone formation, individuals should drink enough fluid to produce at least 2 quarts of urine each day.

Many kidney stones are able to pass out of the body without physician intervention. Stones that cause lasting symptoms or other complications may require treatment, including **lithotripsy**. There are two types of lithotripsy, extracorporeal shock wave lithotripsy and percutaneous ultrasonic lithotripsy. Both procedures involve passing shock waves through the body that will cause the stone to break down. Other procedures require surgical intervention to either retrieve or disintegrate the stone. Stones that do not pass can either cause infection, or, if they completely block the ureter, hydronephrosis, which can eventually cause kidney damage.

Polycystic Kidney Disease

Polycystic kidney disease (PKD) is a disorder in which clusters of cysts develop primarily within the kidneys. Cysts are noncancerous (benign) round sacs of waterlike fluid. The disease is not limited to the kidneys, although the kidneys usually are the most severely affected organs. The disease can cause cysts to develop in your liver, pancreas, membranes that surround your brain and central nervous system, and seminal vesicles. PKD affects more than 12 million people worldwide. The disease varies greatly in its severity, and some complications are preventable. Regular checkups can lead to treatments to reduce damage to your kidneys from complications, such as high blood pressure. The greatest risk for people with polycystic kidney disease is developing high blood pressure. Kidney failure also is common with PKD.

Signs and symptoms of polycystic kidney disease may include high blood pressure, back or side pain related to enlarged kidneys, abdominal pain, an increase in the size of the abdomen, blood in the urine, kidney stones, kidney failure, kidney infections, and headache.

Treating polycystic kidney disease involves dealing with and treating the signs, symptoms, and complications of high blood pressure, pain, bladder and kidney infections, blood in the urine, and kidney failure.

Pyelonephritis

Pyelonephritis is an infection of the kidney and renal pelvis. It may have a sudden onset, or be a chronic condition. Bacteria entering the kidneys from the bladder, usually *E. coli*, causes pyelonephritis. This may be a result of the same mechanisms as seen in cystitis. Sometimes, pyelonephritis is caused by an indwelling urinary

Preparing for Externship

While preparing for externship, it is important for the medical assistant to reinforce his or her professional skills as a member of the health care team. It is especially important to remember that while the medical assistant is at work, the patients are the focus. Skills such as knowing how to properly reach a minor's parents during an emergency and never giving out a patient's personal telephone number are skills the medical assistant should be responsible for knowing as part of completing his or her externship.

Professionalism

catheter and cystoscopy (visualization of the urinary bladder and urethra with a special instrument). Other causes include prostate enlargement and kidney stones. Symptoms of pyelonephritis include back, side, and groin pain; urgency and frequency; pain and burning during urination; fever; nausea and vomiting; and blood and pus in the urine.

Antibiotics are used to treat pyelonephritis. If pyelonephritis is left untreated, scarring may result and could cause permanent kidney damage.

Renal Failure

The two types of renal failure are acute and chronic. **Acute renal failure** occurs when something causes a change in the filtering function of the kidneys, altering the ability of the kidneys to maintain normal body function. A blockage, toxins, or a sudden loss of blood flow to the kidneys can cause acute renal failure. People who have other kidney diseases are at a greater risk for acute renal failure.

There are no immediate signs of acute kidney failure, but, over time, urine output is decreased, resulting in increased fluid buildup in the tissues. Common symptoms include irregular heart rate, **ascites** (fluid in the abdomen), and swelling in the extremities.

In chronic renal failure, there is a gradual and progressive loss of kidney function. Renal failure may be mild or severe. Typically, it takes a period of years for the renal failure to progress. Symptoms may be mild or nonexistent until at least 10 percent of the kidney function is lost. Diabetes and hypertension are the two most common causes of chronic renal failure in the United States. About 2 out of every 1,000 people in the United States have chronic renal failure.

The goal of treatment for chronic renal failure is to identify and treat the reversible causes if the kidney fails. Then, treatment focuses on preventing fluid volume excesses while the kidneys have a chance to heal and resume their normal function. If normal function cannot be regained, then **dialysis** may be necessary (see Figure 29-6). Dialysis uses a filter other than the kidneys to remove toxins and maintain water balance. The two types of dialysis are hemodialysis and peritoneal dialysis. Hemodialysis uses a machine that cleans the blood outside of the body. A specialized catheter, called a shunt, is inserted in the patient's arm or leg. The shunt is accessed with special tubing that carries

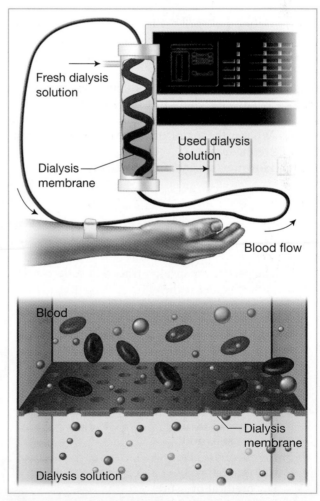

FIGURE 29-6 Dialysis machine showing diffusion of concentrations, which are the same, between the patient's blood and dialysis solution.

the blood to the machines that filter and clean the blood and then return the blood back to the body. Patients receiving hemodialysis must go to a special center three times a week for 2 to 3 hours at a time.

The other type of dialysis is called peritoneal dialysis. Peritoneal dialysis is done through the tissues of the abdomen, where a dialysis fluid is instilled in the stomach, left for a period of time while the membranes in the abdomen filter toxins, and then the fluid is re-moved. These patients can be dialyzed at home or in any environment.

Some patients may receive a kidney transplant, in which a donor kidney is inserted into the patient's body, with the blood vessels and ureters attached to the patient's already existing structures. Kidney transplant recipients must take antirejection drugs for their lifetime following the transplant. Kidney transplants are the second most common transplant in the United States.

SUMMARY

The urinary tract can present many challenges both for the patient and for the medical assistant. One of the most common reasons patients come into the medical office is to seek help for a urinary tract infection.

Oftentimes called the excretory system, the function of the urinary system is to help clean wastes from the bloodstream and then carry those wastes outside the body via the kidneys and bladder, through the urethra.

Chapter Review

COMPETENCY REVIEW

1. Define and spell the terms to learn for this chapter.
2. List the organs of the urinary system.
3. What are the vital functions of the urinary system?
4. Define renal pelvis.
5. In what portion of the kidney is the medulla located?
6. What is the vital function of the nephrons?
7. What are the three processes of urine formation?
8. What is the major organ of the urinary system?
9. Define ureter.
10. How much urine is formed daily?

PREPARING FOR THE CERTIFICATION EXAM

1. The part of the urinary tract that collects urine in the bladder is the
   A. ureter
   B. bladder
   C. urethra
   D. jejunum
   E. renal pelvis

2. The condition in which an individual experiences an involuntary and unpredictable flow of urine is called
   A. constipation
   B. incontinence
   C. dysuria
   D. urethral pressure
   E. anuria

3. A urinary tract disease that causes inflammation of the bladder is
   A. pyelonephritis
   B. glomerulonephritis
   C. polycystic kidney disease
   D. cystitis
   E. renal calculus

4. The anatomical structure that is the functional unit of the kidney is the
   A. nephrons
   B. ureter
   C. bladder
   D. urethra
   E. renal pelvis

continued on next page

5. The anatomical structure of the urinary system that is responsible for carrying urine from the bladder to the outside of the body is the
   A. nephrons
   B. ureter
   C. bladder
   D. urethra
   E. renal pelvis

6. The function of a diuretic is to
   A. treat kidney infections
   B. treat cystitis
   C. remove fluid from the body
   D. add fluid to the body
   E. eliminate kidney stones

7. Chronic renal failure is treated by
   A. lithotripsy
   B. cystoscopy
   C. dialysis
   D. radiology
   E. diuretics

8. Kidney stones are caused by deposits of
   A. mineral salts
   B. proteins
   C. phosphorus
   D. sodium
   E. potassium

9. A procedure that uses a telescopic lens to visualize the urethra and the urinary bladder is called
   A. laparoscopy
   B. cystoscopy
   C. endoscopy
   D. arthroscopy
   E. telescopy

10. A disease that causes a gradual and progressive loss of kidney function is called
    A. acute renal failure
    B. chronic renal failure
    C. polycystic nephritis
    D. cystitis
    E. glomerulonephritis

CRITICAL THINKING

1. During the urinalysis, what substance was found in Mr. Tevia's specimen?

2. If Mr. Tevia had not been able to pass his kidney stone, what would have been a possible treatment for him?

3. What type of dietary instructions should Mr. Tevia receive?

INTERNET ACTIVITY

Use the Internet to learn about types of incontinence and their treatment.

MediaLink More on the urinary system, including interactive resources, can be found on the Student CD-ROM accompanying this textbook.

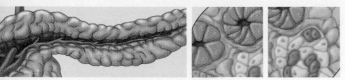

Medical Assistant Role Delineation Chart

HIGHLIGHT indicates material covered in this chapter.

ADMINISTRATIVE

Administrative Procedures

- Perform basic administrative medical assisting functions
- Schedule, coordinate and monitor appointments
- Schedule inpatient/outpatient admissions and procedures
- Understand and apply third-party guidelines
- Obtain reimbursement through accurate claims submission
- Monitor third-party reimbursement
- Understand and adhere to managed care policies and procedures
- *Negotiate managed care contracts*

Practice Finances

- Perform procedural and diagnostic coding
- Apply bookkeeping principles

- Manage accounts receivable
- *Manage accounts payable*
- *Process payroll*
- *Document and maintain accounting and banking records*
- *Develop and maintain fee schedules*
- *Manage renewals of business and professional insurance policies*
- *Manage personnel benefits and maintain records*
- *Perform marketing, financial, and strategic planning*

CLINICAL

Fundamental Principles

- Apply principles of aseptic technique and infection control
- Comply with quality assurance practices
- Screen and follow up patient test results

Diagnostic Orders

- Collect and process specimens
- Perform diagnostic tests

Patient Care

- Adhere to established patient screening procedures
- Obtain patient history and vital signs
- Prepare and maintain examination and treatment areas
- Prepare patient for examinations, procedures and treatments

- Assist with examinations, procedures and treatments
- Prepare and administer medications and immunizations
- Maintain medication and immunization records
- Recognize and respond to emergencies
- Coordinate patient care information with other health care providers
- Initiate IV and administer IV medications with appropriate training and as permitted by state law

GENERAL

Professionalism

- Display a professional manner and image
- Demonstrate initiative and responsibility
- Work as a member of the health care team
- Prioritize and perform multiple tasks
- Adapt to change
- Promote the CMA credential
- Enhance skills through continuing education
- Treat all patients with compassion and empathy
- Promote the practice through positive public relations

Communication Skills

- Recognize and respect cultural diversity
- Adapt communications to individual's ability to understand
- Use professional telephone technique

- Recognize and respond effectively to verbal, nonverbal, and written communications
- Use medical terminology appropriately
- Utilize electronic technology to receive, organize, prioritize and transmit information
- Serve as liaison

Legal Concepts

- Perform within legal and ethical boundaries
- Prepare and maintain medical records
- Document accurately
- Follow employer's established policies dealing with the health care contract
- Implement and maintain federal and state health care legislation and regulations
- Comply with established risk management and safety procedures
- Recognize professional credentialing criteria
- *Develop and maintain personnel, policy and procedure manuals*

Instruction

- Instruct individuals according to their needs
- Explain office policies and procedures
- Teach methods of health promotion and disease prevention
- Locate community resources and disseminate information
- *Develop educational materials*
- *Conduct continuing education activities*

Operational Functions

- Perform inventory of supplies and equipment
- Perform routine maintenance of administrative and clinical equipment
- Apply computer techniques to support office operations
- *Perform personnel management functions*
- *Negotiate leases and prices for equipment and supply contracts*

- *Denotes advanced skills.*

SOURCE: Reprinted by permission of the American Association of Medical Assistants from the AAMA Role Delineation Study: Occupational Analysis of the Medical Assisting Profession.

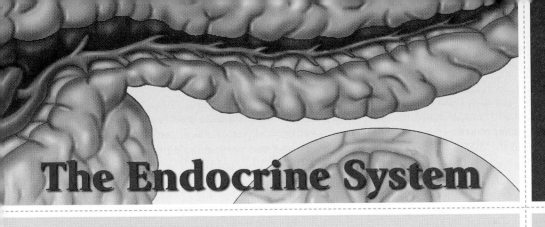

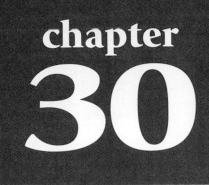

chapter 30

The Endocrine System

Learning Objectives

After completing this chapter, you should be able to:

- Define and spell the terms to learn for this chapter.
- Describe the primary glands of the endocrine system.
- Explain the vital function of the endocrine system.
- State the primary functions of the endocrine glands.
- Identify and state the functions of the various hormones secreted by the endocrine glands.
- Identify and explain common disorders associated with the endocrine system.

Terms to Learn

acromegaly
Addison's disease
cardiomegaly
Cushing's disease
diabetes mellitus
dwarfism
exophthalmos

gestational diabetes
gigantism
goiter
Graves' disease
Hashimoto's thyroiditis
hyperthyroidism
hypothyroidism

insulin-dependent diabetes mellitus (IDDM)
lipolysis
myxedema
non–insulin-dependent diabetes mellitus (NIDDM)

Case Study

12-YEAR-OLD FORREST DISER PRESENTED to the pediatrician's office with a 2-month history of weight loss, fatigue, polyuria, and polydipsia. Family history is significant for several relatives with type 1 diabetes mellitus. In the office, the patient was found to have hyperglycemia with a fasting blood sample, and glucosuria on a urine dipstick test. He was admitted to the hospital, where type 1 diabetes mellitus was diagnosed. After 3 days, he was discharged from the hospital on an insulin protocol of twice a day insulin injections and glucose monitoring. The patient and his family were educated on diet, exercise, symptoms of hypoglycemic coma, and the long-term complications of diabetes mellitus. He was placed on a 2,000-calorie diabetic diet with three meals and two snacks a day.

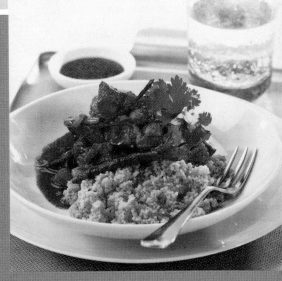

he endocrine system is made up of glands and the hormones they secrete. The primary glands of the endocrine system include the pituitary, pineal, thyroid, parathyroid, islets of Langerhans, adrenals, ovaries in the female, and testes in the male.

The vital function of this system is the production and regulation of hormones. A hormone is the chemical substance that regulates different body function. Hormones are the chemical messengers that regular growth, development, mood, tissue function, metabolism, and sexual function in both males and females.

Many disorders are associated with a hypersecretion or hyposecretion of hormones of the endocrine system.

Controlling the secretion of specific hormones can help treat many of those hormonal conditions or disorders.

The nervous system works closely with the endocrine system in the maintenance of homeostasis. For example, the hypothalamus, which is located in the lower central part of the brain, is the link between the endocrine and nervous systems. The nerve cells in the hypothalamus control the pituitary gland by producing chemicals that suppress or stimulate hormone secretions from the pituitary. The hypothalamus synthesizes and secretes releasing hormones such as thyrotropin-releasing hormone (TRH) and gonadotropin-releasing hormone (GTRH), and releasing factors such as corticotropin-releasing hormone (CRF), growth hormone-releasing factor (GHRF),

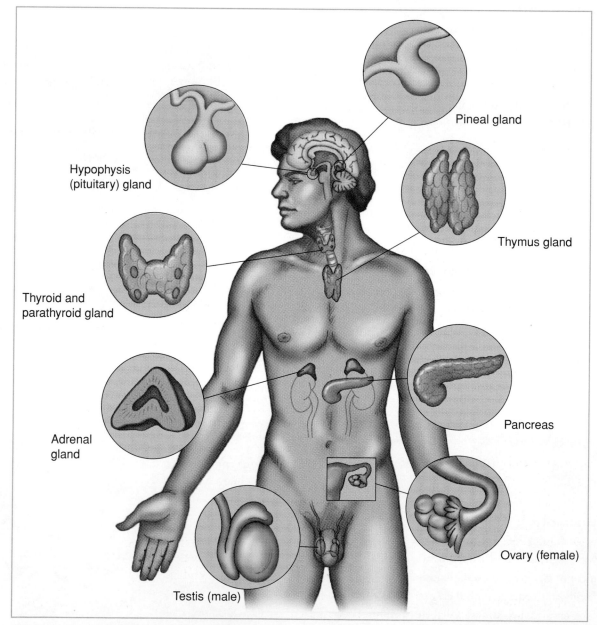

FIGURE 30-1   The primary glands of the endocrine system.

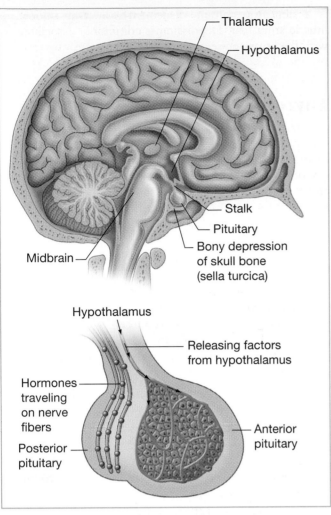

FIGURE 30-2   The pituitary gland and its relation to the brain.

gans, sex glands, the thyroid gland, and the adrenal cortex. The hormones produced in the anterior lobe of the pituitary gland include the following:

- Growth hormone (also called somatotrophic hormone)—essential for the growth and development of bones, muscles, and other organs. Growth hormone enhances protein synthesis, decreases glucose use, and promotes the destruction of fats (**lipolysis**). Hyposecretion of this hormone results in dwarfism; conversely, hypersecretion leads to gigantism during early life, and acromegaly in adults.

- Adrenocorticotropin I—essential for the growth and development of the middle and inner parts of the adrenal cortex. The glucocorticoids cortisol and corticosteroid are secreted by the adrenal cortex.

- Thyroid-stimulating hormone—controls the growth and development of the thyroid gland. It also stimulates the production of thyroxine and triiodothyronine, influencing the body's metabolic processes and metabolism.

- Follicle-stimulating hormone—a gonadotropic hormone that is responsible for stimulating the growth of ovarian follicles in females and the production of sperm in males.

prolactin-releasing factor (PRF), and melanocyte-stimulating releasing factor (MRF). The secretion of the hormones norepinephrine and epinephrine is also controlled by the hypothalamus, which exerts direct nervous control over the anterior pituitary and the adrenal medulla. Figure 30-1 illustrates the primary glands of the endocrine system.

Pituitary Gland

The pituitary gland (see Figure 30-2), is located near the base of the brain in a small depression of the sphenoid bone called the sella turcica. It is attached to the hypothalamus by the infundibulum stalk. The pituitary, which consists of both an anterior lobe and a posterior lobe, is called the master gland of the body, because it regulates all of the other endocrine glands.

Anterior Lobe

The adenohypophysis or anterior lobe (see Figure 30-3) secretes several hormones that are essential for the growth and development of bones, muscles, other or-

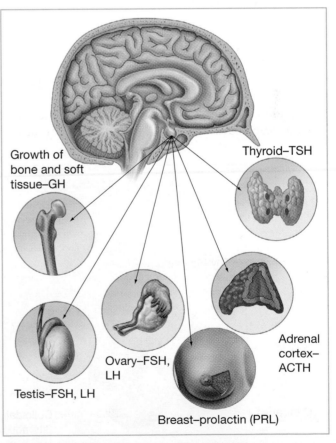

FIGURE 30-3   The anterior pituitary gland and its target organs.

- Luteinizing hormone—gonadotropic hormone that is responsible for the maturation process in the ovarian follicles and for stimulating the development of the corpus luteum in the female. In the male, LH is responsible for the production of testosterone.

- Prolactin (also known as lactogenic hormone)—a gonadotropic hormone that stimulates the mammary glands to produce milk after childbirth.

- Melanocyte-stimulating hormone—controls skin pigmentation. The deposit of melanin helps protect skin after exposure to sunlight.

Posterior Lobe

The posterior lobe of the pituitary gland is also known as the neurohypophysis. It secretes two hormones:

- Antidiuretic hormone (ADH)—also known as vasopressin, it is responsible for stimulating the reabsorption of water by the kidneys, so that less fluid is eliminated. In doing this, the blood pressure can be elevated. If this hormone is undersecreted, a condition known as diabetes insipidus will result.

- Oxytocin—responsible for stimulating the uterus for contraction during labor and childbirth and for stimulating the mammary glands to release milk after delivery.

Pineal Gland

The pineal gland is located at the posterior end of the corpus callosum in the brain. It secretes melatonin and serotonin. Melatonin is released at night and helps with sleep and the release of gonadotropin. Serotonin is a neurotransmitter, vasoconstrictor, and smooth muscle stimulant. Depression is commonly associated with the hormone serotonin.

Thyroid Gland

Located in the neck, the thyroid gland is responsible for metabolism (see Figure 30-4). It is located anterior to the trachea, just below the thyroid cartilage. The thyroid is approximately 5 cm long and 3 cm wide, and weighs about 30 grams. The thyroid gland is responsible for secreting three hormones:

- Thyroxine (T_4)—essential for the maintenance and regulation of the basal metabolic rate (BMR). Thyroxine influences growth and development, both physical and mental, as well as the metabolism of fats, proteins, carbohydrates, water, vitamins, and minerals. In thyroid dysfunction, it can be replaced with medications. Disorders resulting from hyposecretion of thyroxine include cretinism, myxedema, and Hashimoto's disease.

- Triiodothyronine (T_3)—influences the BMR.

- Calcitonin—influences bone and calcium metabolism. During infancy, if there is not enough calcitonin, cretinism may occur, causing mental retardation. Myxedema and Hashimoto's disease are also results of hyposecretion of calcitonin, along with its companion hormones, T_3 and T_4.

Hypersecretion of T_3 and T_4 is called *hyperthyroidism* (thyrotoxicosis). Other disorders resulting from hypersecretion of T_3 and T_4 include Graves' disease, exophthalmic goiter, toxic goiter, and Basedow's disease.

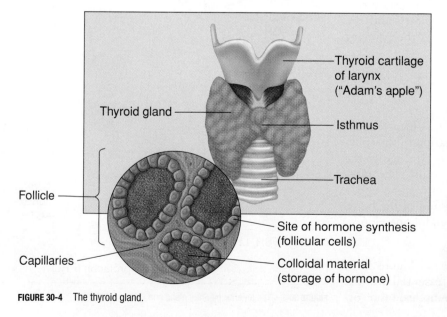

FIGURE 30-4 The thyroid gland.

Labels: Thyroid gland; Thyroid cartilage of larynx ("Adam's apple"); Isthmus; Trachea; Site of hormone synthesis (follicular cells); Colloidal material (storage of hormone); Follicle; Capillaries

Parathyroid Glands

The four parathyroid glands are located around the dorsal and lower aspect of the thyroid gland (see Figure 30-5). Each parathyroid gland is about 6 mm in diameter and weighs about 0.033 grams. The parathyroids secrete parathormone (PTH). PTH is responsible for the maintenance of normal serum calcium levels, along with that of phosphorus. Hyposecretion of PTH may result in hypoparathyroidism, causing tetany (twitching of muscles or nerves). Hypersecretion of PTH may result in hyperparathyroidism, which can result in osteoporosis, kidney stones, and hypercalcemia.

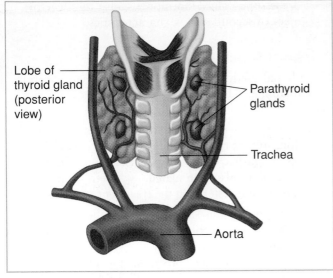

FIGURE 30-5 Parathyroid glands.

Pancreas (Islets of Langerhans)

The islets of Langerhans are small clusters of cells located within the pancreas (see Figure 30-6). Three types of cells make up the islets of Langerhans: the alpha, beta, and delta cells. The alpha cells secrete the hormone glucagon, which helps break down glycogen to glucose, increasing blood sugar. The beta cells secrete the hormone insulin, which lowers blood sugar. Normal fasting blood sugar is 70 to 110 mg/dL. In individuals who do not produce enough insulin, a synthetic insulin can be injected subcutaneously to help control the blood sugar. Hyposecretion of insulin results in diabetes mellitus. Hypersecretion results in hyperinsulinemia. The delta cells secrete somatostatin, which suppresses the release of glucagon and insulin.

Adrenal Glands

The adrenal glands are located on top of each kidney (see Figure 30-7). Each gland is triangle shaped and consists of an outer portion (cortex) and an inner portion (medulla).

Adrenal Cortex

The adrenal cortex secretes the groups of hormones called glucocorticoids (cortisol and corticosterone), mineralocorticoids (aldosterone), and androgens. These hormones are essential to life, and are described here:

- Cortisol—the principal steroid secreted by the cortex. It is responsible for regulating carbohydrate, protein, and fat metabolism. It also stimulates the output of glucose from the liver, increasing the blood sugar level. Cortisol also promotes the transport of amino acids into extracellular tissue for energy stores, and it influences the effectiveness of the catecholamines such as dopamine, epinephrine, and norepinephrine. The final critical function of cortisol is as an anti-inflammatory. Hyposecretion of cortisol may result in Addison's disease. Hypersecretion of cortisol may result in Cushing's disease.

- Corticosterone—essential for the normal use of carbohydrates, the absorption of glucose, and gluconeogenesis.

- Aldosterone—the principal mineralocorticoid secreted by the adrenal cortex. Aldosterone is essential in regulating electrolyte and water balance by promoting sodium and chloride retention and potassium excretion. A reduced plasma volume may result from hyposecretion of aldosterone. Hypersecretion of the hormone may result in primary aldosteronism.

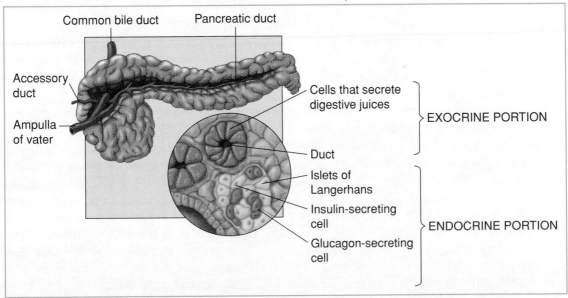

FIGURE 30-6 The pancreas—an endocrine and exocrine gland.

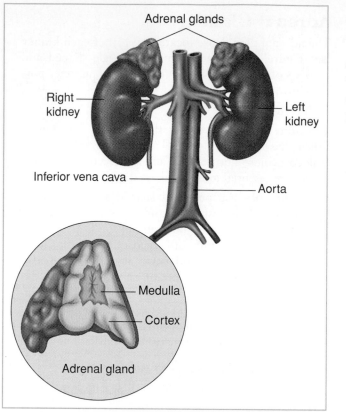

FIGURE 30-7 The adrenal glands.

- Androgens—Androgens are hormones that promote the development of male characteristics. The two main hormones are testosterone and an-

drosterone. These hormones cause the development of secondary sex characteristics.

Adrenal Medulla

The adrenal medulla synthesizes, secretes, and stores catecholamine. The primary catecholamines are dopamine, epinephrine, and norepinephrine:

- Dopamine—responsible for causing vasoconstriction, so that the blood pressure is increased. As a result, cardiac output is increased, and urine production is also stimulated. Synthetic dopamine can be administered in the treatment of shock.

- Epinephrine—also known as adrenaline, this catecholamine is responsible for the "fight or flight" syndrome, as regulated by the sympathetic nervous system. In times of stress, epinephrine causes peripheral vasoconstriction, dilation of the pupils, decreased salivation, decreased GI motility, and increased heart rate. It also elevates the blood pressure and dilates the bronchial tubes. It helps the body to get ready to flee in times of emergency. Epinephrine can be synthetically produced and administered in emergency situations, such as cardiac arrest or allergic reaction.

- Norepinephrine—also acts on the sympathetic nervous system by causing vasoconstriction, elevating systolic and diastolic blood pressure, and increasing the heart rate and cardiac output, while also increasing glycogenolysis.

Lifespan
Considerations

Management of diabetes in children is somewhat challenging, because diet, exercise, and medication must be continually adjusted to meet the changing needs of the growing child.

THE CHILD

- *Most of the structures and glands of the endocrine system develop during the first 3 months of pregnancy. During pregnancy, the hormones that cross the placental barrier protect the fetus. Because of maternal hormones, both male and female newborns may have swelling of the breasts and genitalia.*

- *Excessive production of growth hormone (GH) can cause gigantism. Insufficient production can cause dwarfism. The anterior lobe of the pituitary produces growth hormone.*

- *Diabetes mellitus is the most common endocrine system disorder of childhood. The rate of diabetes is highest among 5- to 7-year-olds and 11- to 13-year-olds. Individuals with childhood-onset diabetes mellitus typically lack the ability to secrete insulin.*

THE OLDER ADULT

- *The number of tissue receptors decreases with age, diminishing the body's response to hormones. Also, when the elderly develop diabetes, they typically have the ability to produce insulin, but not in sufficient quantities to manage blood sugar adequately.*

- *Other risk factors associated with the older adult and the development of diabetes, include age-related insulin resistance, heredity, decreased physical activity, multiple diseases, polypharmacy, obesity, and life stressors.*

- *Other changes in older adults include a decrease in estrogen production in females as a result of menopause, resulting in increased risk of heart disease and increased occurrence of osteoporosis.*

Ovaries

The ovaries produce estrogens and progesterone (see Figure 30-8). Estrogen is the female sex hormone secreted by the graafian follicles of the ovaries. Progesterone is secreted by the corpus luteum and is a steroid hormone. These hormones are needed for promoting the growth, development, and maintenance of secondary female sex organs and characteristics. Other functions of these hormones include uterine pregnancy preparation and mammary gland preparation, and they also play a vital role in a woman's emotional well-being and sexual drive.

Testes

The testes are located in the male scrotum and produce the male hormone testosterone, which is essential for the normal growth and development of the male accessory sex organ (see Figure 30-9). Testosterone is necessary for the reproductive act of copulation.

Placenta

Only present during pregnancy, the placenta produces chorionic gonadotropin hormone, estrogen, and progesterone. Besides acting as an endocrine gland, the placenta is the spongy structure that joins the mother and the child and provides the blood supply between the two.

Gastrointestinal Mucosa

The mucosa of the pyloric area of the stomach secretes the hormone gastrin. Gastrin stimulates gastric acid secretion in the stomach, gallbladder, pancreas, and small intestine.

Secretin is secreted by the mucosa of the duodenum and jejunum. Secretin stimulates pancreatic juice, bile, and intestinal secretions. Pancreozymin-cholecystokinin, which stimulates the pancreas, is also secreted by duodenal mucosa, as is enterogastrone, a hormone that regulates gastric secretions.

Thymus Gland

The thymus gland is actually composed of lymphoid tissue and is located in the mediastinal cavity, in front of and above the heart (see Figure 30-10). The thymus is part of the lymphatic system, but also functions as an endocrine gland by releasing thymosin and thymopoietin. Thymosin promotes the maturation of T lymphocytes. Thymopoietin influences the production of lymphocyte precursors and aids in their process of becoming T lymphocytes.

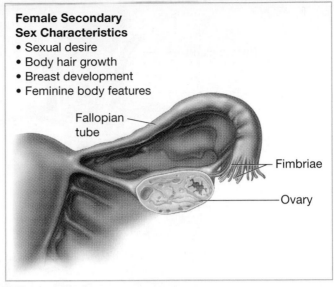

Female Secondary Sex Characteristics
- Sexual desire
- Body hair growth
- Breast development
- Feminine body features

Fallopian tube

Fimbriae

Ovary

FIGURE 30-8 Structure and functions of the ovary.

Common Disorders Associated with the Endocrine System

A variety of diseases are related to disorders of the endocrine system (see Table 30-1). Most are treated medically; however, there are a few surgical options.

Acromegaly

Acromegaly is a hormonal disorder that results when the pituitary gland produces excess growth hormone (GH). It most commonly affects middle-aged adults and can result in serious illness and premature death. The most serious health consequences of acromegaly are diabetes mellitus, hypertension, and increased risk of cardiovascular disease.

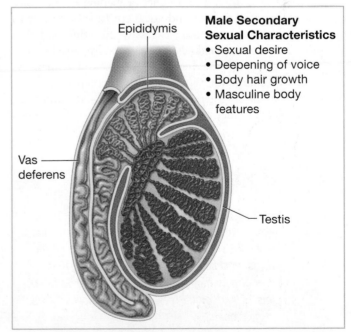

Epididymis

Male Secondary Sexual Characteristics
- Sexual desire
- Deepening of voice
- Body hair growth
- Masculine body features

Vas deferens

Testis

FIGURE 30-9 Structure and function of male testes.

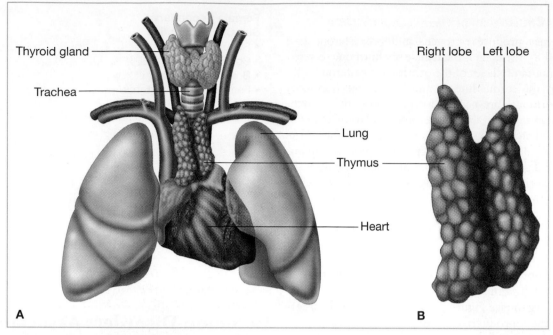

FIGURE 30-10 The thymus gland: (A) appearance and position; (B) with anatomical structures.

Common symptoms of acromegaly are the abnormal growth of the hands and feet. Soft tissue swelling of the hands and feet is often an early feature, with patients noticing a change in ring or shoe size. Gradually, bony changes alter the patient's facial features: the brow and lower jaw protrude, the nasal bone enlarges, and spacing of the teeth increases. Overgrowth of bone and cartilage often leads to arthritis. When tissue thickens, it may trap nerves, causing carpal tunnel syndrome, characterized by numbness and weakness of the hands. Other symptoms of acromegaly include thick, coarse, oily skin; skin tags; enlarged lips, nose, and tongue; deepening of the voice due to enlarged sinuses and vocal cords; snoring due to upper airway obstruction; excessive sweating and skin odor; fatigue and weakness; headaches; impaired vision; abnormalities of the menstrual cycle and sometimes breast discharge in women; and impotence in men. There may be enlargement of body organs, including the liver, spleen, kidneys, and heart.

Preparing for Externship

Part of preparing for externship is examining your own values, how you work with others, and how you view others. As a professional, all patients must be treated with equal respect, regardless of how they might treat you. Learning to do this is part of the process of developing as a professional.

The goals of treatment for acromegaly are to reduce GH production to normal levels, to relieve the pressure that the growing pituitary tumor exerts on the surrounding brain areas, to preserve normal pituitary function, and to reverse or ameliorate the symptoms of acromegaly. Currently, treatment options include surgical removal of the tumor, drug therapy, and radiation therapy of the pituitary.

Addison's Disease

Addison's disease occurs when the cortex of the adrenal gland is damaged, decreasing the production of adrenocortical hormones. This is usually an autoimmune disease, where the body attacks itself. Other causes of Addison's disease include infection of the adrenal glands, cancer, or hemorrhage into the glands.

Addison's disease can occur at any age, including infancy, and is equally prevalent in both men and women. It is rare, occurring in 1 in 100,000 Americans. Signs and symptoms of Addison's disease include weight loss, anorexia, weakness and lethargy, increased pigmentation of the skin and mucous membranes, hypoglycemia, joint and muscle aches, persistent fever, nausea, vomiting, diarrhea, and abdominal discomfort.

Most of the signs and symptoms occur over several months; however, they may occasionally appear quite suddenly. Addison's disease is diagnosed by blood and urine tests that measure the amount of corticosteroid hormones present. With a diagnosis of Addison's disease, the level of corticosteroids is very low.

Treatment consists of replacement of adrenocortical hormones and supplemental sodium. The patient and family are taught the importance of lifelong treatment

TABLE 30-1   **Disorders of the Endocrine System**

Disorder	Description
Acidosis	Excessive acidity of bodily fluids due to the accumulation of acids, as in diabetic acidosis.
Acromogaly	Chronic disease of middle-aged persons that results in an elongation and enlargement of the bones of the head and extremities. There can also be mood changes.
Addison's disease	A disease resulting from a deficiency in adrenocortical hormones. There may be an increased pigmentation of the skin, generalized weakness, and weight loss.
Adenoma	A neoplasm or tumor of a gland.
Cretinism	Congenital condition due to a lack of thyroid, which may result in arrested physical and mental development.
Cushing's syndrome	Set of symptoms that result from hypersecretion of the adrenal cortex. This may be the result of a tumor of the adrenal glands. The syndrome may present symptoms of weakness, edema, excess hair growth, skin discoloration, and osteoporosis.
Diabetes insipidus (DI)	Disorder caused by the inadequate secretion of the antidiuretic hormone ADH by the posterior lobe of the pituitary gland. There may be polyuria and polydipsia.
Diabetes mellitus (DM)	Chronic disorder of carbohydrate metabolism which results in hyperglycemia and glycosuria. Type 1 diabetes mellitus (IDDM) involves insulin dependency, which requires that the patient take daily injections of insulin. Type 2 (NIDDM) patients may not be insulin dependent.
Diabetic retinopathy	Secondary complication of diabetes mellitus (DM) that affects the blood vessels of the retina, resulting in visual changes and even blindness.
Dwarfism	Condition of being abnormally small. It may be the result of a hereditary condition or an endocrine dysfunction.
Gigantism	Excessive development of long bones of the body due to overproduction of the growth hormone by the pituitary gland.
Goiter	Enlargement of the thyroid gland.
Graves' disease	Disease that results from an overactivity of the thyroid gland and can result in a crisis situation. Also called hyperthyroidism.
Hashimoto's disease	A chronic form of thyroiditis.
Hirsutism	Condition of having an excessive amount of hair on the body. This term is used to describe females who have the adult male pattern of hair growth. Can be the result of a hormonal imbalance.
Hypercalcemia	Condition of having an excessive amount of calcium in the blood.
Hyperglycemia	Having an excessive amount of glucose (sugar) in the blood.
Hyperkalemia	Condition of having an excessive amount of potassium in the blood.
Hyperthyroidism	Condition that results from overactivity of the thyroid gland. Also called Graves' disease.
Hypothyroidism	Result of a deficiency in secretion by the thyroid gland. This results in a lowered basal metabolism rate with obesity, dry skin, slow pulse, low blood pressure, sluggishness, and goiter. Treatment is replacement with synthetic thyroid hormone.

(continued)

TABLE 30-1   Disorders of the Endocrine System *(continued)*

Disorder	Description
Ketoacidosis	Acidosis due to an excess of ketone bodies (waste products) that can result in death for the diabetic patient if not reversed.
Myasthenia gravis	Condition in which there is great muscular weakness and progressive fatigue. There may be difficulty in chewing and swallowing and drooping eyelids. If a thymoma is causing the problem, it can be treated with removal of the thymus gland.
Myxedema	Condition resulting from a hypofunction of the thyroid gland. Symptoms can include anemia, slow speech, enlarged tongue and facial features, edematous skin, drowsiness, and mental apathy.
Thyrotoxicosis	Condition that results from overproduction of the thyroid gland. Symptoms include a rapid heart action, tremors, enlarged thyroid gland, exophthalmos, and weight loss.
von Rechlinghausen's disease	Excessive production of parathyroid hormone that results in degeneration of the bones.

and intramuscular hydrocortisone injections. The patient needs to always carry medical identification.

Cushing's Disease

Cushing's disease is a rare disorder than develops when there is too much cortisol (see Figure 30-11). ACTH releases cortisol as a result of stimulation of the pituitary. Symptoms of Cushing's syndrome include weight gain, skin changes, and fatigue. Results of the disease include diabetes, high blood pressure, depression, and osteoporosis. Cushing's disease can cause death if it is not treated. Treatments include surgery and radiation.

Legal
and Ethical Issues

Each state has its own laws *regarding individuals with diabetes driving school buses and other forms of public transportation. It is important to understand the regulations in your state. In some states, if there is evidence that the diabetes is controlled, then the individual may be allowed to drive one of these means of transportation. These individuals do typically need regular monitoring with the appropriate documentation sent to the authorities. The medical assistant is often integral in maintaining these records.*

Diabetes Mellitus

Patients with diabetes mellitus have an inability to produce enough insulin to properly control their blood sugar levels. Insulin is a hormone that converts sugar and starches into the energy that the body needs.

Diabetes is a silent disease, especially adult-onset diabetes, which may not be detected until it has become advanced. According to the American Diabetes Association, approximately 11.1 million people have been diagnosed with diabetes, but an estimated 5.9 million individuals are undiagnosed.

Classic symptoms of diabetes are polyuria (frequent urination), polydipsia (excessive thirst), and polyphagia (excessive hunger). Other symptoms include weakness, weight loss, lethargy, anorexia, irritability, dry skin, vaginal yeast infections in women, recurrent infections, and abdominal cramps.

There are three types of diabetes. Juvenile diabetes is also known as type 1 diabetes. This is typically diagnosed in children who cannot produce sufficient quantities if any, of insulin. These individuals are typically dependent on insulin injections for the duration of their life. Type 1 diabetes is also known as **insulin-dependent diabetes mellitus (IDDM)**.

Type 2 diabetes is also known as **non–insulin-dependent diabetes mellitus (NIDDM)** or adult-onset diabetes. Typically, type 2 diabetes is diagnosed later in life and is the most common form of the disease. It results from insulin resistance combined with a relative insulin deficiency. There is a very strong correlation between obesity and type 2 diabetes. People who are

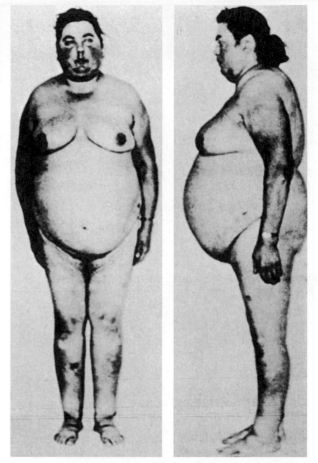

FIGURE 30-11 Cushing's syndrome patient showing round, red face; stocky neck; and marked obesity of the trunk with protruding abdomen. Note bruises on trunk and legs and also stretch marks. Note fat pads above the collar bone and on the back of the neck, which produces the "buffalo hump."

overweight may make sufficient insulin for their ideal body weight, but their body cannot make enough insulin to compensate for extra weight.

Type 2 diabetes is treated with diet and exercise, along with the administration of oral hypoglycemic medications to help control the blood sugar levels. It may also be possible to prevent type 2 diabetes with modest lifestyle changes, including healthy diet choices, exercise, and weight management.

Gestational diabetes is pregnancy-related diabetes. Typically, this type of diabetes disappears after the pregnancy is completed, but occasionally precipitates ongoing type 2 diabetes. During pregnancy, this pa-

tient may have to monitor her diet and blood sugar, and she may need to give herself insulin injections on a daily basis.

Dwarfism

Dwarfism refers to a group of conditions characterized by shorter than normal skeletal growth. This shortness can be manifested in the arms and legs or trunk. More than 300 conditions can cause abnormal skeletal growth and dwarfism. Achondroplasia is the most common type of short-limb dwarfism, occurring in 1 in 25,000 children with both sexes at equal risk. This type of skeletal dysplasia (abnormal skeletal growth) is usually diagnosed at birth.

The majority of children born with the disorder have average-sized parents. The child may experience a delay in developing motor skills, such as controlling the movements of the head, but intellectual development is normal in children with achondroplasia. The average final height for a person with this condition is 130 cm for men and 125 cm for women. Short-statured people lead normal, fulfilled lives. Achieving higher levels of

Professionalism

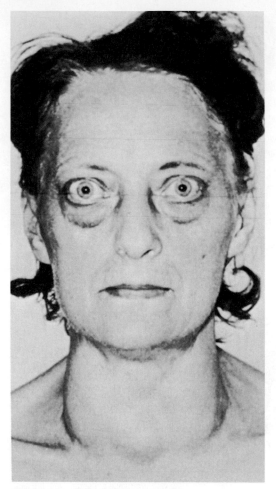

FIGURE 30-12 A patient with exophthalmos.

growth plates, which causes overgrowth of the long bones and very tall stature. The vertical growth in height that marks this condition is also accompanied by growth in muscles and organs, which makes the child extremely large for his or her age. The disorder can also delay puberty.

The cause of excess growth hormone secretion is most often a pituitary gland tumor. Gigantism may also be caused by an underlying medical condition such as multiple endocrine neoplasia. Pituitary tumors are never malignant (cancerous). If excessive secretion of growth hormone occurs after normal bone growth has stopped, the condition is known as acromegaly. Treatments for gigantism include radiation therapy and surgical removal of the tumor.

Hyperthyroidism

In hyperthyroidism, the thyroid hormone levels are elevated. The symptoms of elevated thyroid levels include nervousness, heart palpitations, tremors, sweating, increased activity in the intestinal tract, changes in menstruation, and weight loss. Sometimes, there is a feeling of anxiousness or restlessness, along with changes in the fingernails and hair. Palpitations may be presented, along with possible enlargement of the heart. A condition known as exophthalmos may also affect the eyes. In this disease, the eyeball may protrude beyond its normal protective orbit when the tissues behind swell (see Figure 30-12).

education and career and personal ambitions is not limited by stature.

The physical characteristics of a person born with achondroplasia include a trunk of normal length; disproportionately short arms and legs; bowed legs; reduced joint mobility in the elbow, while other joints seem overly flexible, or "double jointed," because of loose ligaments; shortened hands and feet; large head; flat midface and crowded teeth, because of a small upper jaw; prominent forehead; and flattened bridge of the nose.

There is no cure for achondroplasia. Treatment focuses on the prevention, management, and treatment of medical complications as well as social and family support. Surgery may be advised to relieve pressure on the nervous system, generally at the base of the skull and lower back, or to open obstructed airways by removing the adenoids. Dental and orthodontic work may be necessary to correct malocclusion and ensure dental health.

Gigantism

Gigantism is an excessive secretion of growth hormone during childhood before the closure of the bone

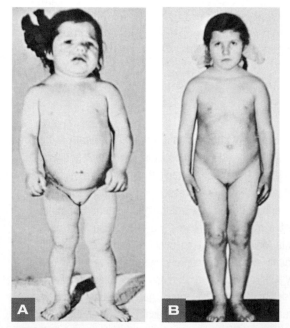

FIGURE 30-13 (A) A 6-year old child with congenital hypothyroidism, cretinism, exhibiting marked mental and physical retardation. (B) The same patient after 3 years of thyroxine therapy, which resulted in a spurt of growth and regression of pathological manifestations. Mental retardation is delayed.

Graves' disease is the most common cause of hyperthyroidism. It is an autoimmune disorder when the antibodies produced by the immune system stimulate the thyroid to produce too much thyroxine. Other forms of hyperthyroidism may be caused by thyroiditis (inflammation of the thyroid gland) or benign or malignant tumors.

Hyperthyroidism can lead to a rapid heart rate, atrial fibrillation, and congestive heart failure. Other complications include osteoporosis (weak, brittle bones), bulging red or swollen eyes, sensitivity to light or blurring and double vision.

Hyperthyroidism is treated with antithyroid medications, radioactive iodine to destroy the thyroid, or surgery (thyroidectomy). If the thyroid is removed or destroyed, then lifelong thyroid replacement therapy must be initiated.

Hypothyroidism

In hypothyroidism, the thyroid does not produce adequate amounts of the thyroid hormones. Because hypothyroidism develops slowly, only about half of the 7 million cases in the United States are diagnosed early. Figure 30-13 shows an example of a child born with hypothyroidism.

Symptoms initially tend to be subtle, including fatigue, decreased concentration, intolerance to cold environments, constipation, loss of appetite, muscle cramping, stiffness, and weight gain. Other symptoms may include hair loss, dry skin, and nail changes. Untreated hypothyroidism can lead to other conditions because the constant stimulation to release more thyroid hormones can cause the thyroid gland to enlarge. This condition is called a goiter (see Figure 30-14). The most common cause of a goiter is Hashimoto's thyroiditis, an autoimmune inflammation of the thyroid. If hypothyroidism goes untreated, there is an associated risk of heart disease, due to the high levels of low-density lipoproteins (LDL—bad cholesterol) that can occur. Cardiomegaly (an enlarged heart) can also occur.

Other complications of hypothyroidism include depression, decreased sexual desire, and slowed mental functioning. Myxedema is a rare, life-threatening condition that is a result of long-term, untreated hypothyroidism (see Figure 30-15). The symptoms of myxedema include intense cold intolerance and drowsiness followed by profound lethargy and unconsciousness. A myxedema coma can be triggered

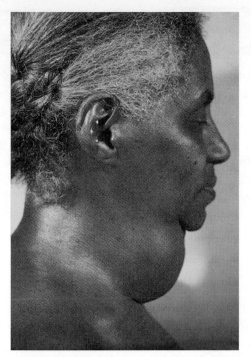

FIGURE 30-14   Goiter.

by sedatives, infection, or other stress. Emergency treatment should be initiated immediately if these symptoms are observed.

Typical treatment for hypothyroidism involves the daily use of a synthetic thyroid hormone called levothyroxine (Synthroid, Levothroid). This oral hormone reduces the symptoms of hypothyroidism, especially in the areas of fatigue, weight loss, and decrease of cholesterol levels. This medication must be taken on a routine basis; it should be monitored regularly with blood work and the dosage adjusted as necessary. Thyroid supplementation is a lifelong therapy.

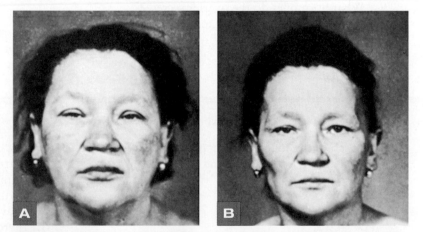

FIGURE 30-15   (A) A 62-year-old patient with myxedema exhibiting marked edema of the face and a somnolent look. The hair is stiff and without luster. (B) The same patient after 3 months of treatment with thyroxine.

Patients with endocrine disorders need to be carefully taught how to use their medications to supplement or replace the hormones that their body is not providing or to counter the effects of the overproduction of hormones. These medications are typically taken for the duration of their life, even when they feel well. Patients need to understand the ramifications of changing their dosage regimen, as well as symptoms of inadequate or excessive medications. Oftentimes, diet and exercise are an integral part of the treatment for patients with endocrine disorders. Type 1 diabetic patients may be treated with multiple daily insulin injections, or they may be given an insulin pump that continually administers small quantities of insulin and can be adjusted as their needs change. Patients and their families need to be comfortable with the regulation of their insulin and the mechanics of the pump.

SUMMARY

The endocrine system releases the hormones that keep the body in its proper balance, helping to maintain homeostasis. These hormones regulate growth, development, mood, tissue function, metabolism, and sexual function. This is achieved by a close working relationship with the nervous system.

Chapter Review

COMPETENCY REVIEW

1. Define and spell the terms to learn for this chapter.
2. What is the vital function of the endocrine system?
3. Why is the pituitary gland known as the master gland of the body?
4. What hormones are secreted by the thyroid gland?
5. What is the function of insulin?
6. What are the four functions of cortisol?
7. Name three functions of the hormone epinephrine.
8. Name the catecholamines synthesized, secreted, and stored by the adrenal medulla.
9. What hormones do the ovaries secrete?
10. Name two hormones secreted by the thymus.

PREPARING FOR THE CERTIFICATION EXAM

1. Which of the following organs/structures is/are NOT found in the endocrine system?
   A. pineal
   B. ovaries
   C. thymus
   D. testes
   E. spleen

2. Graves' disease is a result of the dysfunction of what structure?
   A. pituitary
   B. thymus
   C. ovary
   D. thyroid
   E. adrenal gland

continued on next page

3. The endocrine gland that is responsible for stimulating growth with the growth hormone (GH) is the
   A. parathyroid
   B. pancreas
   C. pituitary posterior lobe
   D. pituitary anterior lobe
   E. adrenal cortex

4. The result of inadequate secretion of the antidiuretic hormone from the pituitary gland is
   A. diabetes insipidus
   B. diabetes mellitus
   C. tetany
   D. exophthalmos
   E. Addison's disease

5. A chronic form of thyroiditis is
   A. myasthenia gravis
   B. myxedema
   C. Graves' disease
   D. Hashimoto's disease
   E. ketoacidosis

6. One of the leading causes of type 2 diabetes is
   A. excessive secretion of insulin
   B. obesity
   C. pancreatectomy
   D. high-protein diets
   E. inadequate control of type 1 diabetes

7. Individuals with hypothyroidism should expect to take medications to treat the disorder for
   A. 1–2 weeks
   B. 10 days
   C. 1 year
   D. 5 years
   E. the remainder of their lives

8. The function of aldosterone is
   A. development of male secondary sex characteristics
   B. development of female secondary sex characteristics
   C. water and electrolyte balance
   D. to suppress the release of glucagon and insulin
   E. to regulate the release of gonadotropin

9. The islets of Langerhans are found in the
   A. parathyroid glands
   B. anterior pituitary
   C. gastric mucosa
   D. pancreas
   E. posterior pituitary

10. Excessive secretion of growth hormone (GH) will result in
    A. exophthalmos
    B. dwarfism
    C. Simmonds' disease
    D. Cushing's syndrome
    E. gigantism

CRITICAL THINKING

1. List the symptoms that were indicative of the final diagnosis.
2. What is the difference between type 1 diabetes and type 2 diabetes?
3. Can this patient stop taking his insulin? Why?
4. This patient wants to play baseball with his friends. What adjustments will he need to make to be able to participate?

INTERNET ACTIVITY

Do an Internet search to learn about support groups for individuals with diabetes. What kind of support is available for people with this disorder?

MediaLink More on the endocrine system, including interactive resources, can be found on the Student CD-ROM accompanying this textbook.

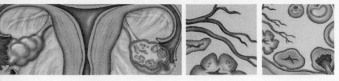

Medical Assistant Role Delineation Chart

ADMINISTRATIVE

Administrative Procedures

- Perform basic administrative medical assisting functions
- Schedule, coordinate and monitor appointments
- Schedule inpatient/outpatient admissions and procedures
- Understand and apply third-party guidelines
- Obtain reimbursement through accurate claims submission
- Monitor third-party reimbursement
- Understand and adhere to managed care policies and procedures
- *Negotiate managed care contracts*

Practice Finances

- Perform procedural and diagnostic coding
- Apply bookkeeping principles

- Manage accounts receivable
- *Manage accounts payable*
- *Process payroll*
- *Document and maintain accounting and banking records*
- *Develop and maintain fee schedules*
- *Manage renewals of business and professional insurance policies*
- *Manage personnel benefits and maintain records*
- *Perform marketing, financial, and strategic planning*

CLINICAL

Fundamental Principles

- Apply principles of aseptic technique and infection control
- Comply with quality assurance practices
- Screen and follow up patient test results

Diagnostic Orders

- Collect and process specimens
- Perform diagnostic tests

Patient Care

- Adhere to established patient screening procedures
- Obtain patient history and vital signs
- Prepare and maintain examination and treatment areas
- Prepare patient for examinations, procedures and treatments

- Assist with examinations, procedures and treatments
- Prepare and administer medications and immunizations
- Maintain medication and immunization records
- Recognize and respond to emergencies
- Coordinate patient care information with other health care providers
- Initiate IV and administer IV medications with appropriate training and as permitted by state law

GENERAL

Professionalism

- Display a professional manner and image
- Demonstrate initiative and responsibility
- Work as a member of the health care team
- Prioritize and perform multiple tasks
- Adapt to change
- Promote the CMA credential
- Enhance skills through continuing education
- Treat all patients with compassion and empathy
- Promote the practice through positive public relations

Communication Skills

- Recognize and respect cultural diversity
- Adapt communications to individual's ability to understand
- Use professional telephone technique

- Recognize and respond effectively to verbal, nonverbal, and written communications
- Use medical terminology appropriately
- Utilize electronic technology to receive, organize, prioritize and transmit information
- Serve as liaison

Legal Concepts

- Perform within legal and ethical boundaries
- Prepare and maintain medical records
- Document accurately
- Follow employer's established policies dealing with the health care contract
- Implement and maintain federal and state health care legislation and regulations
- Comply with established risk management and safety procedures
- Recognize professional credentialing criteria
- *Develop and maintain personnel, policy and procedure manuals*

Instruction

- Instruct individuals according to their needs
- Explain office policies and procedures
- Teach methods of health promotion and disease prevention
- Locate community resources and disseminate information
- *Develop educational materials*
- *Conduct continuing education activities*

Operational Functions

- Perform inventory of supplies and equipment
- Perform routine maintenance of administrative and clinical equipment
- Apply computer techniques to support office operations
- *Perform personnel management functions*
- *Negotiate leases and prices for equipment and supply contracts*

- *Denotes advanced skills.*

SOURCE: Reprinted by permission of the American Association of Medical Assistants from the AAMA Role Delineation Study: Occupational Analysis of the Medical Assisting Profession.

chapter 31

The Reproductive System

Learning Objectives

After completing this chapter, you should be able to:

- Define and spell the terms to learn for this chapter.

- Explain the purpose and function of the female reproductive system.

- Identify the structures of the female reproductive system and briefly explain the function of each.

- Explain the menstrual cycle.

- Explain the purpose and function of the male reproductive system.

- Identify the male external organs of reproduction and explain the function of each.

- Identify and state the function of the testes, epididymis, ductus deferens, seminal vesicles, prostate gland, bulbourethral glands, and the urethra.

- List common disorders associated with the female and male reproductive systems.

Terms to Learn

- benign prostatic hyperplasia (BPH)
- breast cancer
- cervical cancer
- cervicitis
- circumcision
- dysmenorrhea
- endometriosis
- epididymitis
- episiotomy
- erectile dysfunction (ED)
- fibrocystic breast disease
- hydrocele
- hysterectomy
- myomectomy
- ovarian cancer
- ovarian cysts
- ovulation
- pelvic inflammatory disease (PID)
- perineum
- premenstrual syndrome (PMS)
- prostate cancer
- sexually transmitted infection (STI)
- urethritis
- uterine cancer
- uterine fibroids
- vaginitis

Case Study

MARK SANSONE IS AN 85-YEAR-OLD MAN seen in the clinic with complaints of difficulty with urination. He needs to urinate often, especially at night; has difficulty starting his stream; has urgency; and has experienced a decrease in the size and force of his stream. The physician does a full physical on Mr. Sansone, including a PSA test, urinalysis, and digital rectal exam. He is diagnosed with benign prostatic hyperplasia and given a prescription. Mr. Sansone is to follow up with the physician in 6 months.

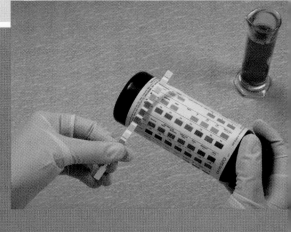

Female Reproductive System

The female reproductive system consists of the ovaries, which are the primary sex organs, and the accessory sex organs, which include the fallopian (uterine) tubes, the uterus, the vagina, the vulva, and the breasts (see Figure 31-1). The vital function of the female reproductive system is to perpetuate the species through sexual (germ cell) reproduction.

Uterus

The uterus is a hollow, pear-shaped, muscular organ located in the anterior portion of the pelvic cavity, between the sacrum and the symphysis pubis, above the bladder and in front of the rectum. There are three identifiable areas: the upper portion, called the body, the central portion, which is called the isthmus, and the neck, which is called the cervix. The fundus is the bulging surface of the body extending from the internal os (mouth) of the cervix upward above the fallopian tube. A number of ligaments support the uterus and hold it in place: two broad ligaments, two round ligaments, and two uterosacral ligaments. There are also ligaments that attach the uterus to the bladder. The normal position of the uterus is tilted, with the cervix pointing toward the sacrum and the fundus toward the suprapubic region. Generally, the normal uterus is about 8 cm long and 2.5 cm thick (see Figure 31-2).

The uterine wall has three layers: the perimetrium (the outer wall), the myometrium (the muscular middle layer), and the endometrium (the mucous membrane lining the inner surface). The endometrium is composed of columnar epithelium and connective tissue and is supplied with arterial blood. The endometrium undergoes marked changes in response to hormonal stimulation during the menstrual cycle.

The uterus has three primary functions. It is the site for cyclic discharge of blood fluid as evidenced by the changes in the endometrium in response to hormonal changes. It is also the site of nourishment and protection of the fetus during pregnancy. Finally, during labor, the myometrium contracts rhythmically to expel the fetus from the uterus.

As a result of weakness of any of the supporting ligaments, the uterus may become malpositioned. This may be caused by trauma, a disease process in the uterus, or as a result of multiple pregnancies. The more common abnormal positions of the uterus include anteflexion, which is the bending forward of the uterus at its body and neck; retroflexion, which is the bending backward of the uterus at any angle with the cervix unchanged from its normal position; anteversion, which is the process of turning the fundus toward the pubis, with the cervix tilted up toward the sacrum; and retroversion, which is the process of turning the uterus backward, with the cervix pointing forward toward the symphysis pubis.

Fallopian Tubes

The fallopian tubes, also called the uterine tubes or the oviducts, extend laterally from either side of the uterus near each ovary. Their function is to serve as ducts to move the ovum from the ovary to the uterus and to move sperm from the uterus toward the ovary. Each tube is about 11.5 cm long and 6 mm wide and is composed of three layers. The serous layer is the

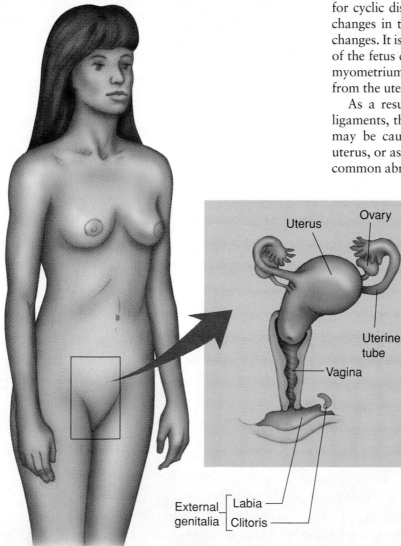

Uterus

Ovary

Uterine tube

Vagina

External genitalia { Labia
Clitoris

FIGURE 31-1 The female reproductive system.

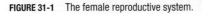

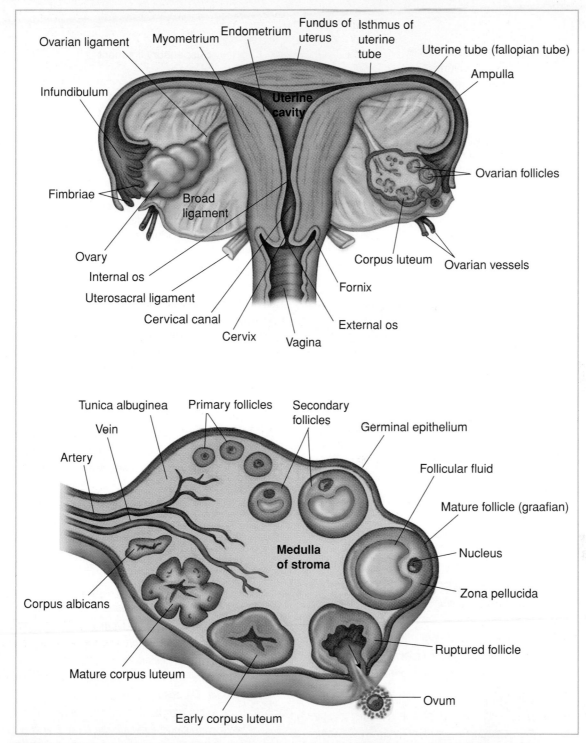

FIGURE 31-2 The uterus, ovaries, and associated structures, with expanded view of a mammalian ovary showing stages of graafian follicle and ovum development.

outermost layer made of connective tissue. The middle layer is the muscular layer, made of circular and longitudinal smooth muscle. The mucosa is the inner layer, consisting of simple columnar epithelium.

The isthmus is the constricted portion of the tube nearest the uterus. The tube extends laterally from the isthmus to the ampulla, where it widens. The tube continues to widen until it gains a funnel-shaped opening at the infundibulum called the ostium. Each ostium is surrounded by fimbriae, finger-like processes that help propel the ovum toward the tube after discharge from the uterus.

Ovaries

The two ovaries, located on either side of the uterus, are almond-shaped organs attached to the uterus by

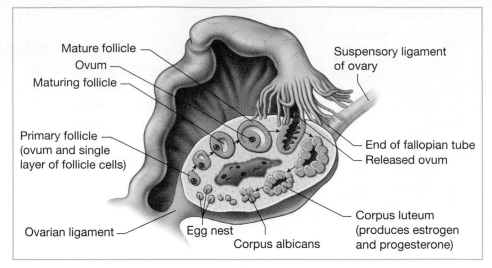

Mature follicle
Ovum
Maturing follicle

Primary follicle
(ovum and single
layer of follicle cells)

Ovarian ligament

Egg nest

Corpus albicans

Suspensory ligament
of ovary

End of fallopian tube
Released ovum

Corpus luteum
(produces estrogen
and progesterone)

FIGURE 31-3 The ovary.

the ovarian ligament (see Figure 31-3). They lie close to the fimbriae of the fallopian tubes. The anterior border of each ovary is connected to the posterior layer of the broad ligament by the mesovarium. On the sides, they are attached by the suspensory liga- ments. Each ovary is about 4 cm long, 2 cm wide, and 1.5 cm thick.

There are two distinct microscopic divisions of the ovary: the cortex (the outer layer) and the medulla (in- ner layer). The cortex contains small secretory sacs

Lifespan
Considerations

THE CHILD
- Every child develops according to his or her own biological clock. Puberty is triggered when the pituitary gland signals the body to release hormones. Hormones in turn stimulate the growth and development of the reproductive organs. Estrogen and testosterone spur the development of the child's secondary sex characteristics, such as breast development in girls and the growth of facial hair in boys. Fluctuating levels of hormones may also bring on adolescent mood swings.

THE OLDER ADULT
- The most dramatic age-related changes in the reproductive system occur with women at menopause when their estrogen production ceases and they lose their capacity to reproduce. The menopause in which the cycle of ovulation ceases occurs between the ages of 45 and 52 years.
- The lower estrogen levels also cause atrophic changes in the uterus and vagina. The uterine lin- ing thins and the elasticity decreases. Vaginal se- cretions are reduced. Common symptoms include hot flashes, palpitations, irritability, headaches, depression, fatigue, weight gain, insomnia, night sweats, forgetfulness, and inability to concentrate. The vaginal walls become thinner and less elastic and there is a decrease in lubrication.

- In the years following menopause, the circulating follicle-stimulating hormone (FSH) and luteinizing hormones (LH) are greatly increased. Over subse- quent years, FSH and LH levels fall slowly before leveling off about 30 years after menopause. These hormonal changes cause a relaxation of lig- aments and a loss of muscular tone that alter the contour of the breast. Women also face an in- creased risk for osteoporosis, heart attack, stroke, and possibly Alzheimer's disease.

- In men, the decline in reproductive ability is more gradual. The testes secrete testosterone and pro- duce spermatozoa. With aging, the rate of sperm production slows although there are few changes in sperm number so this does not affect fertility. However, there may be an increase in chromoso- mal abnormalities. By the age of 85 there is a 35 percent decrease in the level of testosterone and a reduction in the size of the testes. The amount of fluid ejaculated remains the same. Declining levels of testosterone may be partly responsible for losses in muscle strength.

called follicles, which hold the ova in differing stages of development. The different stages are the primary, growing, and graafian. The ovarian medulla contains connective tissue, nerves, blood and lymphatic vessels, and some smooth muscles at the hilus.

The functions of the ovaries are to produce ova (eggs, or reproductive cells) and to produce hormones. The activity of the ovaries is controlled by the anterior lobe of the pituitary, which produces the gonadotropic hormones, FSH (follicle-stimulating hormone) and luteinizing hormone (LH). FSH is instrumental in the development of the follicle nurturing the ovum. Luteinizing hormone stimulates the development of the corpus luteum, a small mass of cells that develops after the release of the ovum. Each month, a graafian follicle ruptures on the ovarian cortex, and an ovum releases into the pelvic cavity and into the fallopian tube. This process is known as **ovulation**. In the average normal woman, more than 400 ova may be produced during the reproductive years.

The hormones estrogen and progesterone are also produced by the ovaries. These two hormones play key roles in the reproductive system. Estrogen is the female sex hormone secreted by the follicles. Progesterone is a steroid hormone secreted by the corpus luteum. Both hormones are responsible for promoting growth, development, and maintenance of the female secondary sex characteristics and organs. They prepare the uterus for pregnancy, promote development of the mammary glands, and play a major role in a woman's emotional well-being and sexual drive.

Vagina

The vagina is a musculomembranous tube extending from the vestibule to the uterus. Typically, the vagina is 10 to 15 cm in length and is situated between the bladder and the rectum. It is lined by mucous membrane and squamous epithelium. There is a fold of membrane called the hymen that partially covers the external opening of the vagina.

The vagina has three basic functions. It is the organ of female copulation, the passageway for discharge of menstruation, and the passageway for the birth of the fetus.

Vulva

The vulva consists of the five organs that comprise the external female genitalia. These include the following structures:

- Mons pubis: The pad of fatty, triangular-shaped fatty tissue that is covered with hair after puberty. It is the rounded area over the symphysis pubis.

- Labia majora: The two folds of adipose tissue that are lip-like structures lying on either side of the vaginal opening.

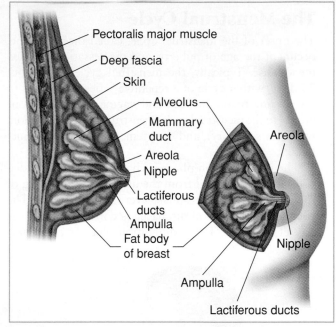

FIGURE 31-4 The breast.

- Labia minora: The two thin folds of skin within the labia majora enclosing the vestibule.

- Vestibule: The cleft between the labia minora, approximately 4 to 5 cm long and about 2 cm wide. There are four structures in the vestibule: the urethra (the external opening of the urinary system), the vagina, and the two excretory glands of the Bartholin's glands.

- Clitoris: Small organ of sensitive erectile tissue that is analogous to the penis of the male.

Between the vulva and the anus is an external region known as the **perineum**, which is composed of muscle covered with skin. Sometimes during labor, this area is incised by the physician in a process called **episiotomy**, which is performed in order to prevent tearing of the perineum during delivery.

Breast

The breasts, or mammary glands, are compound alveolar structures consisting of 15 to 12 glandular tissue lobes separated by septa of connecting tissue (see Figure 31-4). The areola is the dark, pigmented area found in the skin of each breast, and the nipple is the elevated area in the center of the areola. During pregnancy, the areola changes from pinkish in color to a darker brown or reddish color. The areola is supplied with a row of small sebaceous glands that secrete an oil that keeps it resilient. The lactiferous glands consist of 20 to 24 glands in the areola of the nipple and during lactation will provide milk to a suckling infant. Prolactin is the hormone produced by the anterior lobe of the pituitary that stimulates the mammary glands to produce milk after childbirth. The other hormones that play a role in milk production include insulin and glucocorticoids.

The Menstrual Cycle

The onset of the menstrual cycle, called the menarche, occurs at the age of puberty, and the cessation is called menopause. Typically, the menstrual cycle lasts about 28 days, with a cycle of a repetitive series of changes to the uterine tissue, breasts, and vagina. There are four phases to the menstrual cycle: menstruation, proliferation, luteal (or secretory), and the premenstrual (or ischemic) phases.

The menstruation phase is characterized by the discharge of blood fluid from the uterus by a shedding of the endometrium. This phase averages 4 to 5 days. The first day of the blood discharge is considered the first day of the cycle. The proliferation phase is characterized by the thickening and vascularization of the endometrium, along with the maturing of the ovarian follicle. This phase begins on about the fifth day of the cycle and lasts until the eruption of the graafian follicle, about day 14.

The luteal or secretory phase is characterized by the continued thickening of the endometrium, while the glands in the endometrium become tortuous, and by the appearance of coiled arteries in the tissue. The endometrium becomes edematous (swollen and fluid filled). During this phase, the body is preparing for a possible pregnancy by getting the endometrium ready to support the early developmental phase of an embryo. The corpus luteum in the ovary is developing and secreting progesterone at this time. The progesterone level is at its highest during this phase, and the estrogen level begins to decrease.

During the premenstrual, or ischemic, phase, the coiled arteries become constricted, the endometrium becomes anemic and begins to shrink, and the corpus luteum decreases in functional activity. This phase lasts about 2 days and ends with the onset of menstruation.

Male Reproductive System

The male reproductive system consists of the testes; various ducts; the urethra; accessory glands, which include the bulbourethral, prostate, and the seminal vesicles; and the supporting structures and accessory sex organs, the scrotum and the penis (see Figure 31-5). The vital function of the male reproductive system is to provide the sperm cells necessary to fertilize the ovum, thereby perpetuating the species.

External Organs

In the male, the scrotum and the penis are the external organs of reproduction. The scrotum is a pouch-like structure, located behind the penis. It is suspended from the perineal region and is divided into two sacs by a septum, one containing each of the two testes along with the epididymis, the connecting tube to the rest of the reproductive system. The tissues of the scrotum have fibers of smooth muscle that contract in the absence of sufficient heat, giving the scrotum a wrinkled appearance. This contractile action brings the testes closer to the perineum, helping them to absorb sufficient body heat to maintain the viability of the spermatozoa.

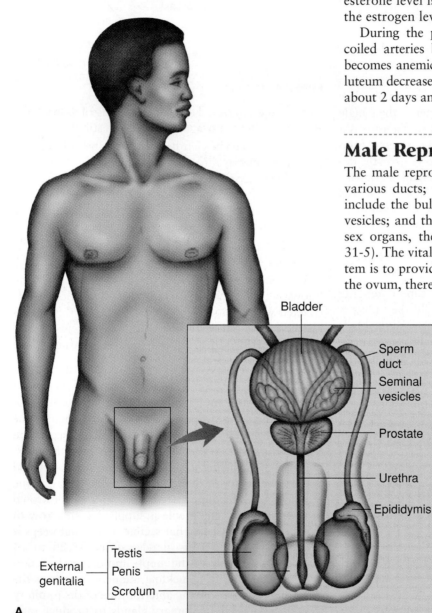

FIGURE 31-5 (A) The male reproductive system: sperm duct, seminal vesicles, prostate, urethra, epididymis, and external genitalia.

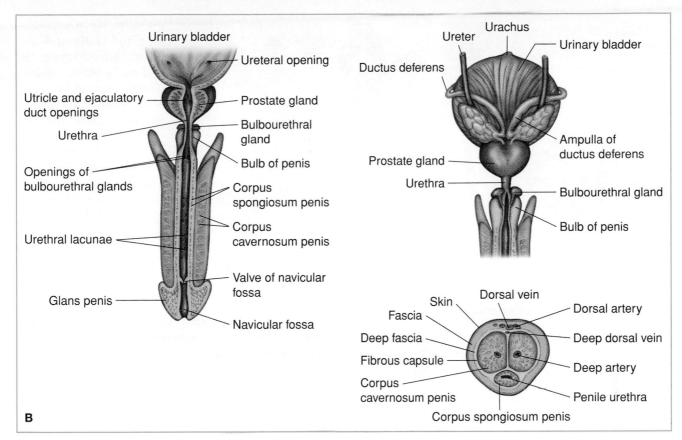

FIGURE 31-5 (B) The structures of the bladder, prostate gland, and penis.

The penis is the male external sex organ and is composed of erectile tissue and covered with skin. The size and shape of the penis varies with an average erect penis being about 15 to 20 cm in length. There are three longitudinal columns of erectile tissues capable of significant enlargement when engorged with blood, such as during sexual stimulation. Two of these columns are called the *corpora cavernosa penis*. The third column is called the *corpus spongiosum*. The corpus spongiosum extends at its distal end into the glans penis, the cone-shaped head at the end of the penis, and the site of the urethral orifice. The penis is covered with a loose fold of skin called the foreskin or prepuce. The foreskin contains glands that secrete a lubricating fluid called smegma. During a procedure called a **circumcision**, the foreskin is removed. This is often performed for medical, cultural, or religious reasons.

The erectile state in the penis occurs when sexual stimulation causes large quantities of blood from dilated arteries supplying the penis to fill the cavernous spaces in the erectile tissue. When the arteries constrict, the pressure on the veins in the area is reduced, allowing more blood to leave the penis than can enter it, allowing it to return to its previous size. The functions of the penis are to serve as the male organ for intercourse or copulation, and as the site of the orifice for the elimination of urine and semen from the body.

Internal Organs

The two oval-shaped organs located in the scrotum are called the testes. Each testes is about 4 cm long and 2.5 cm wide. The interior of each is divided into about 250 wedge-shaped lobes by fibrous tissues. The seminiferous tubules are located within each lobe of the testes. This is the site of the development of the spermatozoa, the male reproductive cells (see Figure 31-6). Other cells within the testes produce the male sex hormone, testosterone. Testosterone is responsible for the development of the normal secondary sex characteristics during puberty. Testosterone also places a vital role in the erection process and is necessary for the reproductive act. Additionally, it also affects the growth of hair on the face, muscular development, and vocal timbre. The seminiferous tubules form a network in the testes and they connect with the efferent ductus to leave the testes and enter the epididymis.

Each testes is connected to the epididymis, a coiled tube lying in the posterior aspect of the testes. Each epididymis is between 13 and 20 feet in length, but is coiled into a space that is less than 5 cm in length, and ends at the ductus deferens. The function of the epididymis is the maturation of sperm and is the first part of the duct system through which the sperm pass in their travels to the urethra.

The ductus deferens (vas deferens) is a slim, muscular tube that is about 45 cm in length and is continuous

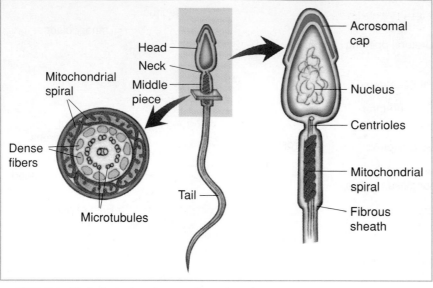

FIGURE 31-6 The basic structure of a spermatozoon (sperm).

Prostate Gland

The prostate gland is about 4 cm wide and weighs about 20 grams. It wraps around the urethra, similar to a donut wrapping around a straw. It is composed of glandular, connective, and muscular tissue and lies behind the urinary bladder. It surrounds the first 2.5 cm of the urethra and secretes an alkaline fluid that aids in maintaining the viability of the spermatozoa.

Bulbourethral Glands (Cowper's Glands)

The bulbourethral glands are two small, pea-sized glands located inferior to the prostate and on either side of the urethra. A 2.5-cm duct connects them with the wall of the urethra, where they can secrete a mucous secretion into the seminal fluid before ejaculation.

with the epididymis. It is the excretory duct of the testes and extends from the point adjacent to the testes and enters the abdomen at the inguinal canal. A duct from the seminal vesicle joins the ductus deferens at the inguinal canal. Between the testes and the internal inguinal ring (part of the abdomen), the ductus deferens is contained within a structure known as the spermatic cord. The spermatic cord also contains arteries, veins, lymphatic vessels, and nerves.

The two seminal vesicles are connected by a narrow duct to the ductus deferens, which then forms the ejaculatory duct, a short tube that penetrates the base of the prostate gland and opens into the prostate portion of the urethra. The seminal vesicles produce an alkaline fluid that becomes part of the seminal fluid or semen.

Urethra

The male urethra is approximately 20 cm long, and is divided into three sections: the prostatic, the membranous, and the penile. The urethra extends from the bladder to the urethral orifice at the end of the penis. The functions of the urethra in the male are the expulsion of urine and semen from the body.

Common Disorders Associated with the Female Reproductive System

Disorders that may affect the proper functioning of the reproductive system range from abnormal hormone secretion and breast diseases, to sexually transmitted infections, the presence of cancerous tissue in a region, and all inflammations, infections, and disorders in between. Many of those problems frequently affect fertility and the actual process of being able to reproduce. (see Table 31-1 lists common disorders and pathology of the female reproductive system).

Breast Cancer

Breast cancer is cancer arising in breast tissue (see Figure 31-7). Although it is primarily a disease of women, about 1 percent of breast cancers occur in men. It is the most common type of cancer in women and is the second leading cause of death by cancer in women, following only lung cancer.

The breasts are made of fat, glands, and connective (fibrous) tissue. They have several lobes, which are divided into lobules and end in the milk glands. Tiny ducts run from the many tiny glands, connect together, and end in

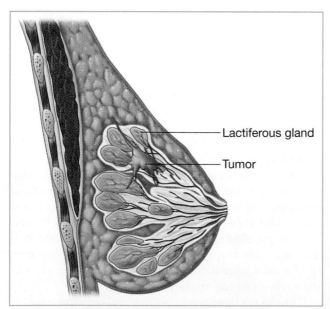

FIGURE 31-7 Breast cancer. Tumor is growing within a milk gland.

TABLE 31-1 Disorders of the Female Reproductive System

Disorder	Description
Abruptio placenta	An emergency condition in which the placenta tears away from the uterine wall before the 20th week of pregnancy. This requires immediate delivery of the baby.
Amenorrhea	An absence of menstruation, which can be the result of many factors, including pregnancy, menopause, and dieting.
Breech presentation	Position of the fetus within the uterus in which the buttocks or feet are presented first for delivery rather than the head.
Carcinoma *in situ*	Malignant tumor that has not extended beyond the original site.
Cervical cancer	A malignant growth in the cervix of the uterus. This is an especially difficult type of cancer to treat, and causes 5 percent of the cancer deaths in women. Pap tests have helped to detect early cervical cancer.
Cervical polyps	Fibrous or mucous tumor or growth found in the cervix of the uterus. These are removed surgically if there is a danger that they will become malignant.
Cervicitis	Inflammation of the cervix of the uterus.
Choriocarcinoma	A rare type of cancer of the uterus that may occur following a normal pregnancy or abortion.
Condyloma	A wart-like growth on the external genitalia.
Cystocele	Hernia or outpouching of the bladder that protrudes into the vagina. This may cause urinary frequency and urgency.
Dysmenorrhea	Painful cramping that is associated with menstruation.
Eclampsia	Convulsive seizures and coma occurring between the 20th week of pregnancy and the first week of postpartum.
Ectopic	A fetus that becomes abnormally implanted outside the uterine cavity. This is a condition requiring immediate surgery.
Endometrial cancer	Cancer of the endometrial lining of the uterus.
Fibroid tumor	Benign tumor or growth that contains fiber-like tissue. Uterine fibroid tumors are the most common tumors in women.
Mastitis	Inflammation of the breast, which is common during lactation but can occur at any age.
Menorrhagia	Excessive bleeding during the menstrual period. Can be either in the total number of days or the amount of blood or both.
Ovarian carcinoma	Cancer of the ovary.
Ovarian cyst	Sac that develops within the ovary.
Pelvic inflammatory disease (PID)	Any inflammation of the female reproductive organs, generally bacterial in nature.
Placenta previa	When the placenta has become attached to the lower portion of the uterus and, in turn, blocks the birth canal.

(continued)

TABLE 31-1 **Disorders of the Female Reproductive System** *(continued)*

Disorder	Description
Preeclampsia	Toxemia of pregnancy that if untreated can result in true eclampsia. Symptoms include hypertension, headaches, albumin in the urine, and edema.
Premature birth	Delivery in which the infant (neonate) is born before the 37th week of gestation (pregnancy).
Premenstrual syndrome (PMS)	Symptoms that develop just prior to the onset of a menstrual period, which can include irritability, headache, tender breasts, and anxiety.
Prolapsed uterus	A fallen uterus that can cause the cervix to protrude through the vaginal opening. It is generally caused by weakened muscles from vaginal delivery or as a result of pelvic tumors pressing down.
Rh factor	A condition that can develop in a baby when the mother's blood type is Rh negative and the father's is Rh positive. The baby's red blood cells can be destroyed as a result of this condition. Treatment is early diagnosis and blood transfusion.
Salpingitis	Inflammation of the fallopian tube or tubes.
Spontaneous abortion	Loss of a fetus without any artificial aid. Also called a miscarriage.
Stillbirth	Birth in which the fetus dies before or at the time of delivery.
Toxic shock syndrome	Rare and sometimes fatal staphylococcus infection that generally occurs in menstruating women.
Tubal pregnancy	Implantation of a fetus within the fallopian tube instead of the uterus. This requires immediate surgery.
Vaginitis	Inflammation of the vagina, generally caused by a microorganism.

the nipple. These ducts are where 80 percent of breast cancers occur. Cancer may also develop in the lobules. Another type of breast cancer is inflammatory breast cancer. The most serious cancers are metastatic cancers, meaning that the cancer has spread from the place where it started into other tissues. The most common place for breast cancer to metastasize is into the lymph nodes under the arm or above the collarbone on the same side as the cancer. Other common sites of breast cancer metastasis are the brain, the bones, and the liver.

Family history has long been known to be a risk factor for breast cancer. The risk is highest if the affected relative developed breast cancer at a young age or if she is a close relative such as a mother, sister, daughter, or aunt. Hormonal influences also play a role in the development of breast cancer. Women who start their periods at an early age or experience a late menopause have a higher risk of developing breast cancer. Conversely, being older at your first menstrual period and early menopause tend to protect one from breast cancer.

Early breast cancer has no symptoms, and it is not painful. Most breast cancer is discovered before symptoms are present, either by finding an abnormality on a mammography or feeling a breast lump. A lump located under the arm or above the collarbone that does not go away may be an indication of the presence of breast cancer. Other possible symptoms are breast discharge, nipple inversion, or changes in the skin overlying the breast.

Most breast lumps are not cancerous; however, all breast lumps should be evaluated by a physician. Breast discharge is a common problem and is rarely a symptom of cancer. Discharge is of most concern if it is from only one breast or if it is bloody. In any case, all breast discharge should also be evaluated. Nipple inversion is a common variant of normal nipples, but nipple inversion that is a new development can be of concern. And any changes in the skin of the breast that include redness, changes in texture, and puckering should also be evaluated.

In this disease, patient preference plays a major role in decisions regarding treatment, and treatment depends on several factors, including the type of breast cancer, the hormone receptor status of the tumor, the stage of the tumor, the size of the breast, and the person's general health, age, and menstrual status (has or has not been through menopause). Radiation therapy is used to kill tumor cells if there are any left after surgery. Chemotherapy may also be used to kill the cancer cells or stop them from growing. Hormonal therapy may also be given.

Surgery is the mainstay and, in many cases, the best form of therapy for breast cancer. The choice as to which type of surgery is based on a number of factors, including the size and location of the tumor, the type of tumor, and the person's overall health and personal wishes. Breast-sparing surgery, such as a lumpectomy, is often possible. Other more radical treatment may include a simple mastectomy, a modified radical mastectomy, and, in the most severe cases, a radical mastectomy, which is complete removal of the breast.

Cervical Cancer

Cervical cancer is the rapid, uncontrolled growth of severely abnormal cells on the cervix. There are two main types of cervical cancer: squamous cell (epidermoid) cervical cancer and adenocarcinoma cervical cancer. Fortunately, when detected at an early stage, cervical cancer is highly curable. Pap test screening, when done regularly, is the single most important tool for preventing cervical cancer because it can detect abnormal cervical cell changes before they become cancerous, when treatment is most effective.

Several factors may play a role in causing cervical cancer. These include smoking or a history of smoking, having an impaired immune system, such as from having human immunodeficiency virus (HIV) or human papillomavirus (HPV), and using birth control pills for more than 5 years.

Because abnormal cervical cell changes rarely cause symptoms, it is important to have regular Pap test screening. As cervical cell changes progress to cervical cancer, symptoms may develop. These often include abnormal vaginal bleeding or a significant unexplained change in your menstrual cycle pain during sexual intercourse, and abnormal vaginal discharge containing mucus that may be tinged with blood. Symptoms that may occur when cervical cancer has progressed may include anemia because of abnormal vaginal bleeding, ongoing pelvic, leg, or back pain, urinary problems because of blockage of a kidney or ureter, leakage of urine or fecal content into the vagina because an abnormal opening (fistula) has developed between the vagina and the bladder or rectum, and weight loss.

Cervical cancer detected in its early stages can be cured with treatment and close follow-up. The treatment may include surgery to remove the cancer, radiation therapy to treat other organs affected by the cancer, or chemotherapy to treat cancer that has spread or metastasized. The treatment may be a single

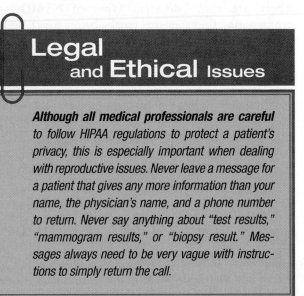

Cultural Considerations

It should never be assumed that a patient is going to seek curative measures when diagnosed with a specific syndrome. Some cultures do not condone treatment for cancer or other disorders for personal or religious reasons, and the medical assistant must respect, and not judge, the individual for his or her choice. This can be difficult to do, especially when the diagnosis is an easily cured disorder. It is the patient's choice, and not the medical assistant's.

therapy or a combination of any of these. The choice of treatment and the long-term outcome depend on the type and stage of cancer. A person's age, overall health, quality of life, and desire to be able to have children are almost always considered.

Cervicitis

Cervicitis is an inflammation of the cervix. Most cases are caused by infection with sexually transmitted infections, including gonorrhea and chlamydia. Most often, there are no signs and symptoms, and the patient may first learn of the condition as a result of a Pap test or a biopsy for another condition. If symptoms are present, they may include vaginal discharge that is grayish or yellow, possibly with an odor; frequent, painful urination; pain during intercourse; and vaginal bleeding after intercourse, between menstrual periods, or after menopause.

Legal and Ethical Issues

Although all medical professionals are careful to follow HIPAA regulations to protect a patient's privacy, this is especially important when dealing with reproductive issues. Never leave a message for a patient that gives any more information than your name, the physician's name, and a phone number to return. Never say anything about "test results," "mammogram results," or "biopsy result." Messages always need to be very vague with instructions to simply return the call.

Successful treatment of cervicitis involves addressing the cause of the inflammation. In most cases, antibiotics are used to clear an underlying bacterial infection. If the cause is viral, such as genital herpes, the treatment is an antiviral medication. However, antiviral medication does not cure herpes, which is a chronic condition. The person's sexual partner may also be treated to prevent reinfection.

Dysmenorrhea

Dysmenorrhea is the presence of painful cramps during menstruation. More than half of all girls and women suffer from some form of dysmenorrhea, which is often associated with a dull or throbbing pain that usually centers in the lower midabdomen, radiating toward the lower back or thighs. Menstruating women of any age can experience cramps, and while the pain may be only mild for some women, others may experience severe discomfort that can significantly interfere with everyday activities for several days each month.

In addition to cramping, some women may experience nausea and vomiting, diarrhea, irritability, sweating, or dizziness. Cramps usually last for 2 or 3 days at the beginning of each menstrual period, and many women often notice their painful periods disappear after they have their first child. This is probably due to the stretching of the opening of the uterus or because the birth improves the uterine blood supply and muscle activity.

Dysmenorrhea is controlled by treating the underlying disorder. This may include the use of nonsteroidal anti-inflammatory drugs (NSAIDs), which prevent or decrease the formation of prostaglandins. For more severe pain, prescription-strength ibuprofen (Motrin) is available. These drugs are usually begun at the first sign of the period and taken for a day or two. There are many different types of NSAIDs, and women may find that one works better for them than the others.

New studies of a drug patch containing glyceryl trinitrate to treat dysmenorrhea suggest that it also may help ease pain. Other treatments may include simply changing the position of the body, changes in dietary intake of fibers, fats, calcium, and carbohydrates, and using visualization and guided imagery to help relieve and ease the cramps. Aromatherapy and massage may ease pain for some women. Others find that imagining a white light hovering over the painful area can actually lessen the pain for brief periods. Acupuncture and Chinese herbs are other popular alternative treatments for cramps.

Endometriosis

Endometriosis occurs when the endometrium, which is the tissue that lines the inside of the uterus, travels outside the uterus. In a women with endometriosis, the tissue is found in the pelvis or abdominal cavity. This tissue reacts to the changing levels of estrogen, but cannot be sloughed off with the tissues inside the uterus. This tissue still causes bleeding and forms scars and adhesions. Typically, this is what causes daily or monthly cyclic pain.

Symptoms of endometriosis include blood in the urine, difficulty urinating, dyspareunia (painful intercourse), heavy menstrual bleeding, irregular periods, nausea and vomiting, pelvic pain after intercourse or exercise, and dysmenorrhea. The symptoms of endometriosis tend to decrease after menopause, when the involved tissues shrink.

Although the cause of endometriosis is unknown, several theories have been proposed. One theory is that delayed childbearing increases the risk for endometriosis. Another is that during menstruation, some of the endometrial tissue backs up through the fallopian tubes into the abdomen. Genetics may also play a role.

Early diagnosis and treatment may limit cell growth and help prevent adhesions, while pregnancy, oral contraceptives, and other hormones seem to delay its onset. Treatment with medication focuses on treating the discomfort. Surgery is generally reserved for women with severe endometriosis. Conservative surgery will attempt to remove or destroy all of the endometriotic tissue existing outside the uterus, remove adhesions, and restore the pelvic anatomy. More extensive surgery will be done for women with severe symptoms or disease and no desire to bear children. Typically, a total **hysterectomy** (removal of the uterus, ovaries and fallopian tubes along with any adhesions) will be performed. Hormonal replacement will be lifelong after the removal of the ovaries.

Fibrocystic Breast Disease

Fibrocystic breast disease involves common, benign changes in the tissues of the breast (see Figure 31-8). The condition is so commonly found in normal breasts, it is believed to be a normal variant. Other related terms that refer to this disorder include mammary dysplasia, benign breast disease, and diffuse cystic mastopathy. The cause is not completely understood; however, the changes are believed to be associated with ovarian hormones since the condition usually subsides with menopause and may vary in consistency during the menstrual cycle.

The incidence of fibrocystic breast disease is estimated to be more than 60 percent of all women. It is common in women between the ages of 30 and 50, and rare in postmenopausal women. The risk factors may include family history and diet. Symptoms may range from mild to severe, and frequently include a dense, irregular and bumpy "cobblestone" consistency in the breast tissue, breast discomfort that is persistent or that occurs intermittently, and a feeling of fullness in the breasts. There may also be premenstrual tenderness and swelling and nipple sensation changes, such as itching.

Treatment of this disorder often involves self-care, dietary restrictions to eliminate caffeine, performing a breast self-exam monthly, and wearing a well-fitted bra to provide good breast support. Oral contraceptives may also be prescribed because they often decrease the symptoms.

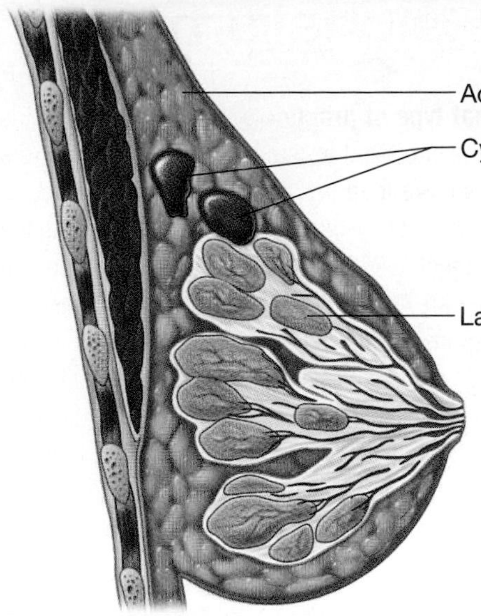

Ovarian Cancer

Ovarian cancer starts in the cells of the ovary or ovaries. There are three main types of ovarian cancer, depending on the type of cell where the cancer starts: epithelial cell cancer, which starts in the outer covering of the ovary and is the most common type of ovarian cancer; germ cell tumors that start in the egg cells within the ovary and generally occur in younger women, even in children; and stromal tumors, which start in the cells that form the structural framework of the ovary. Ovarian cancer can develop for a long time without causing any signs or symptoms. When symptoms do start, they are often vague and easily mistaken for more common illnesses. Most women with ovarian cancer have advanced disease at the time of their diagnosis.

Symptoms of early-stage ovarian cancer frequently include mild abdominal discomfort or pain, abdominal swelling, change in bowel habits, feeling full after a light meal, indigestion, gas, an upset stomach, a feeling that the bowel has not completely emptied, nausea and vomiting, constant tiredness, pain in lower back or leg, abnormal menstrual or vaginal bleeding, more frequent urination, and pain during intercourse. Symptoms of advanced ovarian cancer may cause a buildup of fluid in the abdomen, shortness of breath and a dry persistent cough, nausea and vomiting, abdominal tumors, and weight loss.

Treatment is based on the type, grade, and stage of the cancer, and it may include surgery to remove the tumor and some surrounding tissue, radiation therapy, and chemotherapy. Complementary therapies, such as medi-

FIGURE 31-8 Fibrocystic breast disease.

- Adipose
- Cysts
- Lactiferous gland

tation and supportive therapies, are also encouraged as part of the treatment for ovarian cancer. Alternative therapies, such as traditional Chinese medicines or special diets, are sometimes used; however, their effectiveness in the treatment of cancer is not completely known.

Ovarian Cysts

Ovarian cysts are sacs filled with fluid or a semisolid material that develops on or within the ovary. Typically, ovarian cysts are not disease related and disappear on their own. During the days preceding ovulation, a follicle grows. At the time of expected ovulation, the follicle fails to rupture and release an egg. Instead of being reabsorbed, the fluid within the follicle persists and forms a cyst. Functional cysts usually disappear within 60 days without treatment and are relatively common. They occur most often during childbearing years, that is, puberty to menopause, but may occur at any time. No known risk factors have been identified. Functional ovarian cysts should not to be confused with other disease conditions involving ovarian cysts, specifically benign cysts of different types that must be treated to resolve, true ovarian

Patient Education

When caring for a patient dealing with a disorder or a condition of the reproductive system, the medical assistant has a responsibility to be knowledgeable about the structures affected by these disorders and, just as important, to be knowledgeable about the emotional and psychosocial aspects associated with many of these disorders. As a member of the health care team, your role is to provide the patient with basic information that will assist him or her in understanding how to live with the situation. Oftentimes, this involves teaching the patient about lifestyle changes, nutrition, and how to deal with change and new challenges that directly affect their lifestyles.

Professionalism

tumors, including ovarian cancer, or hormonal conditions such as polycystic ovarian disease.

Oftentimes, there are no symptoms; however, if symptoms are present, they generally include constant, dull aching pelvic pain, pain with intercourse or pelvic pain during movement, pelvic pain shortly after beginning or ending a menstrual period, and abdominal bloating or distention.

Functional ovarian cysts generally disappear within 60 days without any treatment. Oral contraceptive pills may be prescribed to help establish normal cycles and decrease the development of functional ovarian cysts. Ovarian cysts that do not appear to be functional may require surgical removal by laparoscopy or exploratory laparotomy. Surgical removal is often necessary if a cyst is larger than 6 cm or that persists for longer than 6 weeks. Other medical treatment may be recommended if other disorders are found to be the cause of ovarian cysts, such as polycystic ovary disease.

Pelvic Inflammatory Disease

The most common and serious complication of sexually transmitted infections (STIs) among women is **pelvic inflammatory disease (PID)**. This condition is an infection of the upper genital area and occurs when disease-carrying organisms migrate upward from the urethra and cervix into the upper genital area. PID can affect the uterus, ovaries, and fallopian tubes. If untreated this disease can cause scarring, which can lead to infertility, tubal pregnancy, chronic pelvic pain, and other serious consequences.

Many different organisms can cause PID, but most cases are associated with gonorrhea and genital chlamydial infections, two common STIs. After a period of time, the infection spreads to other cells and organs, causing more infection and scarring.

The major symptoms of PID are lower abdominal pain and abnormal vaginal discharge. Other symptoms such as fever, pain in the right upper quadrant, painful intercourse, and irregular menstrual bleeding may also be present. PID may be very painful, or may have few if any symptoms even though it can seriously damage the reproductive organs.

Premenstrual Syndrome

Premenstrual syndrome (PMS) is a condition affecting women that may cause annoying symptoms including constipation, diarrhea, nausea, anorexia, appetite cravings, headache, backache, muscular aches, edema, insomnia, clumsiness, malaise, irritability, indecisiveness, mental confusion, and depression. There is no specific known cause, but it is believed that there is a relationship to the amount of prostaglandin and estrogen produced (see Figure 31-9). It is estimated that 85 percent of women who menstruate are affected by PMS. However, only 5 to 10 percent of menstruating women are severely impaired by PMS. There is no known reason why some women are affected, while others are not.

Some recommendations may help to decrease the severity of PMS symptoms. These include eating a healthy diet high in vegetables and fruits and low in starches, sugars, sodium, fat, caffeine, and alcohol; performing regular aerobic exercise; including enough vitamins and minerals, especially B vitamins, calcium, and magnesium in the diet; and using relaxation therapy and stress management techniques. Some herbal treatments have also been reported as helpful, including chasteberry and black cohosh. Medications may be used to help decrease and control the symptoms of PMS as well.

Sexually Transmitted Infections

Sexually transmitted infection (STI) is a term used to describe more than 20 different infections that are transmitted through exchange of semen, blood, and other body fluids; or by direct contact with the affected body areas of people with STIs. Sexually transmitted infections are also called venereal diseases. The Centers for Disease Control and Prevention (CDC) has reported

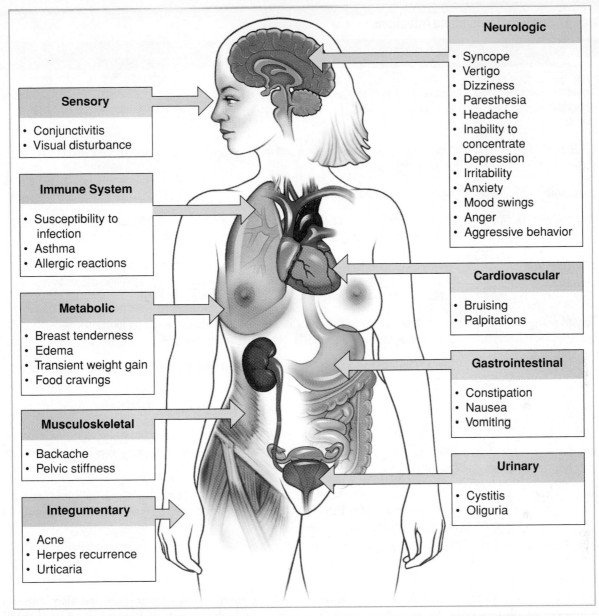

Sensory
- Conjunctivitis
- Visual disturbance

Immune System
- Susceptibility to infection
- Asthma
- Allergic reactions

Metabolic
- Breast tenderness
- Edema
- Transient weight gain
- Food cravings

Musculoskeletal
- Backache
- Pelvic stiffness

Integumentary
- Acne
- Herpes recurrence
- Urticaria

Neurologic
- Syncope
- Vertigo
- Dizziness
- Paresthesia
- Headache
- Inability to concentrate
- Depression
- Irritability
- Anxiety
- Mood swings
- Anger
- Aggressive behavior

Cardiovascular
- Bruising
- Palpitations

Gastrointestinal
- Constipation
- Nausea
- Vomiting

Urinary
- Cystitis
- Oliguria

FIGURE 31-9   Multisystem effects of premenstrual syndrome.

that 85 percent of the most prevalent infectious diseases in the United States are sexually transmitted. The rate of STIs in this country is 50 to 100 times higher than that of any other industrialized nation. One in four sexually active Americans will be affected by an STI at some time in his or her life. They can have very painful long-term consequences as well as immediate health problems. They can cause birth defects, blindness, bone deformities, brain damage, cancer, heart disease, infertility and other abnormalities of the reproductive system, mental retardation, and death. Some of the most common and potentially serious STIs in the United States include chlamydia, human papillomavirus (HPV), genital herpes, gonorrhea, syphilis, and HIV infection.

The symptoms of STIs vary somewhat according to the disease agent, the sex of the patient, and the body systems affected. Some are easy to identify, while others produce infections that may either go unnoticed for some time or are easy to confuse with other diseases. Syphilis in particular can be confused with disorders ranging from infectious mononucleosis to allergic reactions to prescription medications. In addition, the incubation period of STIs varies. Some produce symptoms close enough to the time of sexual contact, often less than 48 hours. Others may have an even longer incubation period, so that the patient may not recognize the early symptoms as those of a sexually transmitted infection. Some symptoms of STIs that affect the genitals and reproductive organs include bleeding not associated with menstruating, abnormal vaginal discharge, vaginal burning, itching, pain in the pelvic area while having sex, discharge from the tip of the penis, swelling of the lymph nodes near the groin area, and in males and females, painful or burning sensations when urinating.

TABLE 31-2 Sexually Transmitted Infections

Disease	Description
Acquired immune deficiency syndrome (AIDS)	The final stage of infection from the human immunodeficiency virus (HIV). At present there is no cure.
Candidiasis	A yeast-like infection of the skin and mucous membranes that can result in white plaques on the tongue and vagina.
Chancroid	Highly infectious nonsyphilitic ulcer.
Chlamydial infection	Parasitic microorganism causing genital infections in males and females. Can lead to pelvic inflammatory disease (PID) in females and eventual infertility.
Genital herpes	Growths and elevations of warts on the genitalia of both males and females that can lead to cancer of the cervix in females. These painful vesicles on the skin and mucosa erupt periodically and can be transmitted through the placenta or at birth.
Genital warts	Growths and elevations of warts on the genitalia of both males and females that can lead to cancer of the cervix in females. There is currently no cure.
Gonorrhea	Sexually transmitted inflammation of the mucous membranes of either sex. Can be passed on to an infant during the birth process.
Hepatitis	Infectious, inflammatory disease of the liver. Hepatitis B and C types are spread by contact with blood and bodily fluids of an infected person.
Syphilis	Infectious, chronic, venereal disease that can involve any organ. May exist for years without symptoms.
Trichomoniasis	Genitourinary infection that is usually without symptoms (asymptomatic) in both males and females. In women the disease can produce itching and/or burning, a foul-smelling discharge, and results in vaginitis.

Both men and women may also develop skin rashes, sores, bumps, or blisters near the mouth or genitals. Other symptoms of STIs are systemic, which means that they affect the body as a whole. These symptoms may include fever, chills, and similar flu-like symptoms, skin rashes over large parts of the body, arthritis-like pains or aching in the joints, and throat swelling and redness that lasts for 3 weeks or longer.

Although self-care can relieve some of the pain and symptoms of STIs, other symptoms often require immediate medical attention, such as antibiotics, which are used to treat gonorrhea, chlamydia, syphilis, and other STIs caused by bacteria. What is most important to note is that the risk of becoming infected with an STI can be reduced or eliminated by changing certain personal behaviors. Abstaining from sexual relations or maintaining a mutually monogamous relationship with a partner are considered legitimate options. Avoiding sexual contact with partners who are known to be infected with an STI, whose health status is unknown, who abuse drugs, or who are involved in prostitution are also considered ways in which the risk of becoming infected with an STI can be decreased or eradicated completely. (See Table 31-2 for more information about sexually transmitted infections.)

Uterine Cancer

Uterine cancer (endometrial cancer) starts in the cells of the lining of the uterus. In most cases, it develops in the glandular tissue of the endometrium and is called adenocarcinoma. If the cancer is found and treated early, treatment is usually very successful. There is no single cause of uterine cancer; however, some factors appear to increase the risk of developing it. These include age, particularly in women over 50, obesity, childlessness, reaching menopause later than average, prolonged use of medications with the hormone estrogen, and the taking of the drug tamoxifen.

Many of the signs and symptoms of uterine cancer may be associated with other disorders of the female reproductive system. These frequently include bleeding between menstrual periods, heavy bleeding or spotting during periods or after menopause, bleeding after intercourse, and a foul discharge. Other symptoms may include a yellow watery discharge, cramping pain, pressure in the abdomen or pelvis, back, or legs, and discomfort over the pubic area.

Treatment of uterine cancer will depend on the type, grade, and stage of the cancer. These treatments may include any one, or a combination of, surgery, radiation therapy, or chemotherapy.

Uterine Fibroids

Uterine fibroids are benign growths or tumors made up of muscle cells and other tissues that grow within the wall of the uterus (see Figure 31-10). Fibroids can grow as a single growth or as a cluster of tumors. They can be seed sized or the size of a grapefruit. They are common in women of childbearing age, and African-American women are more likely to get them than women of other racial groups. African-American women also tend to get fibroids at an earlier age than do women of other races. There also appears to be a higher risk for fibroids with women who are overweight or obese. Women who have given birth appear to be at a lower risk for fibroids. There is no known cause of uterine fibroids and they can be frustrating to endure because there are few treatment options.

The symptoms that may occur with uterine fibroids include heavy bleeding or painful periods; bleeding between periods, feeling of fullness in the pelvic area, frequent urination, pain during sex, lower back pain, and reproductive problems, including infertility or early onset of labor. Although the cause of fibroids is unknown, it may be a combination of hormones, genetics and environmental factors. Fibroids usually shrink or disappear after menopause, but not always.

Patients who have mild symptoms may only require over-the-counter medications for pain relief and relief of inflammation. Those who require more relief may require *gonadotropin releasing hormone agonists* (GnRHa). These drugs will decrease the size of the fibroids. Side effects can include hot flashes, depression, insomnia, decreased libido, and joint pain. *Antihormonal* agents may stop or slow the growth of fibroids. These drugs only offer temporary relief from the symptoms of the fibroids, because the symptoms will restart as soon the therapy is discontinued.

Two types of surgery are used to treat fibroids. A **myomectomy** removes the fibroids without taking the healthy tissue of the uterus. This may be done either by laparotomy or as an open surgery. A hysterectomy removes the entire uterus.

Vaginitis

Vaginitis is an inflammation of the vagina that can result in discharge, itching, or pain. The cause is usually

a change in the normal balance of vaginal bacteria or an infection. Vaginitis can also result from reduced estrogen levels after menopause. The most common types of vaginitis are bacterial vaginitis, yeast infections, trichomoniasis, and atrophic vaginitis. The signs and symptoms of vaginitis may include any change in color, odor, or amount of discharge from the vagina, vaginal itching or irritation, pain during intercourse, painful urination, and light vaginal bleeding.

Treatment depends on the type of vaginitis, present. For bacterial vaginitis, vaginal gels or creams may be prescribed. Yeast infections are usually treated with

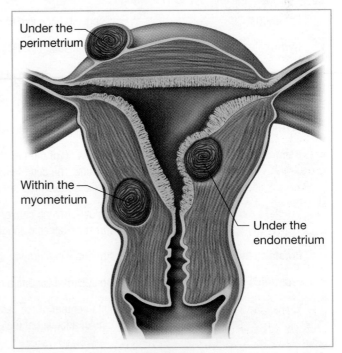

Under the perimetrium

Within the myometrium

Under the endometrium

FIGURE 31-10 Types of uterine fibroid tumors.

antifungal creams or suppositories. Trichomoniasis is frequently treated with Flagyl (metronidazole). And atrophic vaginitis is generally treated with estrogen.

Common Disorders Associated with the Male Reproductive System

The male reproductive system is essential to reproduction. It is also related to the male excretion, or urinary, system, and many of the disorders affect both systems. Conditions range from inflammatory, such as epididymitis, and infectious diseases, such as those classified as STIs, to other, more life-threatening diseases and disorders such as prostate cancer and testicular cancer. (See Table 31-3 for more information about disorders of the male reproductive system.)

Benign Prostatic Hyperplasia

Benign prostatic hyperplasia (BPH), also known as benign prostatic hypertrophy, is an enlargement of the

TABLE 31-3 Disorders of the Male Reproductive System

Disorder	Description
Anorchism	A congenital absence of one or both testes.
Aspermia	The lack of, or failure to, eject sperm.
Azoospermia	Absence of sperm in the semen.
Balanitis	Inflammation of the skin covering the glans penis.
Benign prostatic hypertrophy	Enlargement of the prostate gland commonly seen in males over age 50.
Carcinoma of the testes	Cancer of one or both testes.
Cryptorchidism	Failure of the testes to descend into the scrotal sac before birth. Generally, the testes will descend permanently before the boy is 1 year old. A surgical procedure called an orchidopecy may be required to bring the testes down into the scrotum permanently and secure them permanently. Failure of the testes to descend could result in sterility in the male.
Epididymitis	Inflammation of the epididymis that causes pain and swelling in the inguinal area.
Epispadias	Congenital opening of the male urethra on the dorsal surface of the penis.
Hydrocele	Accumulation of fluid within the testes.
Hypospadias	Congenital opening of the male urethra on the underside of the penis.
Impotence	Inability to copulate due to inability to maintain an erection or to achieve orgasm.
Perineum	In the male, the external region between the scrotum and the anus.
Phimosis	Narrowing of the foreskin over the glans penis that results in difficulty with hygiene. The condition can lead to infection or difficulty with urination. The condition is treated with circumcision, the surgical removal of the foreskin.
Prostate cancer	A slow-growing cancer that affects a large number of males after age 50. The PSA (prostate-specific antigen) test is used to assist in early detection of this disease.
Prostatic hyperplasia	Abnormal cell growth within the prostate.
Prostatitis	An inflamed condition of the prostate gland that may be the result of infection.
Varicocele	Enlargement of the veins of the spermatic cord that commonly occurs on the left side of adolescent males. This seldom needs treatment.

prostate gland that may occur in men who are 50 years of age and older (see Figure 31-11). By age 60, four out of five men may have an enlarged prostate. As the prostate enlarges, it compresses the urethra, thereby restricting the normal flow of urine. The restriction generally causes a number of symptoms, including a condition known as prostatism. Prostatism is any collection of the prostate gland that interferes with the flow of urine from the bladder.

Symptoms usually include a weak or hard-to-start urine stream; a feeling that the bladder is not empty; a need to urinate often, especially at night; a feeling of urgency (the sudden need to urinate right away); abdominal straining; interruption of the stream; acute urinary retention; and recurrent urinary infections.

Treatment for BPH may include drug therapy, nonsurgical procedures, and surgery. Medications either work by reducing the size of the prostate (finasteride) or by relaxing the smooth muscle of the prostate and the bladder neck to improve urine flow and reduce bladder outlet obstruction.

Epididymitis

Epididymitis is an inflammation or infection of the epididymis, which is the long coiled tube attached to the upper part of each testicle, and where mature sperm are stored before ejaculation. It is the most common cause of pain in the scrotum. The acute form is usually associated with the most severe pain and swelling. If symptoms last for more than 6 weeks after treatment begins, the condition is considered chronic.

Epididymitis can occur any time after the onset of puberty, but is most common between the ages of 18 and 40. Factors that increase the risk of developing epididymitis include infection of the bladder, kidney, prostate, or urinary tract, the presence of other recent illness, a narrowing of the urethra, and use of a urethral catheter.

Although epididymitis can be caused by the same organisms that cause some STIs or occur after prostate surgery, the condition is generally due to pus-generating bacteria associated with infections in other parts of the body. It can also be caused by injury or infection of the scrotum or by irritation from urine that has accumulated in the vas deferens. It is characterized by sudden redness and swelling of the scrotum. The affected testicle is hard and sore, and the other testicle may feel tender. The patient has chills and fever and usually has acute **urethritis**, or inflammation of the urethra. Enlarged lymph nodes in the groin may also cause scrotal pain that intensifies throughout the day and may become so severe that walking normally becomes impossible.

Because this disorder that affects both testicles can make a man sterile, antibiotic therapy must be initiated as soon as symptoms appear. To prevent reinfection, medication must be taken exactly as prescribed, even if

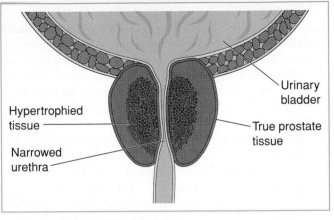

FIGURE 31-11   Benign prostatic hyperplasia.

the patient's symptoms disappear or he begins to feel better. Over-the-counter anti-inflammatories can relieve pain but should not be used without the approval of a family physician or urologist. Bed rest is also recommended until symptoms subside, and patients are advised to wear athletic supporters when they resume normal activities. If pain is severe, a local anesthetic such as lidocaine (Xylocaine) may be injected directly into the spermatic cord.

Erectile Dysfunction

Erectile dysfunction (ED) is the inability to achieve or maintain an erection sufficient for sexual intercourse. It occurs when not enough blood is supplied to the penis, when the smooth muscle in the penis fails to relax, or when the penis does not retain the blood that flows into it. According to studies at the National Institutes of Health, 5 percent of men have some degree of erectile dysfunction at age 40, and approximately 15 to 25 percent at age 65 and older. Although the likelihood of erectile dysfunction increases with age, it is not an inevitable part of aging. About 80 percent of erectile dysfunction has a physical cause that can be addressed.

Risk factors for ED include hypertension, hyperlipidemia, endocrine disorders, low testosterone, thyroid disease, diabetes, coronary artery disease, peripheral vascular disease, anemia, medications, smoking, alcohol abuse, surgical procedures, neurological conditions, and psychiatric illness.

ED can affect relationships and men should discuss the issue with their partners as well as seek medical advice. A medical evaluation is done when a man expresses his concern about his condition with his physician. Underlying causative factors should be treated.

Treatment may include medication therapy, medication changes, or other treatments that include devices (the vacuum constriction device), urethral and penile injection therapies, and surgical therapies, including a penile prosthesis.

Hydrocele

A hydrocele is a painless buildup of watery fluid around one or both testicles that causes the scrotum or groin area to swell. Although this swelling may be unsightly and uncomfortable, it is not painful and generally is not dangerous. A hydrocele can be present at birth (congenital) or can develop after birth (acquired). With a congenital hydrocele, the normal process of testicle migration and closure of the space around the testicles is interrupted. The space may not close, or the closure may be delayed. A hydrocele occurs when fluid from the abdominal cavity fills this space.

The symptom of a congenital hydrocele is a swollen scrotum or groin area. The scrotum may have a bluish tinge. The swelling is painless, may be soft or firm, and cannot be reduced by changing its position or gently pushing it up. It may also be small in the morning and gradually increase in size throughout the day, and may be translucent. If pain is present, it may indicate the presence of an inguinal hernia, injury to the testicles, or some other problem.

For a congenital hydrocele that remains the same size or gets smaller, aggressive treatment is not recommended. It generally will go away by age 1 or 2. The focus should be on watching the hydrocele for any changes. However, surgery generally is necessary if a hydrocele varies in size, does not go away by the age of 1 or 2, comes and goes, or feels firm.

Prostate Cancer

Prostate cancer is a malignant tumor that grows in the prostate gland. It is the most common cancer found in American men. By age 50, one in four American men have some cancerous cells in the prostate gland. By age 80, the ratio increases to one in two. The average age of diagnosis is 70. Prostate cancer is the second leading cause of cancer death in men, exceeded only by lung cancer. However, only 1 in 32 men with a diagnosis of cancer actually dies from prostate cancer.

Prostate cancer can grow slowly for many years, but it occasionally will grow quickly and spread (metastasize) to other parts of the body. Men may or may not have symptoms of prostate cancer. For those who do, the more common symptoms are dull pain in the lower pelvic area; general pain in the lower back, hips, and upper thighs; blood in the urine or semen; dribbling when urinating; erectile dysfunction; frequent urination, especially at night; painful urination and/or ejaculation; smaller stream of urine or urgent need to urinate; and loss of appetite and weight. If the cancer has spread to other parts of the body, there may be persistent bone pain, occasional nerve loss, or a loss of bladder function.

Some risk factors that are associated with prostate cancer these include advanced age, eating a diet that is high in animal fats, being of the African and Northern European ethnic group, the presence of a family history of cancer, and a history of vasectomy, smoking, or cadmium exposure.

Depending on the type and stage of the prostate cancer, treatment options may include any one or all of the following: chemotherapy, cryosurgery to freeze cancer cells, external radiation to the prostate and pelvis, hormone therapy, radioactive implants in the prostate, surgery to remove part of all of the prostate and the surrounding tissue, surgical removal of the testes to block testosterone production, and watchful waiting and monitoring only. Hormone and chemotherapy are used for men with advanced cancer. The focus of hormone therapy is to reduce the body's production of testosterone, which should slow the growth of the cancer.

SUMMARY

The reproductive system functions both for reproduction and maintaining the secondary sex characteristics for both males and females. The female reproductive system is cyclic, with an approximate 28-day cycle as the body prepares itself for reproduction. The male reproductive system produces sperm on a regular basis and is not reliant on any cycle for reproduction.

Chapter Review

COMPETENCY REVIEW

1. Define and spell the terms to learn for this chapter.
2. What is another term for the fallopian tube?
3. What are the three identifiable areas of the uterus?
4. What is the function of the ovaries?
5. What are the three functions of the vagina?

6. What are the two principal hormones in the female reproductive system?
7. What is the vital function of the male reproductive system?
8. What are the two functions of the penis?
9. What are the two functions of the male urethra?
10. What is the function of the seminal vesicles?

PREPARING FOR THE CERTIFICATION EXAM

1. A condition that is caused when the endometrium travels outside the uterus is called
   A. pelvic inflammatory disease
   B. endometriosis
   C. sexually transmitted infection (STIs)
   D. myometriosis
   E. salmonella infection

2. The most common complication of an STI is
   A. pelvic inflammatory disease
   B. endometriosis
   C. myometriosis
   D. ovarian dysfunction
   E. fallopian tube dysfunction

3. The male reproductive system does NOT include the
   A. ureters
   B. urethra
   C. vas deferens
   D. prostate
   E. testes

4. The upper portion of the uterus is called the
   A. fundus
   B. corpus
   C. ovum
   D. cervix
   E. vulva

5. The more common abnormal positions of the uterus include all of the following EXCEPT
   A. anteversion
   B. retroversion
   C. anteflexion
   D. retroflexion
   E. introversion

6. Surgical removal of the fallopian tube and ovary is called
   A. panhysterosalpingo-oophorectomy
   B. oophorectomy
   C. salpingo-oophorectomy
   D. panhysterectomy
   E. laparoscopy

7. The male sperm, in the form of semen, are nourished by a fluid in the
   A. seminal vesicles
   B. epididymis
   C. prostate gland
   D. urethra
   E. vas deferens

8. The vas deferens in the male reproductive system is also known as the
   A. vasectomy
   B. ductus deferens
   C. spermatic cord
   D. scrotum
   E. phimosis

9. The testes produce
   A. progesterone
   B. estrogen
   C. testosterone
   D. oxytocin
   E. prolactin

10. The hormone that stimulates the production of milk in a mother postdelivery is
    A. progesterone
    B. estrogen
    C. testosterone
    D. oxytocin
    E. Prolactin

CRITICAL THINKING

1. Why did the physician include a PSA and digital rectal exam for Mr. Sansone.
2. If Mr. Sansone has BPH, does he have prostate cancer?
3. Why was Mr. Sansone having difficulty starting his stream of urine and having urgency to urinate?

INTERNET ACTIVITY

Do an Internet search of the National Breast Cancer Foundation and other breast cancer awareness organizations. Research the following regarding breast cancer: cancer myths, early detection, and up-and-coming research.

MediaLink More on the repoductive system, including interactive resources, can be found on the Student CD-ROM accompanying this textbook.

APPENDIX I:
Abbreviations and Symbols

a	ampere; anode; anterior; aqua; area; artery
AB, Ab	abortion; abnormal; antibody
ABC	aspiration biopsy cytology
ABG	arterial blood gases
ABLB	alternate binaural loudness balance
ABO	blood group
ABR	auditory brainstem response
AC	air conduction; anticoagulant
a.c.	before meals
ACAT	automated computerized axial tomography
Acc.	accommodation
ACG	angiocardiography
Ach	acetylcholine
ACL	anterior cruciate ligament
ACLS	advanced cardiac life support
ACR	American College of Rheumatology
ACS	American Cancer Society
ACTH	adrenocorticoptropic hormone
AD	right ear (O) (auris dexter); Alzheimer's Disease; advance directive
ADA	American Diabetes Association
ad lib	as desired; freely
adeno-CA	adenocarcinoma
ADH	antidiuretic hormone
ADHD	attention-deficit hyperactivity disorder
ADL	activities of daily living
ADP	adenosine diphosphate
AE	above the elbow
AF	atrial fibrillation
AFB	acid-fast bacillus (TB organism)
AFP	alpha-fetoprotein
A/G	albumin/globulin ratio
Ag	antigen
AGN	acute glomerulonephritis
AH	abdominal hysterectomy
AHF	antihemophilic factor VIII
AHG	antihemophillic globulin factor VIII
AI	aortic insufficiency; artificial insemination
AIDS	acquired immune deficiency syndrome
AIH	artificial insemination homologous
AK	above knee

AKA	above-knee amputation
alk phos	alkaline phosphatase
ALD	aldolase
ALL	acute lymphocytic leukemia
ALS	amyotropic lateral sclerosis
ALT	argon laser trabeculoplasty; alanine aminotransferase
AMA	American Medical Association
AMD	age-related macular degeneration
AMI	acute myocardial infarction
AML	acute myelogenous leukemia
Angio	angiogram
ANS	autonomic nervous system
A&P	auscultation and percussion; anatomy and physiology
AP, AP view	anterior-posterior; anteroposterior view
APB	atrial premature beat
APTT	activated partial thromboplastin time
ARC	AIDS-related complex
ARD	acute respiratory disease
ARDS	acute respiratory distress syndrome
ARF	acute respiratory failure; acute renal failure
ARMD	age-related macular degeneration
AROM	active range of motion
AS	aortic stenosis; arteriosclerosis; left ear (X)
ASCVD	arteriosclerotic cardiovascular disease
As, Ast, astigm	astigmatism
Ascus	atypical squamous cells of undetermined significance
ASD	atrial septal defect
ASH	asymmetrical septal hypertrophy
ASHD	arteriosclerotic heart disease
ASL	American Sign Language
Astigm.	astigmatism
AST	aspartate aminotransferase
ATN	acute tubular necrosis
ATP	adenosine triphosphate
AU	both ears (auris unitas)
AV, A-V	atrioventricular; arteriovenous
AVMs	arteriovenous malformations
AVR	aortic valve replacement

Ba	barium
BAC	blood alcohol concentration
BaE	barium enema
baso	basophil
BBB	bundle branch block (L for left; R for right)
BBT	basal body temperature
BC	bone conduction
BE	barium enema
BG, bG	blood glucose; blood sugar
b.i.d.	twice a day
BIN, bin	twice a night
BK	below knee
BKA	below-knee amputation
BM	bowel movement
BMD	bone mineral density (test)
BMR	basal metabolic rate
BNO	bladder neck obstruction
BP	blood pressure
BPH	benign prostatic hypertrophy
Broncho	bronchoscopy
BRP	bathroom privileges
BS	breath sounds; bowel sounds; blood sugar
BSE	breast self-examination
BSI	body systems isolation
BSP	bromsulphalein
BT	bleeding time
BUN	blood urea nitrogen
BX, bx	biopsy
c̄	with (cum)
C1, C2, etc.	first cervical vertebra, second cervical vertebra, etc.
C&S	culture and sensitivity
CA	cancer; carcinoembryonic antigen
Ca	calcium; cancer
CABG	coronary artery bypass graft
CAD	coronary artery disease
CAM	complementary and alternative medicines
cap	capsule
CAPD	continuous ambulatory peritoneal dialysis
CAT, CT	computerized axial tomography
cath	catheterization
CBC	complete blood count
CBD	common bile duct
CBS	chronic brain syndrome
cc	cubic centimeter
CC	clean-catch urine specimen; cardiac catheterization; chief complaint

CCU	coronary care unit; cardiac care unit
CD4	protein on T-cell helper lymphocyte
CDC	Centers for Disease Control and Prevention
CDH	congenital dislocation of the hip
CEA	carcinoembryonic antigen
CF	cystic fibrosis
CGL	chronic granulocytic leukemia
c.gl.	correction with glasses
CGN	chronic glomerulonephritis
CHD	congestive heart disease
chemo	chemotherapy
CHF	congestive heart failure
CHO	carbohydrate
chol	cholesterol
Ci	curie
Cib	food (cibus)
CIC	coronary intensive care
CIN	cervical intraepithelial neoplasia
CIS	carcinoma in situ
CK	creatine kinase
CL, Cl	chloride
CLL	chronic lymphocytic leukemia
cm	centimeter
CMG	cystometrogram
CML	chronic myelogenous leukemia
CMP	cardiomyopathy
CNS	central nervous system
c/o	complains of
CO	cardiac output
CO$_2$	carbon dioxide
COLD	chronic obstructive lung disease
COPD	chronic obstructive pulmonary disease
CP	cerebral palsy; chest pain
CPD	cephalopelvic disproportion
CPK	creatine phosphokinase
CPM	continuous passive motion
CPR	cardiopulmonary resuscitation
CPS	cycles per second
CR	computerized radiography
CRF	chronic renal failure
CS, C-section	cesarean section
C&S	culture and sensitivity
C-section	cesarean section (surgical delivery)
CSF	cerebrospinal fluid
C-spine	cervical spine film
CT	computed tomography
CTA	clear to auscultation
CTS	carpal tunnel syndrome
CUC	chronic ulcerative colitis
CV	cardiovascular
CVA	cerebrovascular accident
CVD	cardiovascular disease
CVP	central venous pressure
CVS	chorionic villus sampling

CWP	childbirth without pain
Cx	cervix
CXR	chest x-ray
cyl.	cylindrical lens
cysto	cystoscopic exam
/d	per day
D	diopter (lens strength)
dB, db	decibel
DBS	deep brain stimulation
D/C	discontinue
D&C	dilatation and curettage
D&E	dilation and evacuation
dc	discontinue
DC	discharge
DCIS	ductal carcinoma in situ
DDS	Doctor of Dental Surgery; dorsal cord stimulation
decub	decubitus
Derm	dermatology
DES	diethylstilbestrol
DHT	dihydrotestosterone
DI	diabetes insipidus; diagnostic imaging
diff	differential
dil	dilute; diluted
DJD	degenerative joint disease
DM	diabetes mellitus
DNA	deoxyribonucleic acid
DNR	do not resuscitate
DO	doctor of osteopathy
DOA	dead on arrival
DOB	date of birth
DOE	dyspnea upon exertion
DPT	diphtheria, pertussis, tetanus injection
DRE	digital rectal examination
DRGs	diagnostic related groups
DSA	digital subtraction angiography
DTaP	diphtheria, tetanus and pertussis (vaccine)
DTR	deep tendon reflex
DT's	delerium tremens
DUB	dysfunctional uterine bleeding
DVA	distance visual acuity
DVT	deep vein thrombosis
Dx	diagnosis
EBV	Epstein-Barr virus
ECC	endocervical curettage
ECCE	extracapsular cataract extraction
ECF	extracellular fluid; extended care facility
ECG; EKG	electrocardiogram
ECHO	echocardiogram
E. coli	Escherichia coli
ECSL	extracorporeal shockwave lithotriptor
ECT	electroconvulsive therapy
ED	erectile dysfunction
EDC	estimated date of confinement
EEG	electroencephalogram
EENT	eyes, ears, nose, throat
EGD	esophagogastroduodenoscopy

ELISA	enzyme-linked immunosorbent assay
EM	emmetropia (normal vision)
EMG	electromyography
ENG	electronystagmography
ENT	ear, nose, and throat
EOM	extraocular movement
eosin, eos	eosinophil
ERCP	endoscopic retrograde cholangiopancreatography
ERT	estrogen replacement therapy; external radiation therapy
ERV	expiratory reserve volume
ESR, SR	erythrocyte sedimentation rate
ESL, ESWL	extracorporeal shock-wave lithotripsy
ESR, SR, sed rate	erythrocyte sedimentation rate; sedimentation rate
ESRD	end-stage renal disease
EST	electroshock therapy
ET	endotracheal; endotracheal
ETF	eustachian tube function
F	Fahrenheit
FACP	Fellow, American College of Physicians
FACS	Fellow, American College of Surgeons
FBS	fasting blood sugar
FDA	Food and Drug Administration
FEF	forced expiratory flow
FEKG	fetal electrocardiogram
FEV	forced expiratory volume
FH	family history
FHR	fetal heart rate
FHS	fetal heart sound
FHT	fetal heart tone
FMS	fibromyalgia syndrome
FROM	full range of motion
FS	frozen section
FSH	follicle-stimulating hormone
FTA-ABS	fluorescent treponemal antibody absorption
FTND	full-term normal delivery
5-FU	5-fluorouracil
FUO	fever of undetermined origin
FVC	forced vital capacity
FX, fx	fracture
g	gram
Ga	gallium
GB	gallbladder
GC	gonorrhea
GCSF	granulocyte colony-stimulating factor
GERD	gastroesophageal reflux disease
GGT	gamma-glutamyl transferase
GH	growth hormone
GI	gastrointestinal

GIFT	gamete intrafallopian transfer	HTN	hypertension	kg	kilogram
GnRF	gonadotropin-releasing factor	Hx	history	KS	Kaposi's sarcoma
		hypo	hypodermic	KUB	kidneys, ureters, bladder
GOT	glutamic oxaloacetic transaminase	Hz	Hertz	kV	kilovolt
		IBD	inflammatory bowel syndrome	kW	kilowatt
Gpi	globus pallidus			L, l	liter
GPT	glutamic pyruvic transaminase	IBS	irritable bowel syndrome	L1, L2, etc.	first lumbar vertebra, second lumbar vertebra, etc.
gr	grain	IC	intracardiac; interstitial cystitis	LA	left atrium
grav I	first pregnancy	ICCE	intracapsular cataract cryoextraction	L&A	light and accommodation
GSW	gunshot wound			lab	laboratory
gtt	drops (guttae)	ICF	intracellular fluid	LAC	laceration; long arm cast
GTT	glucose tolerance test	ICP	intracranial pressure	LAK	lymphokine-activated killer (cells)
GU	genitourinary	ICSH	interstitial cell-stimulating hormone	LAT, lat	lateral
gyn, gyne	gynecology	ICU	intensive care unit	lb	pound
h	hour	ID	intradermal	LB	large bowel
H	hypodermic; hydrogen	I&D	incision and drainage	LBBB	left bundle branch block
H&L	heart & lungs	IDDM	insulin-dependent diabetes mellitus	LBW	low birth weight
HAA	hepatitis-associated antigen			LCIS	lobular carcinoma in situ
HAV	hepatitis A virus	Ig	immunoglobins (IgA, IgD, IgE, IgG, IgM)	LD	lactate dehydrogenase
HBIG	hepatitis B immune globulin			LDH	lactic dehydrogenase
HBOT	hyperbaric oxygen therapy	IH	infectious hepatitis	LDL	low-density lipoproteins
HBP	high blood pressure	IHSS	idiopathic hypertropic subaortic stenosis	LE	left eye; lupus erythematosus; lower extremity
HBV	hepatitis B virus	IL-2	interleukin-2		
HCG	human chorionic gonadotropin	IM	intramuscular	LEDs	light-emitting diodes
HCl	hydrochloric acid	inj	injection	LES	lower esophageal sphincter
HCO3	bicarbonate	I&O	intake and output	LGI	lower gastrointestinal series
HCT, Hct, crit	hematocrit	IOL	intraocular pressure	LH	luteinizing hormone
HCV	hepatitis C virus	IOP	intraocular pressure	LH-RH	luteinizing hormone-releasing hormone
HD	hemodialysis; Hodgkin's disease	IPD	intermittent peritoneal dialysis	LIF	left iliac fossa
HDL	high-density lipoproteins	IPPB	intermittent positive pressure breathing	liq	liquid; fluid
HDN	hemolytic disease of the newborn	IQ	intelligence quotient	L K & S	liver, kidney, and spleen
HDS	herniated disk syndrome	IR	interventional radiologist	ll	left lateral
HEENT	head, eyes, ears, nose and throat	IRDS	infant respiratory distress syndrome	LLC	long leg cast
		IRT	internal radiation therapy	LLE	left lower extremity
HF	heart failure	IRV	inspiratory reserve volume	LLL	left lower lobe
Hg	mercury	IS	intercostal space	LLQ	left lower quadrant
HgB, Hb, Hgb, HGB	hemoglobin	ITP	idiopathic thrombocytopenia purpura	LMP	last menstrual period
HGH	human growth hormone	IU	international unit	LOM	limitation of motion
HIV	human immunodeficiency virus (causes AIDS)	IUD	intrauterine device	LP	lumbar puncture
		IUGR	intrauterine growth rate; intrauterine growth retardation	LPE	laser peripheral iridotomy
HLA	human leukocyte antigen			LPF	low-power field
HMD	hyaline membrane disease	IV	intravenous	LRQ	lower right quadrant
HNP	herniated nucleus pulposa (herniated disk)	IVC	intravenous cholangiogram; inferior vena cava; intraventricular catheter	L, lt	left
				LTH	lactogenic hormone
H2O	water			LUE	left upper extremity
Hpd	hematoporphyrin derivative	IVCD	intraventricular conduction delay	LUL	left upper lobe
H. pylori	*Heliocobacter pylori*	IVF	in vitro fertilization	LUQ	left upper quadrant
HPV	human papillomavirus	IVP	intravenous pyelogram	LV	left ventricle
HRT	hormone replacement therapy	IVS	interventricular septum	LVAD	left ventricular assist device
		IVU	intravenous urogram	lymph	lymphocyte
h.s.	at bedtime	J	joule	M	molar; thousand; muscle
HSG	hysterosalpingography	JNC	Joint National Committee	m	male; meter; minim
HSO	hysterosalpingoophrectomy	JVP	jugular venous pulse	mA	milliampere
HSV	herpes simplex virus			mAs	milliampere second
HSV-2	herpes simplex virus-2	K	potassium	MBC	minimal breathing capacity
Ht	height	KB	knee bearing	MCH	mean corpuscular hemoglobin
HT	hypermetropia (hyperopia)	KD	knee disarticulation	MCHC	mean corpuscular hemoglobin concentration
HTLV	human T-cell leukemia-lymphoma virus			mCi	millicurie
				MCV	mean corpuscular volume
				MD	medical doctor; muscular dystrophy

mEq	milliequivalent	NPUAP	National Pressure Ulcer Advisory Panel	Pe tube	polyethylene tube placed in the eardrum
mets	metastases	NSAIDs	nonsteroidal anti-inflammatory drugs	PFT	pulmonary function test
MG	myasthenia gravis			PGH	pituitary growth hormone
mg	milligram (0.001 gram)	NSR	normal sinus rhythm	pH	acidity or alkalinity of urine
MH	marital history	n&v	nausea and vomiting	PH	past history
MI	myocardial infarction; mitral insufficiency	NVA	near visual acuity	PID	pelvic inflammatory disease
MICU	mobile intensive care unit	O	pint	PIF	prolactin release-inhibiting factor
MIF	melanocyte-stimulating hormone release-inhibiting factor	O₂	oxygen	PKU	phenylketonuria
		OA	osteoarthritis	PM, pm	afternoon, evening
mix astig	mixed astigmatism	OB	obstetrics	PMH	past medical history
mL, ml	milliliter	OB-GYN	obstetrics and gynecology	PMI	point of maximal impulse
mm	millimeter (0.001 meter; 0.039 inch)	OC	oral contraceptive	PMN, seg, poly	polymorphonuclear neutrophil
		OCD	obsessive-compulsive disorder		
mmHg	millimeters of mercury				
mMol	millimole	OCG	oral cholecystography	PMP	previous menstrual period
MMR	measles, mumps, and rubella (vaccine)	OCPs	oral contraceptive pills	PMR	physical medicine and rehabilitation
		od	once a day		
mol wt	molecular weight	OD	right eye (oculus dexter); overdose	PMS	premenstrual syndrome
mono	mononucleosis; monocyte			PND	paroxysmal nocturnal dyspnea; postnasal drip
MR	mitral regurgitation	OHS	open heart surgery		
MRI	magnetic resonance imaging	OM	otitis media	PNS	peripheral nervous system
MS	musculoskeletal; mitral stenosis; multiple sclerosis	O&P	ova and parasites	P.O.	per os (by mouth)
		ophth.	ophthalmology	PP	postprandial (after meals)
MSH	melanocyte-stimulating hormone	OR	operating room	PPD	purified protein derivative (tuberculin test)
		ortho	orthopedics		
MTX	methotrexate	os	mouth opening; bone	PPI	proton pump inhibitors
mV	millivolt	OS	left eye (oculus sinister)	pr	per rectum
MV	minute volume	OTC	over the counter	PRF	prolactin-releasing factor
MVA	motor vehicle accident	Oto	otology	prn	as required; as needed
MVP	mitral valve prolapse	OU	both eyes (oculi unitas); each eye (oculus uterque)	PROM	passive range of motion
MVV	maximal voluntary ventilation			prot.	protocol
		OV	office visit	PSA	prostate specific antigen
MY	myopia	oz	ounce	pt	patient; pint
				PT	prothrombin time
n	nerve	P	pulse; phosphorus	PTC	percutaneous transhepatic cholangiography
Na	sodium	PA	posteroanterior view (radiology); pernicious anemia		
NAD	no apparent distress			PTCA	percutaneous transluminal coronary angioplasty
NANBH	non-A, non-B hepatitis virus	PAC	premature arterial contraction		
				PTH	parathyroid hormone
NB	newborn	PAP	pulmonary arterial pressure; Papanicolaou test	PTS	permanent threshold shift
nCi	nanocurie			PTT	partial thromboplastin time
NCU	nongonococcal urethritis	para I	first delivery	PUD	peptic ulcer disease
NCV	nerve conduction velocity	PAT	paroxysmal atrial tachycardia	PUL	percutaneous ultrasonic lithotropsy
NED	no evidence of disease				
NIDDM	non-insulin-dependent diabetes mellitus	Path	pathology	PVC	premature ventricular contraction
		PBI	protein bound iodine		
NG	nasogastric (tube)	p.c.	after meals (post cibum)	PVD	peripheral vascular disease
NGU	nongonococcal urethritis	PCL	posterior cruciate ligament		
NH₄	ammonia	PCP	Pneumocystis carinii pneumonia	q	every
NHL	non-Hodgkin's lymphoma			qam, qm	every morning
NHLBI	National Heart, Lung and Blood Institute	PCV	packed cell volume (hematocrit)	q.d.	daily
				qh	every hour
NICU	neonatal intensive care unit	PD	peritoneal dialysis	q2h	every 2 hours
NIDDM	non-insulin-dependent diabetes mellitus	PDR	Physicians' Desk Reference	q.i.d.	four times a day
		PE	physical examination; pulmonary embolism	qns	quantity not sufficient
NIH	National Institute of Health			qpm, qn	every night
		PEEP	positive end-expiratory pressure	qs	quantity sufficient
NMR	nuclear resonance imaging			qt	quart
NPDL	nodular, poorly differentiated lymphocytes	PEG	percutaneous endoscopic gastrostomy; pneumoencephalogram		
				R	roentgen; respiration; right
NPH	neutral protamine Hegedorn (insulin)	PERLA	pupils equal, react to light and accommodation	RA	rheumatoid arthritis; radium; right arm
NPO	nothing by mouth (nil per os)			rad	radiation absorbed dose
		PET	positron emission tomography	RAI	radioactive iodine
NPT	nocturnal penile tumescence			RAIU	radioactive iodine uptake
				RBC	red blood cell

RD	respiratory disease	SLE	systemic lupus erythematosus	TNF	tumor necrosis factor
RDA	recommended daily allowance (dietary allowance)	SMBG	self-monitoring of blood glucose	TNM	tumor, nodes, metastases
				TNS	transcutaneous nerve stimulation
RDS	respiratory distress syndrome	SMD	senile macular degeneration	top	topically
RE	right eye	SOB	shortness of breath	TPA	*Treponema pallidum* agglutination (test)
REM	rapid eye movement	SOM	serous otitis media		
Rh	Rhesus (factor)	sono	sonogram, sonography	TPA, tPA	tissue plasminogen activator
RIA	radioimmunoassay	SOP	standard operating procedure		
RIF	right iliac fossa			TPN	total parenteral nutrition
RL	right lateral	sp gr, SG	specific gravity	TPR	temperature, pulse, respiration
RLL	right lower lobe	SPP	suprapublic prostatectomy		
RLQ	right lower quadrant	SR	sedimentation rate	tr, tinct	tincture
RML	right middle lobe; right mediolateral (episiotomy)	ss	one half	TSE	testicular self-exam
		st	stage (of disease)	TSH	thyroid-stimulating hormone
RNA	ribonucleic acid	ST	esotropia		
R/O	rule out	staph	staphylococcus	TSS	toxic shock syndrome
ROM	range of motion; read only memory	stat	immediately	TTH	thyrotropic hormone
		STD	skin test done; sexually transmitted diseases	TTS	temporary threshold shift
RP	retrograde pyelogram			TUIP	transurethral incision of the prostate
RPM	revolutions per minute	STH	somatotropin hormone		
RQ	respiratory quotient	strep	streptococcus	TUMP	transurethral microwave thermotherapy
RT	radiation therapy	STS	serologic test for syphilis		
RUL	right upper lobe	STSG	split-thickness skin graft	TUNA	transurethral needle ablation
RUQ	right upper quadrant	Subcu, Subq	subcutaneous		
RV	right ventricle	SVC	superior vena cava	TUR, TURP	transurethral resection of the prostate
Rx	take thou; prescribe; treatment; therapy	SVD	spontaneous vaginal delivery		
		SVT	supraventricular tachycardia	TV	tidal volume
		Sx	signs, symptoms	TX, Tx	traction; treatment; transplant
s̄	without	syr	syrup		
S1	first heart sound			U	units
S2	second heart sound	T	temperature	U/A	urinalysis
SA, S-A	sinoatrial	T1, T2, etc.	first thoracic vertebra, second thoracic vertebra, etc.	UC	urine culture; uterine contractions
SAC	short arm cast				
SAD	seasonal affective disorder			UCHD	usual childhood diseases
SAH	subarachnoid hemorrhage	T_3	triiodothyronine; third thoracic vertebra	UE	upper extremity
SALT	serum alanine aminotransferase			UG	urogenital
		T_3RU	triiodothyronine resin uptake	UGI	upper gastrointestinal (x-ray) series
SARS	severe acute respiratory syndrome				
		T_4	thyroxine; fourth thoracic vertebra; T-cell lymphocyte	U&L, U/L	upper and lower
SAST	serum aspartate aminotransferase			ULQ	upper left quadrant
		T_7	free thyroxine index; seventh thoracic vertebra	ung	ointment
SBE	subacute bacterial endocarditis			URI	upper respiratory infection
		T_8	T-cell lymphocyte (cytotoxic or killer cell)	URQ	upper right quadrant
SBFT	small-bowel follow-through			u/s	ultrasound
		T&A	tonsillectomy and adenoidectomy	USP	United States Pharmacopeia
SC, sc, subq	subcutaneous				
SCD	sudden cardiac death	tab	tablet	UTI	urinary tract infection
SCLE	subacute cutaneous lupus erythematosus	TAH	total abdominal hysterectomy	UV	ultraviolet
				UVR	ultraviolet radiation
SD	shoulder disarticulation; standard deviation	TB	tuberculosis		
		TBW	total body weight	v	vein
SEE-2	Signing Exact English	TENS	transcutaneous electrical nerve stimulation	VA	visual acuity
seg, poly	polymorphonuclear neutrophil			VC	vital capacity
		TFS	thyroid function test	VCD	vacuum constriction device
segs	segmented (mature RBCs)	THA	total hip arthroplasty	VCG	vectorcardiogram
SG	skin graft; specific gravity	THR	total hip replacement	VCU, VCUG	voiding cystourethrogram
s.gl.	without correction or glasses	TIA	transient ischemic attack		
SGOT	serum glutamic oxaloacetic transaminase	t.i.d.	three times a day	VD	venereal disease
		TIMS	topical immunomodulators	VDRL	Venereal Disease Research Laboratory (syphilis test)
SGPT	serum glutamic pyruvic transaminase	TIPS	transjugular intrahepatic portosystemic shunt		
				VF	visual field
sh	shoulder	TJ	triceps jerk	VHD	ventricular heart disease
SH	serum hepatitis	TKA	total knee arthroscopy	VLDL	very low-density lipoproteins
SIDS	sudden infant death syndrome	TKR	total knee replacement		
		TLC	total lung capacity	vol	volume
SK	streptokinase	TMJ	temporomandibular joint	vol %	volume percent

VMA	vanillylmandelic acid	WNL	within normal limits	XRT	radiation therapy
VP	vasopressin	WPW	Wolff-Parkinson-White syndrome	XT	exotropia
VPB	ventricular premature beat	wt	weight	XX	female sex chromosomes
VS	vital signs	w/v	weight by volume	XY	male sex chromosomes
VSD	ventricular septal defect			YAG	yttrium-aluminum-garnet (laser)
VT	ventricular tachycardia	x	multiplied by		
		XM	cross match for blood (type and cross match)	YOB	year of birth
WBC	white blood cell			yr	year
WDWN	well developed, well nourished	XP	xeroderma pigmentosum		
		XR	x-ray	z	atomic number

CHARTING ABBREVIATIONS AND SYMBOLS

aa	of each	FHT	fetal heart tones	qm	every morning (quaque mane)
ac	before meals (ante cibum)	GB	gallbladder		
AD	right ear (auris dextra)	GI	gastrointestinal	qn	every night (quaque nocte)
ADL	activities of daily living	GU	genitourinary	R	right; respiration
ad lib	as desired	h, hr	hour	RBC	red blood cell; red blood (cell) count
adm	admission	hpf	high power field		
AE	above elbow	hs	hour of sleep; bedtime (hora somni)	Rh	Rhesus blood factor (Rh + or Rh −)
AJ	ankle jerk				
AK	above knee	hypo	hypodermic injection	RLQ	right lower quadrant
alt dieb	every other day	ICU	intensive care unit	R/O	rule out
alt hor	every other hour	IM	intramuscular	ROM	range of motion
alt noc	every other night	I&O	intake and output	RUQ	right upper quadrant
AM, am	before noon (ante meridiem); morning	IU	international unit	SC, sc, subq	subcutaneous
		IV	intravenous	SOB	shortness of breath
AMA	against medical advice	L	left	SOS	if necessary (si opus sit)
AMB	ambulate; ambulatory	L&A	light and accommodation	stat	immediately
ant	anterior	LAT	lateral	Sx	signs, symptoms
AP	anteroposterior	L&W	living and well	T, temp	temperature
A-P	anterior-posterior	LLQ	left lower quadrant	tabs	tablets
approx	approximately	LMP	last menstrual period	TC&DB	turn, cough, deep breathe
AQ, aq	water	LOA	left occipitoanterior	tid	three times a day
ASAP	as soon as possible	LPF	low power field (10x)	tinct	tincture
AS or LE	left ear (auris sinistra)	LUQ	left upper quadrant	TPN	total parenteral nutrition
AV	atrioventricular	MTD	right ear drum (membrana tympani dexter)	trans	transverse
BE	below elbow			ULQ	upper left quadrant
bid	twice a day	MTS	left ear drum (membrana tympani sinister)	ung	ointment
bin	twice a night			URQ	upper right quadrant
BK	below knee	neg	negative	VS	vital signs
BM	bowel movement	NG	nasogastric	WBC	white blood cell; white blood (cell) count
BMR	basal metabolic rate	NPO	nothing by mouth		
BRP	bathroom privileges	NS	normal saline	WM, BM	white male, black male
C	Centigrade, Celsius or calorie (kilocalorie)	OD	right eye (oculus dexter)	WF, BF	white female, black female
		OP	outpatient		
caps	capsules	OR	operating room	×	times, power
CBR	complete bed rest	OS or OL	left eye (oculus sinister, oculus laevus)	−	negative
CC	chief complaint; clean catch (urine)			+	positive
		OU	each eye (oculus uterque)	F	female
CCU	cardiac (coronary) care unit	P	pulse	M	male
		PA	posteroanterior	+/−	positive or negative
c/o	complains of	pc	after meals (post cibum)	*	birth
cont	continue	PI	present illness	†	death
dc	discontinue	po	by mouth (per os)	%	percent
DC	discharge from hospital	PO	postoperative	#	number; pound
DNA	does not apply	PM, pm	afternoon or evening (post meridiem)	&	and
DNR	do not resuscitate			<	less than
DNS	did not show	prn	as necessary, as required, when necessary	=	equal
Dr	doctor			>	greater than
D/W	dextrose in water	q	every (quaque)	?	question
Dx	diagnosis	qd	every day (quaque die)	@	at
EOM	extraocular movement	qh	every hour (quaque hora)	^	increase
ER	emergency room	q2h	every 2 hours	™	trade mark
Ex	examination	q4h	every 4 hours	©	copyright
F	Fahrenheit	qid	four times a day (quarter in die)	®	registered
FHS	fetal heart sounds			¶	paragraph

APPENDIX II:
Glossary of Word Parts

PREFIXES

a	no, not, without, lack of, apart	end	within, inner	neo	new
ab	away from	endo	within, inner	nulli	none
ad	toward, near	ep	upon, over, above		
ambi	both	epi	upon, over, above	olig	little, scanty
an	no, not, without, lack of	eso	inward	oligo	little, scanty
ana	up	eu	good, normal		
ant	against	ex	out, away from	pan	all
ante	before	exo	out, away from	par	around, beside
anti	against	extra	outside, beyond	para	beside, alongside, abnormal
apo	separation			per	through
astro	star-shaped	hemi	half	peri	around
auto	self	heter	different	poly	many, much, excessive
		hetero	different	post	after, behind
bi	two, double	homo	similar, same	pre	before
bin	twice	homeo	similar, same, likeness, constant	primi	first
brachy	short			pro	before
brady	slow	hydr	water	proto	first
		hydro	water	pseudo	false
cac	bad	hyp	below, deficient	pyro	fire
cata	down	hyper	above, beyond, excessive		
centi	a hundred	hypo	below, under, deficient	quadri	four
chromo	color			quint	five
circum	around	in	in, into, not		
con	with, together	infra	below	re	back
contra	against	infer	below	retro	backward
		inter	between		
de	down, away from	intra	within	semi	half
deca	ten	ir (in)	into	sub	below, under, beneath
di (a)	through, between			supra	above, beyond
dia	through, between	macro	large	super	above, beyond
dif	apart, free from, separate	mal	bad	sym	together
dipl	double	mega	large, great	syn	together, with
di (s)	two, apart	meso	middle		
dis	apart	meta	beyond, over, between, change	tachy	fast
dys	bad, difficult, painful			tetra	four
		micro	small	trans	across
ec	out, outside, outer	milli	one-thousandth	tri	three
ecto	out, outside, outer	mon (o)	one		
em	in	mono	one	ultra	beyond
en	within	multi	many, much	uni	one

WORD ROOTS/COMBINING FORMS

abdomin	abdomen	aden	gland	alveol	small, hollow air sac
abort	to miscarry	aden/o	gland	ambyl	dull
absorpt	to suck in	adhes	stuck to	ambul	to walk
acanth	a thorn	adip	fat	amni/o	lamb
acetabul	vinegar cup	agglutinat	clumping	ampere	ampere
acid	acid	agon	agony	amputat	to cut though
acoust	hearing	agor/a	market place	amyl	starch
acr	extremity, point	albin	white	anastom	opening
acr/o	extremity, point	albumin	protein	andr	man
act	acting	alimentat	nourishment	andr/o	man
actin	ray	all	other	ang	vessel

ang/i	vessel	cartil	gristle	cost	rib
angin	to choke, quinsy	castr	to prune	cost/o	rib
angi/o	vessel	caud	tail	cox	hip
anis/o	unequal	caus	heat	cran/i	skull
ankyl	stiffening, crooked	cavit	cavity	crani/o	skull
an/o	anus	celi	abdomen, belly	creat	flesh
anter/i	toward the front	cellul	little cell	creatin	flesh, creatine
anthrac	coal	centr	center	crine	to secrete
aort	aorta	centr/i	center	crin/o	to secrete
aort/o	aorta	cephal	head	crur	leg
append	appendix	cept	receive	cry/o	cold
arachn	spider	cerebell	little brain	crypt	hidden
arche	beginning	cerebell/o	little brain	cubit	elbow, to lie
arter	artery	cerebr/o	cerebrum	culd/o	cul-de-sac
arter/i	artery	cervic	cervix, neck	curie	curie
arteri/o	artery	cheil	lip	cutane	skin
arthr	joint	chem/o	chemical	cyan	dark blue
arthr/o	joint	chlor/o	green	cycl	ciliary body
artific/i	not natural	chol	gall, bile	cycl/o	ciliary body
aspirat	to draw in	chole	gall, bile	cyst	bladder, sac
atel	imperfect	chol/e	gall, bile	cyst/o	bladder, sac
atel/o	imperfect	choledoch/o	common bile duct	cyt	cell
ather	fatty substance, porridge	chondr	cartilage	cyth	cell
ather/o	fatty substance, porridge	chondr/o	cartilage	cyt/o	cell
atri	atrium	chord	cord		
atri/o	atrium	chori/o	chorion	dacry	tear
aud/i	to hear	choroid	choroid	dactyl	finger or toe
audi/o	to hear	choroid/o	choroid	dactyl/o	finger or toe
auditor	hearing	chromat	color	defecat	to remove dregs
aur	ear	chrom/o	color	dem	people
aur/i	ear	chym	juice	dendr/o	tree
auscultat	listen to	cine	motion	dent	tooth
aut	self	cinemat/o	motion	dent/i	tooth
axill	armpit	circulat	circular	derm	skin
		cirrh	orange-yellow	derm/a	skin
bacter/i	bacteria	cirrh/o	orange-yellow	dermat	skin
balan	glans penis	cis	to cut	dermat/o	skin
bartholin	Bartholin's glands	claudicat	to limp	derm/o	skin
bas/o	base	clavicul	little key	dextr/o	to the right
bil	bile, gall	cleid/o	clavicle	diast	to expand
bil/i	bile, gall	coagul	to clot	didym	testis
bi/o	life	coagulat	to clot	digit	finger or toe
blast/o	germ cell	coccyg/e	tailbone	dilat	to widen
blephar	eyelid	coccyg/o	tail bone	disk	a disk
blephar/o	eyelid	cochle/o	land snail	dist	away from the point of origin
bol	to cast, throw	coit	a coming together		
brach/i	arm	col	colon	diverticul	diverticula
bronch	bronchi	coll/a	glue	dors	backward
bronch/i	bronchi	collis	neck	dors/i	backward
bronchiol	bronchiole	col/o	colon	duct	to lead
bronch/o	bronchi	colon	colon	duoden	duodenum
bucc	cheek	colon/o	colon	dur	dura, hard
burs	a pouch	colp/o	vagina	dur/o	dura, hard
		concuss	shaken violently	dwarf	small
calc	lime, calcium	condyle	knuckle	dynam	power
calc/i	calcium	con/i	dust		
calcan/e	heel bone	conjunctiv	to join together	ech/o	echo
cancer	crab	connect	to bind together	ectop	displaced
capn	smoke	constipat	to press together	eg/o	I, self
capsul	a little box	continence	to hold	ejaculat	to throw out
carcin	cancer	cor	pupil	electr/o	electricity
carcin/o	cancer	coriat	corium	eme	to vomit
card	heart	corne	cornea	embol	to cast, to throw
card/i	heart	corpor	body	emulsificat	disintegrate
cardi/o	heart	corpor/e	body	encephal	brain
carp	wrist	cortic	cortex	encephal/o	brain
carp/o	wrist	cortis	cortex	enchyma	to pour

enter	intestine	gon/o	genitals	lacrim	tear
enucleat	to remove the kernel of	granul/o	little grain, granular	lamin	lamina, thin plate
eosin/o	rose-colored	gravida	pregnant	lamp (s)	to shine
episi/o	vulva, pudenda	gryp	curve	lapar/o	flank, abdomen
equ/i	equal	gynec/o	female	laryng	larynx
erget	work			laryng/e	larynx
erg/o	work	halat	breathe	laryng/o	larynx
eructat	a breaking out	hallux	great (big) toe	later	side
erysi	red	hem	blood	laxat	to loosen
erythr/o	red	hemat	blood	lei/o	smooth
esophag/e	esophagus	hemat/o	blood	lemma	rind, sheath, husk
esophag/o	esophagus	hem/o	blood	lent	lens
esthesi/o	feeling	hemorrh	vein liable to bleed	lept	seizure
estr/o	mad desire	hepat	liver	letharg	drowsiness
eti/o	cause	hepat/o	liver	leuk	white
eunia	a bed	herni/o	hernia	leuk/o	white
excret	sifted out	hidr	sweat	levat	lifter
		hirsut	hairy	libr/i	balance
f(erat)	to bear	hist/o	tissue	lingu	tongue
fasc	a band (fascia)	hol/o	whole	lip	fat
fasci/o	a band (fascia)	horizont	horizon	lipid	fat
femor	femur	humer	humerus	lip/o	fat
fenestrat	window	hydr	water	lith	stone
fibr	fibrous tissue, fiber	hymen	hymen	lith/o	stone
fibrillat	fibrils (small fibers)	hypn	sleep	lob	lobe
fibrin/o	fiber	hyster	womb, uterus	lob/o	lobe
fibr/o	fiber	hyster/o	womb, uterus	lobul	small lobe
fibul	fibula			locat	to place
filtrat	to strain through	icter	jaundice	log	study
fixat	fastened	ile	ileum	log/o	word
flex	to bend	ile/o	ileum	lopec	fox mange
fluor/o	fluorescence	ili	ilium	lord	bending
foc	focus	ili/o	ilium	lucent	to shine
follicul	little bag	illus	foot	lumb	loin
format	a shaping	immun/o	safe, immunity	lumb/o	loin
fungat	mushroom, fungus	infarct	infarct (necrosis of an area)	lump	lump
fus	to pour	infect	infection	lun	moon
		infer/i	below	lymph	lymph, clear fluid
galact/o	milk	inguin	groin	lymph/o	lymph, clear fluid
ganglion	knot	insul	insulin		
gastr	stomach	insulin/o	insulin	malign	bad kind
gastr/o	stomach	integument	covering	mamm/o	breast
gen	formation, produce	intern	within	mandibul	lower jawbone
gene	formation, produce	ionizat	ion (going)	man/o	thin
genet	formation, produce	ion/o	ion	mast	breast
genital	belonging to birth	iont/o	ion	masticat	to chew
gen/o	kind	irid	iris	mast/o	breast
ger	old age	irid/o	iris	maxill	jawbone
gest	to carry	isch	to hold back	maxilla	jaw
gester	to bear	ischi	ischium	maxim	greatest
gigant	giant	is/o	equal	meat	passage
gingiv	gums			meat/o	passage
glandul	little acorn	jaund	yellow	med	middle
gli	glue			medi	toward the middle
gli/o	glue	kal	potassium	medull	marrow
glob	globe	kary/o	cell's nucleus	medull/o	marrow
globin	globule	kel	tumor	melan	black
globul	globe	kerat	cornea	melan/o	black
glomerul	glomerulus, little ball	kerat/o	horn, cornea	men	month
glomerul/o	glomerulus, little ball	keton	ketone	mening	membrane (meninges)
gloss/o	tongue	kil/o	a thousand	mening/i	membrane
gluc/o	sweet, sugar	kinet	motion	mening/o	membrane
glyc	sweet, sugar	kyph	a hump	menise	crescent
glyc/o	glucose, sweet, sugar			men/o	month
glycos	sweet, sugar	labi	lip	ment	mind
gonad	seed	labyrinth	maze	mes	middle
goni/o	angle	labyrinth/o	maze	mes/o	middle

mester	month	orth	straight	physi/o	nature
metr	to measure, womb, uterus	orth/o	straight	pil/o	hair
metr/i	womb, uterus	oscill	to swing	pine	pine cone
micturit	to urinate	oscill/o	to swing	pineal	pineal body
miliar	millet (tiny)	oste	bone	pin/o	to drink
minim	least	oste/o	bone	pituitar	phlegm
mi/o	less, smaller	ot	ear	plak	plate
mit	thread	ot/o	ear	plasma	a thing formed, plasma
mitr	mitral valve	ovar	ovary	plast	a developing
mnes	memory	ovul	ovary	pleur	pleura
mucos	mucus	ovulat	ovary	pleura	pleura
mucus	mucus	ox	oxygen	pleur/o	pleura
muscul	muscle	ox/i	oxygen	plicat	to fold
muscul/o	muscle	oxy	sour, sharp, acid	pneum/o	lung, air
muta	to change			pneumon	lung
mutat	to change	pachy	thick	poiet	formation
my	muscle	pancreat	pancreas	poli/o	gray
myc	fungus	paque	dark	pollex	thumb
myc/o	fungus	palat/o	palate	por	a passage
mydriat	dilation, widen	palliat	cloaked	porphyr	purple
myel	bone marrow, spinal cord	pallid/o	globus, pallidus	poster/i	behind, toward the back
myel/o	marrow	palm	palm	prand/i	meal
my/o	muscle	palpitat	throbbing	presby	old
my/os	muscle	papill	papilla	press	to press
myring	drum membrane	para	to bear	proct	anus, rectum
myring/o	drum membrane	paralyt	to disable, paralysis	proct/o	anus, rectum
myx	mucus	partum	labor	prolif	fruitful
		parturit	in labor	prophylact	guarding
narc/o	numbness	patell	kneecap, patella	prostat	prostate
nas/o	nose	path	disease	prosth/e	an addition
nat	birth	path/o	disease	prot/e	first
nat/o	birth	pause	cessation	proxim	near the point of origin
necr	death	pector	chest	prurit	itching
necr/o	death	pectorat	breast	psych	mind
nephr	kidney	ped	foot, child	psych/o	mind
nephr/o	kidney	ped/i	foot, child	pudend	external genitals
neur	nerve	pedicul	a louse	pulm/o	lung
neur/i	nerve	pelv/i	pelvis	pulmon	lung
neur/o	nerve	pen	penis	pulmonar	lung
neutr/o	neither	penile	penis	pupill	pupil
nid	nest	pept	to digest	purpur	purple
noct	night	perine	perineum	py	pus
nom	law	periton/e	peritoneum	pyel	renal pelvis
norm	rule	phac	lens	pyel/o	renal pelvis
nucl	nucleus	phac/o	lens	pylor	pylorus, gate keeper
nucle	kernel, nucleus	phag	to eat, engulf	py/o	pus
nyctal	blind	phag/o	to eat, engulf	pyret	fever
nystagm	to nod	phak	lentil, lens	pyr/o	heat, fire
		phalang/e	closely knit row		
occlus	to shut up	pharyng/o	pharynx	rach	spine
ocul	eye	pharyng	pharynx	rachi	spine
odont	tooth	phas	speech	radi	radius
olecran	elbow	phen/o	to show	rad/i	radiating out from a center
onc/o	tumor	phe/o	dusky	radiat	radiant
onych	nail	phim	a muzzle	radic/o	spinal nerve root
onych/o	nail	phleb	vein	radicul	spinal nerve root
o/o	ovum, egg	phleb/o	vein	radi/o	ray
oophor	ovary	phon	voice	rect/o	rectum
ophthalm	eye	phone	voice	relaxat	to loosen
ophthalm/o	eye	phon/o	sound	remiss	remit
opt	eye	phor	carrying	ren	kidney
opt/o	eye	phos	light	ren/o	kidney
or	mouth	phot/o	light	respirat	breathing
orch	testicle	phragm	partition	reticul/o	net
orchid	testicle	phragmat/o	partition	retin	retina
orchid/o	testicle	phras	speech		
organ	organ	physic	nature		

retin/o	retina
rhabd/o	rod
rheumat	discharge
rheumat/o	discharge
rhin/o	nose
rhonch	snore
rhytid/o	wrinkle
roent	roentgen
rotat	to turn
rrhyth	rhythm
rrhythm	rhythm
rube/o	red
sacr	sacrum
salping	tube, fallopian tube
salping/o	tube, fallopian tube
salpinx	tube, fallopian tube
sarc	flesh
sarc/o	flesh
scapul	shoulder blade
scler	hardening
scler/o	hardening, sclera
scoli	curvature
scoli/o	curvature
scop	to examine
seb/o	oil
secund	second
semin	seed
seminat	seed
senile	old
senil	old
sept	putrefaction
septic	putrefying
ser (a)	whey
ser/o	whey, serum
sert	to gain
sexu	sex
sial	saliva
sial/o	salivary
sider/o	iron
sigmoid	sigmoid
sigmoid/o	sigmoid
sin/o	a curve
sinus	a hollow curve
situ	place
som	body
somat	body
somat/o	body
somn	sleep
son	sound
son/o	sound
spadias	a rent, an opening
spastic	convulsive
sperm	seed (sperm)
spermi	seed (sperm)
spermat	seed (sperm)
spermat/o	seed (sperm)
sphygm/o	pulse
spin	spine, a thorn
spir/o	breath
splen/o	spleen
spondyl	vertebra
spondyl/o	vertebra
staped	stirrup
steat	fat
sten	narrowing
ster	solid
stern	sternum
stern/o	sternum
sterol	solid (fat)
steth	chest
steth/o	chest
stigmat	point
stom	mouth
stomat	mouth
strabism	a squinting
strict	to draw, to bind
superfic/i	near the surface
super/i	upper
suppress	suppress
surrog	substituted
sympath	sympathy
synov	joint fluid
syst	contraction
system	a composite whole
systol	contraction
tel	end, distant
tele	distant
tempor	temples
tend/o	tendon
tendin	tendon
ten/o	tendon
tenon	tendon
tenos	tendon
tens	tension
tentori	tentorium, tent
terat	monster
testicul	testicle
test/o	testicle
thalass	sea
thel/i	nipple
therm	hot, heat
therm/o	hot, heat
thorac	chest
thorac/o	chest
thorax	chest
thromb	clot
thromb/o	clot
thym	thymus, mind, emotion
thyr	thyroid, shield
thyr/o	thyroid, shield
thyrox	thyroid, shield
tibi	tibia
tinnit	a jingling
toc	birth
tom/o	to cut
ton	tone, tension
ton/o	tone
tonsill	tonsil, almond
topic	place
top/o	place
tors	twisted
tort/i	twisted
tox	poison
toxic	poison
trach/e	trachea
trache/o	trachea
tract	to draw
trephinat	a bore
trich	hair
trich/o	hair
trigon	trigone
trism	grating
trop	turning
troph	a turning
tubercul	a little swelling
tuss	cough
tympan	ear drum
tympan/o	drum
uln	ulna, elbow
uln/o	ulna, elbow
umbilic	navel
ungu	nail
ur	urine
ure	urinate
urea	urea
uret	urine
ureter	ureter
ureter/o	ureter
urethr	urethra
urethr/o	urethra
urin	urine
urinat	urine
urin/o	urine
ur/o	urine
uter	uterus
uter/o	uterus
uve	uvea
vagin	vagina
vag/o	vagus, wandering
varic/o	twisted vein
vas	vessel
vascul	small vessel
vas/o	vessel
vector	a carrier
ven	vein
venere	sexual intercourse
ven/i	vein
ven/o	vein
ventilat	to air
ventr	near or on the belly side of the body
ventricul	ventricle
ventricul/o	little belly
vermi	worm
vers	turning
vertebr	vertebra
vertebr/o	vertebra
vesic	bladder
vesicul	vesicle
vir	virus (poison)
viril	masculine
viscer	body organs
volt	volt
volunt	will
volvul	to roll
vuls	to pull
watt	watt
xanth/o	yellow
xen	foreign material
xer	dry
xer/o	dry
xiph	sword
zo/o	animal
zoon	life

-able	capable	-grade	a step	-penia	lack of, deficiency
-ac	pertaining to	-graft	pencil, grafting knife	-pepsia	to digest
-ad	pertaining to	-gram	a weight, mark, record	-pexy	surgical fixation
-age	related to	-graph	to write, record	-phagia	to eat
-al	pertaining to	-graphy	recording	-phasia	to speak
-algesia	pain			-pheresis	removal
-algia	pain	-hexia	condition	-phil	attraction
-ant	forming			-philia	attraction
-ar	pertaining to	-ia	condition	-phobia	fear
-ary	pertaining to	-iasis	condition	-phoresis	to carry
-ase	enzyme	-ic	pertaining to	-phragm	a fence
-asthenia	weakness	-ide	having a particular	-phraxis	to obstruct
-ate	use, action		quality	-phylaxis	protection
-ate (d)	use, action	-in	chemical, pertaining to	-physis	growth
		-ine	pertaining to	-plakia	plate
-betes	to go	-ing	quality of	-plasia	formation, produce
-blast	immature cell, germ cell	-ion	process	-plasm	a thing formed, plasma
-body	body	-ism	condition	-plasty	surgical repair
		-ist	one who specializes, agent	-plegia	stroke, paralysis
-cele	hernia, tumor, swelling	-itis	inflammation	-pnea	breathing
-centesis	surgical puncture	-ity	condition	-poiesis	formation
-ceps	head	-ive	nature of, quality of	-praxia	action
-cide	to kill			-ptosis	prolapse, drooping
-clasia	a breaking	-kinesia	motion	-ptysis	to spit, spitting
-clave	a key	-kinesis	motion	-puncture	to pierce
-cle	small				
-clysis	injection	-lalia	to talk	-rrhage	to burst forth, bursting forth
-cope	strike	-lemma	a sheath, rind	-rrhagia	to burst forth, bursting forth
-crit	to separate	-lepsy	seizure	-rrhaphy	suture
-culture	cultivation	-lexia	diction	-rrhea	flow, discharge
-cusis	hearing	-liter	liter	-rrhexis	rupture
-cuspid	point	-lith	stone		
-cyesis	pregnancy	-logy	study of	-scope	instrument
-cyst	bladder	-lymph	clear fluid	-scopy	to view, examine
-cyte	cell	-lysis	destruction, to separate	-sepsis	decay
				-sis	condition
-derma	skin	-malacia	softening	-some	body
-dermis	skin	-mania	madness	-spasm	tension, spasm, contraction
-desis	binding	-megaly	enlargement, large	-stalsis	contraction
-dipsia	thirst	-meter	instrument to measure	-stasis	control, stopping
-drome	a course	-metry	measurement	-staxis	dripping, trickling
-dynia	pain	-mnesia	memory	-sthenia	strength
		-morph	form, shape	-stomy	new opening
-ectasia	dilatation			-systole	contraction
-ectasis	dilatation, distention	-noia	mind		
-ectasy	dilation			-taxia	order
-ectomy	surgical excision	-oid	resemble	-therapy	treatment
-edema	swelling	-ole	opening	-thermy	heat
-emesis	vomiting	-oma	tumor	-tic	pertaining to
-emia	blood condition	-omion	shoulder	-tome	instrument to cut
-er	relating to, one who	-on	pertaining to	-tomy	incision
-ergy	work	-one	hormone	-tone	tension
-esthesia	feeling	-opia	eye, vision	-tripsy	crushing
		-opsia	eye, vision	-troph (y)	nourishment, development
-form	shape	-opsy	to view	-trophy	nourishment, development
-fuge	to flee	-or	one who, a doer	-type	type
		-ory	like, resemble		
-gen	formation, produce	-orexia	appetite	-um	tissue
-genes	produce	-ose	like	-ure	process
-genesis	formation, produce	-osis	condition	-uria	urine
-genic	formation, produce	-ous	pertaining to	-us	pertaining to
-glia	glue				
-globin	protein	-paresis	weakness	-y	condition, pertaining to,
-gnosis	knowledge	-pathy	disease		process

Glossary

Number in parentheses ( ) indicates chapter.

abduction Movement of a body part away from the midline. (21)

acne vulgaris A common skin condition that occurs when oil and dead skin cells clog the skin's pores; usually called simply acne. (20)

acromegaly A hormonal disorder that results when the pituitary gland produces excess growth hormone, most commonly affecting middle-aged adults and potentially resulting in serious illness and premature death. (30)

active immunity The introduction of immunity by infection or with a vaccine. (26)

active transport The process in cells that requires energy to transport materials to, from, and within the cell. Active transport mechanisms include phagocytosis and pinocytosis. (19)

acute renal failure A condition that occurs when something, such as a blockage, toxins, or a sudden loss of blood flow, causes a change in the filtering function of the kidneys. (29)

Addison's disease A condition in which the cortex of the adrenal gland is damaged, decreasing the production of adrenocortical hormones, usually resulting from an autoimmune disorder but also caused by infection, cancer, or hemorrhage into the glands. (30)

adduction The movement of a body part toward the midline. (21)

alopecia Baldness or loss of hair. (20)

Alzheimer's disease A progressive, degenerative disease of the brain characterized by loss of memory and other cognitive functions. (23)

amblyopia Also called "lazy eye." A disorder in children caused by the eye muscles being weaker in one eye. (24)

amphiarthrotic joint An articulation, or joint, that permits very slight movement. (21)

amyotrophic lateral sclerosis (ALS) Also called motor neuron disease, Lou Gehrig's disease. A disease of unknown cause that breaks down the nerve cells from the brain to the spinal cord (upper motor neurons) and from the spinal cord to the peripheral nerves (lower motor neurons), which control muscle movement. (23)

anatomical position Term used to describe relationships of the parts of the body. In this position, the body is assumed to be standing, with the feet together, the arms to the side, and the head and eyes and palms of the hands facing forward. (19)

anatomy The study of the structure of an organism. (19)

anemia A condition in which there are insufficient levels of hemoglobin in the red blood cells, caused by decreased healthy red cell production by the bone marrow, increased erythrocyte destruction, or blood loss from heavy menstrual periods or internal bleeding. (25)

aneurysm An abnormal widening or ballooning of a portion of an artery, related to weakness in the wall of the blood vessel. (25)

angioplasty A surgical vessel repair procedure frequently used to reopen blocked coronary arteries. (25)

antagonist A muscle that counteracts, or opposes, the action of another muscle. (22)

antibodies Specialized proteins that lock onto specific antigens. (26)

antigen A foreign substance that invades the body. (26)

aponeurosis A wide, thin, sheetlike tendon, made up of fibrous connective tissue, that typically attaches muscles to other muscles. (22)

appendicitis An inflammation of the appendix caused by a blockage of the inside of the appendix, the lumen, which leads to increased pressure, impaired blood flow, and potentially gangrene and rupture. (28)

appendicular skeleton One of the two divisions of the skeletal system, consisting of the 126 bones, including the extremities, that are not part of the axial skeleton. (21)

arrhythmia An irregular heartbeat caused by a disturbance of normal electrical activity of the heart. The two types are tachycardia, or fast heart rate, and bradycardia, or slow heart rate. (25)

arteriosclerosis Also called hardening of the arteries. A thickening and loss of elasticity of the arteries, occurring over many years during which the arteries develop areas that become hard and brittle due to deposits of calcium. (25)

arthritis Inflammation of one or more joints caused by various disease processes. (21)

articulation Also called a joint. The place where two bones connect, with the positioning of the bones determining the type of movement the joint performs. (21)

ascites Fluid in the abdomen. (29)

asthma A chronic inflammatory condition typically caused when allergens or other irritating substances cause swelling in the lining of the trachea and bronchial tubes, which causes the creation of mucus, which can cause coughing or a sense of struggling to breathe. (27)

astigmatism A condition caused by irregularities of the cornea, leading to blurred images in near or distant vision. (24)

atherosclerosis Narrowing of the vessel lumen of the arteries due to a buildup of fatty material and plaque, thus slowing or stopping the flow of blood, which can lead to cell death in the area supplied by the vessel. It is the leading cause of congestive heart disease. (25)

atmospheric pressure The pressure of the air around us, measured as 760 mmHg at sea level, lower at higher altitudes. (27)

atom The smallest chemical unit of matter. (19)

atria The two upper receiving chambers of the heart. (25)

atrioventricular node Also called the AV node. One of the three areas of specialized neuromuscular tissue that initiate the heartbeat, it is located beneath the endocardium of the right atrium and is a "gatekeeper," responsible for transmitting impulses from the sinoatrial node to the inferior portions of the heart. (25)

atrophy A loss of muscle mass and strength that occurs with the disuse of muscles over time. (22)

audiology The study of hearing disorders. (24)

axial skeleton One of the two divisions of the skeletal system, consisting of 80 bones from the axis of the body, including the skull and vertebral system. (21)

B lymphocytes White blood cells created and matured in the bone marrow that seek out invading organisms and send T lymphocytes to destroy them. (26)

Bell's palsy A weakness or paralysis of the muscles that control expression on one side of the face. (23)

benign prostatic hyperplasia (BPH) Also called benign prostatic hypertrophy. An enlargement of the prostate gland, usually occurring in men older than 50, which compresses the urethra, restricting the normal flow of urine. (31)

bicuspid valve Also called the mitral valve. Valve through which the blood leaves the left atrium of the heart. (25)

bradycardia An abnormally slow heart rate, fewer than 60 beats per minute, which may be regular or irregular. (25)

breast cancer The types are infiltrating ductal, the most common, in which the cancer arises in the tiny ducts that run from the milk glands to the nipple; infiltrating lobular, which develops in the lobules; and inflammatory. (31)

bronchitis Respiratory system disorder in which the mucous membranes in the bronchial passages become inflamed, resulting in mucus, coughing, and breathlessness. (27)

bundle of His Also called the atrioventricular (AV) bundle. One of the three areas of specialized neuromuscular tissue that initiate the heartbeat, it extends from the AV node into the intraventricular septum, where it branches off, sending a branch to each ventricle. (25)

bursitis Inflammation of the bursa, a small sac of fluid that cushions and lubricates an area where joint-related tissues, including bones, tendons, ligaments, muscles, and skin, rub against one another. (21)

cancellous (spongy) bone The reticular tissue that makes up most of the volume of a long bone and that includes the red bone marrow, which manufactures most of the red blood cells found in the body. (21)

cardiac muscle A type of involuntary muscle found in the heart, roughly quadrangular in shape, cross striated, and having a single central nucleus. (22)

cardiomegaly An enlarged heart. (30)

cataract A clouding over the eye's lens that prevents light from entering through it. (24)

cavities Spaces within the body. (19)

cell A basic unit of life that contains the internal organs, of viscera. Comprised of cell membrane, which protects it and regulates the movement of water, nutrients, and wastes; a central nucleus, which contains the cell's DNA (deoxyribonucleic acid) and RNA (ribonucleic acid); and organelles, small structures that help carry out the day-to-day operations of the cell. (19)

cell membrane The membrane that protects the cell from the outside environment and regulates the movement of water, nutrients, and wastes into and out of cells. (19)

cellulitis An acute, spreading bacterial infection below the surface of the skin characterized by redness, warmth, swelling, and pain. It can also cause fever, chills, and enlarged lymph nodes. (20)

cerebrospinal fluid The fluid produced by the choroid plexus in the ventricles of the brain that fills the spinal canal and the subarachnoid space that surround the brain, cushioning the brain and spinal cord and nourishing them with oxygen and glucose. (23)

cervical cancer Cancer of the cervix. The two main types are squamous cell (epidermoid) and adenocarcinoma. (31)

cervicitis An inflammation of the cervix, most often caused by infection with sexually transmitted infections (STIs). (31)

chemotherapy Cancer treatment using drugs. (26)

chronic fatigue syndrome (CFS) Immune system disorder of unknown origin. (26)

chronic obstructive pulmonary disease (COPD) Respiratory system condition comprising primarily two diseases, chronic bronchitis and emphysema, in which the flow of air through the airways and out of the lungs is obstructed. (27)

chronic renal failure A gradual and progressive loss of kidney function, typically as a result of another disease. (29)

cilia Hairlike projections in the nose that increase the surface area of a cell, increasing its ability to trap dust, pollen, and other foreign matter to prevent it from entering the nasal cavity. (19, 27)

circumcision Surgical removal of the foreskin of the penis, performed for religious, cultural, or medical reasons. (31)

circumduction The process of moving a body part in a circular motion. (21)

cirrhosis A potentially life-threatening condition that occurs when the liver is damaged, usually after years of inflammation, by scarring, or fibrosis, that replaces healthy tissue and prevents the liver from working normally. (28)

colitis Inflammation of the large intestine caused by many different disease processes, including infections, primary inflammatory disorders (ulcerative colitis, Crohn's colitis, lymphocytic and collagenous colitis), lack of blood flow (ischemic colitis), and history of radiation to the large bowel. (28)

colorectal cancer Collective term for colon cancer, affecting the large intestine, and rectal cancer, affecting the last eight to 10 inches of the colon. (28)

common cold An infection of the upper respiratory tract caused by any one of a number of viruses and differing from other viral infections by its lack of high fever or significant fatigue. (27)

compact bone The dense, hard layer of bone tissue in a long bone. (21)

complement A group of proteins activated by antibodies that assist in destroying bacteria, viruses, and infected cells. (26)

congestive heart failure (CHF) Also called simply heart failure. A condition in which the heart cannot pump enough blood to the other organs, which can result from such conditions as coronary artery disease, past heart attack, hypertension, heart valve disease due to past rheumatic fever or other cause, primary diseases of the heart muscle itself, heart defects present at birth, and any infection of the heart valves or heart muscle, such as endocarditis or myocarditis. (25)

conjunctivitis Also called pinkeye. An inflammation of the conjunctiva, the tissue that lines the inside of the eyelid, frequently caused by a virus, bacteria, or other irritating substance. (24)

constipation A condition in which stools are difficult to pass, involving straining, a feeling of not completely emptying the bowels, and hard or pellet-like stools. (28)

contact dermatitis An allergic reaction of the skin caused by irritating substances coming in contact with it, often resulting in red, irritated skin and occasionally in vesicles and rash. (20)

corneal abrasion A lesion or abrasion on the cornea as the result of an injury or infection. (24)

coronary heart disease (CHD) Also called coronary artery disease (CAD).

Condition resulting from a narrowing of the coronary arteries that supply blood to the heart, which can lead to a higher risk of heart attack and, potentially, sudden death. (25)

cortex In the kidney, the outer layer, in which the arteries, veins, convoluted tubules, and glomerular capsules are found. (29). In the lymph node, that portion populated mainly by lymphocytes. (26)

Crohn's disease Also called inflammatory bowel disease (IBD). A chronic inflammatory disease of the intestines that primarily causes ulcerations in the lining of the small and large intestines but can affect the digestive system anywhere from the mouth to the anus. (28)

Cushing's disease A rare disorder when too much cortisol is released by ACTH as a result of stimulation of the pituitary. (30)

cyanosis A blue-colored complexion caused by lack of oxygen. (27)

cystic fibrosis (CF) A chronic and progressive respiratory system disorder, usually diagnosed in childhood, in which the mucus becomes thick, dry, and sticky, causing it to build up and clog passages in many organs but primarily in the lungs and pancreas. (27)

cystitis An inflammation of the bladder that usually occurs when bacteria infect the lower urinary tract. Most cases are caused by *Escherichia coli*, a bacterium found in the lower gastrointestinal system. (29)

cytokinesis The separation of the cytoplasm into two parts. (19)

cytoplasm The substance that fills a cell. (19)

decubitus ulcer Also called pressure sores or bedsores. Area of skin and tissue that breaks down when constant pressure is maintained on it. (20)

dermis One of the two layers that compose the skin. (20)

diabetes mellitus A condition in which the body is unable to produce enough insulin to properly control blood sugar levels by converting sugar and starches into energy. The three types are type 1, also known as juvenile diabetes and as insulin-dependent diabetes mellitus (IDDM), type 2, also known as adult-onset and as non–insulin-dependent diabetes mellitus (NIDDM), and gestational diabetes, which occurs during pregnancy. (30)

dialysis A filter other than the kidneys to remove toxins and maintain water balance. The two types are hemodialysis, which uses a machine that cleans the blood outside the body, and peritoneal dialysis, which is done through the tissues of the abdomen, with a dialysis fluid instilled in the stomach, left for a period while the membranes in the abdomen filter toxins, and then removed. (29)

diaphragm A dome-shaped respiratory muscle that divides the ventral cavity into two parts. (19)

diaphysis The shaft of a long bone. (21)

diarrhea An increase in the frequency of bowel movements or a decrease in the form of stool. The two types are acute, which lasts a few days to a week, and chronic, defined usually as lasting more than three weeks. (28)

diarthrotic joint An articulation, or joint, that allows for free movement in a variety of directions. (21)

diastolic blood pressure Pressure recorded in an artery when the left ventricle relaxes. In standard notation it is recorded below the systolic pressure. (25)

dislocation A disconnection of the bones that meet at a joint, usually caused by a sudden impact, such that the bones are no longer in their normal positions. (21)

diverticulitis Inflammation of a small pouch or sac in the wall of the colon, generally caused by stool lodging in the diverticula, that can lead to swelling or rupture. (28)

diverticulosis The condition of having diverticula, or small outpouchings, in the large intestine, most typically in the sigmoid colon, a condition that increases with age because of the weakening of the colon walls. (28)

DNA (deoxyribonucleic acid) The genetic code that coordinates protein synthesis. (19)

dorsiflexion The process of bending a body part backward. (21)

dwarfism A condition characterized by shorter than normal skeletal growth, resulting from more than 300 recognized conditions, with achondroplasia being the most common type of short-limb dwarfism. (30)

dysmenorrhea The presence of abdominal cramps during menstruation. The two types are primary, in which there is no underlying gynecological abnormality, and secondary, in which there is such an abnormality. (31)

dyspnea Difficulty breathing. (25)

eczema Also called atopic dermatitis. A chronic skin condition characterized by scaling, itching rashes and caused by an allergic-type reaction on the skin. (20)

electrolyte Medical/scientific term for salts, specifically an ion that is electrically charged and moves to either a negative (cathode) or positive (anode) electrode. (19)

emphysema A progressive respiratory system disease in which the tissues necessary to support the physical shape and function of the lung are destroyed, primarily causing shortness of breath. (27)

encephalitis An inflammation in the brain, most often caused by viral infections. (23)

endocardium The inner lining of the heart wall. (25)

endometriosis A condition in which the endometrium, the tissue lining the uterus, travels outside the uterus into the pelvis or abdominal cavity. (31)

endomysium The connective tissue covering that surrounds an individual muscle cell. (22)

endosteum The tough connective tissue membrane lining the medullary canal and containing the bone marrow in a long bone. (21)

epidermis One of the two layers that compose the skin. (20)

epididymitis An inflammation or infection of the epididymis, the long coiled tube attached to the upper part of each testicle, where mature sperm are stored before ejaculation. (31)

epilepsy A common neurological disorder in which the nervous system produces intense, abnormal bursts of electrical activity in the brain, which can lead to seizures that temporarily interfere with muscle control, movement, speech, vision, or awareness. (23)

epimysium A thin connective tissue covering muscles. (22)

epiphysis The ends of a developing long bone. (21)

episiotomy An incision in the perineum, the external region between the vulva and the anus, during labor to prevent its tearing during delivery. (31)

erectile dysfunction (ED) The inability to achieve or maintain an erection sufficient for sexual intercourse, resulting from insufficient blood supply, from the smooth muscle failing to relax, or from the penis not retaining the blood that flows into it. (31)

erythrocytes Also called red blood cells. Biconcave cells produced in the red bone marrow that are small enough to pass through capillaries. (25)

eversion The process of turning the body outward. (21)

exophthalmos A condition produced by hyperthyroidism in which the eyeball protrudes beyond its normal protective orbit because of swelling in the tissues behind. (30)

extension The process of straightening a flexed limb. (21)

fascia The connective tissue structure covering the skeletal muscles and separating them from one another. (22)

fascicles Sections into which a muscle is divided. (22)

fibrocystic breast disease Also called mammary dysplasia, benign breast disease, and diffuse cystic mastopathy. A condition that involves common, benign changes in the tissues of the breast. (31)

fibromyalgia A musculoskeletal pain and fatigue disorder with no known cause but with evidence pointing to a genetic predisposition to a neuromuscular/neuroendocrine abnormality that disturbs the usual sensory perception, especially of pain signals. (22)

flexion The process of bending (or curving) the spine. (21)

folliculitis An inflammation or infection of hair follicles that most often appears in areas that become irritated by shaving or the rubbing of clothes or where follicles and pores are blocked by oils and dirt. (20)

gastroesophageal reflux disease (GERD) Condition in which the muscle at the superior portion of the stomach (the cardiac sphincter) does not close tightly or relaxes inappropriately, allowing for a "backwash" of gastric fluids and stomach contents into the esophagus and the throat. (28)

genetics The study of the makeup of animals or plants. (19)

germinal centers The primary resting places for B lymphocytes. (26)

gestational diabetes A condition in which the body is unable to produce enough insulin to properly control blood sugar levels by converting sugar and starches into energy, occurring during pregnancy and typically disappearing afterward but occasionally precipitating ongoing type 2 diabetes. (30)

gigantism A condition in which excessive growth hormone is secreted during childhood, before the closure of the bone growth plates, which causes overgrowth of the long bones, muscles, and organs, usually caused by a pituitary gland tumor. (30)

glaucoma A condition caused by an increase in the amount of pressure in the eye, leading to an excessive amount of aqueous humor, can lead to damage of the optic nerve and eventual blindness. The two basic types are open-angled glaucoma, in which pressure builds up very slowly, and acute-angle closure glaucoma, considered to be much more serious, in which the space between the iris and the cornea decreases, causing a greater degree of pressure to build. (24)

glomerulonephritis Also called glomerular disease. A condition that hampers the kidneys' ability to remove waste and excess fluids and can lead to kidney failure. (29)

goiter An enlarged thyroid gland, most commonly caused by Hashimoto's thyroiditis, an autoimmune inflammation. (30)

gout A disease caused by the formation of crystals in a joint, leading to inflammation. It most commonly seen in men older than 40 and most frequently affects the great toe. (21)

Graves' disease An autoimmune disorder in which the antibodies produced by the immune system stimulate the thyroid to produce too much thyroxine, the most common cause of hyperthyroidism. (30)

Hashimoto's thyroiditis An autoimmune inflammation of the thyroid that causes hypothyroidism and goiter. (30)

hay fever Also called seasonal allergic rhinitis or pollinosis. A seasonal allergy that causes inflammation of the mucous membranes of the nose and eyes. (27)

headache Headache categories differentiated by the International Headache Society (IHS) are migraine, tension, cluster, and posttraumatic. (23)

hearing loss The two most common types are conductive, a temporary condition that may develop when sound waves have no way of being conducted through the ear, and sensorineural, which occurs when neural structures of the ear become damaged, eventually leading to deafness. (24)

heart murmur A condition in which a damaged or diseased valve allows blood to escape and move backward through the valve. (25)

hemostasis The stoppage of bleeding as a result of the smooth muscle at the site of a break causing the vessel wall to contract, creating a spasm that reduces the amount of blood loss and initiates the attachment of platelets to the broken area and to each other there, which forms a plug. (25)

hemoptysis The coughing up of blood. (27)

hemorrhoid A dilated vein in the walls of the anus and sometimes around the rectum, usually caused by untreated constipation but occasionally associated with chronic diarrhea. (28)

hernia An abnormal protrusion of an organ, or part of an organ, through the wall of the body cavity where it is located, the most common types of abdominal hernias being hiatal and inguinal hernias. (28)

herpes simplex An infection that primarily affects the mouth or the genital area. The two different strains are Herpes simplex virus type 1 (HSV-1), the more common, which usually is acquired in childhood and is associated with infections of the lips, mouth, and face, and Herpes simplex virus 2 (HSV-2), which is sexually transmitted. (20)

herpes zoster Also called shingles. An infection caused by the varicella zoster virus that causes a painful rash. The virus first causes chickenpox and then lies dormant in the nerves, but with the potential to reactivate as shingles. (20)

hiatal hernia A condition in which the upper portion of the stomach protrudes into the chest cavity through a weakened or enlarged esophageal hiatus, an opening in the diaphragm normally large enough to accommodate only the esophagus. (28)

hilum The notch in the concave border of each kidney, the entrance for the renal artery and vein, nerves, lymphatic vessels, and the opening for the ureters. (29)

homeostasis The result of an organism's systems working together to maintain balance or equilibrium by adjusting for constant changes. (19)

hordeolum Also called a sty. An inflamed gland of the eyelid, often caused by a bacterial infection, that appears as a pus-filled swelling near the roots of the eyelash. (24)

hydrocele A painless buildup of watery fluid around one or both testicles that causes the scrotum or groin area to swell. (31)

hyperopia Also called farsightedness. Visual distortion caused by the lens focusing behind the retina. (24)

hypertension Also called high blood pressure. Condition in which blood pressure is consistently higher than 140/90, which can lead to kidney failure, stroke, heart attack, peripheral artery disease, and eye damage. (25)

hyperthyroidism A condition in which the thyroid produces excess amounts of hormones, potentially leading to exophthalmos, palpitations, atrial fibrillation, enlargement of the heart, and congestive heart failure. (30)

hypotension Also called low blood pressure. Condition in which blood pressure is consistently lower than 90/60, which can cause inadequate blood flow to the heart, brain, and other vital organs. (25)

hypothyroidism A condition in which the thyroid produces inadequate amounts of hormones, which can lead to an enlarged thyroid gland, a goiter, from the constant stimulation. (30)

hysterectomy A surgical procedure to remove a woman's uterus. The types are complete (total), in which the cervix, fallopian tubes, and ovaries are removed; partial (subtotal), in which the upper part of the uterus is removed but the cervix is not; and radical, in which the uterus, cervix, upper part of the vagina, and supporting tissues are removed. (31)

immune response A series of immune system attacks on organisms and substances that invade the body systems and cause disease. (26)

immune system The tissues, organs, and physiologic processes used by the body to identify abnormal cells and foreign substances and defend against those that might be harmful, including bacteria, microbes, viruses, toxins, and parasites. (26)

impacted cerumen Hardened ear wax that obstructs the auditory canal and can lead to hearing loss or tinnitus. (24)

impetigo A contagious skin infection, found most commonly in children, caused by bacteria that form round, crusted, oozing spots, typically around the nose and mouth. (20)

incontinence The involuntary and unpredictable flow of urine. The three types are stress, the most common, which happens when sneezing, laughing, or the like; urge, which occurs when the bladder contracts without warning; and overflow, which happens when a blockage prohibits normal emptying and the bladder simply overflows. (29)

infectious mononucleosis Also called simply mono and "the kissing disease." A viral infection caused by the Epstein-Barr virus (EBV), part of the herpes family, characterized by an increase in white blood cells that contain a single nucleus and commonly found in young adults. (26)

influenza Also called flu. An illness caused by infection of the respiratory tract by viruses. (27)

inguinal hernia A condition in which tissue or part of the intestine push through a weak spot in the abdominal wall in the groin area, causing a bulge in the groin or scrotum. (28)

insertion In locations at which skeletal muscles attach, the attachment point on the bone that moves. (22)

insulin-dependent diabetes mellitus (IDDM) Also known as type 1 diabetes, juvenile diabetes. A condition in which the body is unable to produce enough insulin to properly control its blood sugar level by converting sugar and starches into energy, typically diagnosed in children. (30)

interstitial cystitis (IC) An inflammation of the bladder wall, the cause of which is unknown. (29)

inversion The process of turning the body inward. (21)

irritable bowel syndrome (IBS) A common intestinal condition characterized by abdominal pain and cramps, diarrhea or constipation or both, gas, bloating, nausea, and other symptoms. (28)

kidney stones Also called renal calculi. Deposits of mineral salts in the kidney, usually benign there, that can pass into the ureter, slowing down or blocking urine flow and irritating the ureter, causing bleeding. (29)

kidneys Paired, bean-shaped organs located at the back of the abdominal cavity and lying on either side of the spinal column in the flank area, against the muscles of the back. (29)

Legionnaire's disease A type of pneumonia or lung infection caused by the *Legionella* germ. (27)

leukemia A malignant cancer of the bone marrow and blood, affecting the white blood cells. The two types are lymphocytic, affecting the lymphoid cells, and myeloid, or myelogenous, affecting the myeloid cells, and the disease can be acute or chronic. (25)

leukocytes Also called white blood cells. Larger blood cells that fight infection and thus contribute to homeostasis. (25, 26)

lipolysis The destruction of fats. (30)

lithotripsy Procedure that involves passing shock waves through the body to break down kidney stones. The two types are extracorporeal shockwave and percutaneous ultrasonic. (29)

lung cancer Types include adenocarcinoma, the most common type, bronchoalveolar cell carcinoma, squamous cell carcinoma, and carcinoid lung cancer. (27)

lymph A clear fluid that travels through the body's arteries, circulating through the tissues to cleanse them and keep them firm and then draining away through the lymphatic system. The lymph nodes are the filters of the system. (25)

lymphedema A condition resulting from an interruption of the normal lymphatic flow. The two types are primary, in which each stage is called by a different name (Milroy's disease or syndrome, Meige lymphedema or lymphedema praecox, lymphedema tarda), and secondary, generally caused by an obstruction of or injury to the lymph system. (26)

lymphocytes White blood cells created in the bone marrow that allow the body to recognize organisms that have invaded it previously. The two kinds are B lymphocytes and T lymphocytes. (26)

lysosomes Organelles that contain enzymes that aid in the digestion of nutrient molecules and other materials. (19)

macular degeneration Deterioration of the central portion of the retina. The two types are dry, in which there is a formation of small yellow deposits (drusen) under the macula, and wet, in which abnormal new blood vessels called subretinal neovascularization grow underneath the retina and the macula. (24)

malignant melanoma A type of cancer arising from the melanocyte cells of the skin, which produce the pigment melanin, that develops when the melanocytes no longer respond to normal control mechanisms of cellular growth. (20)

medulla In the kidney, the middle portion, in which the renal pyramids are found. (29). In the lymph node, the portion primarily made up of macrophages attached to reticular fibers. (26)

medullary canal The narrow space or cavity throughout the length of the diaphysis in a long bone, which contains yellow bone marrow, made of fat cells. (21)

meiosis A two-part cell division process in organisms that reproduce sexually that results in gametes with one-half the number of chromosomes of the parent cell. (19)

Ménière's disease A condition of the inner ear, named after French physician Prosper Ménière who first described it; characterized by vertigo, tinnitus, fluctuating hearing loss, and pressure or pain in the affected ear. (24)

meningitis An infection of the meninges that surround and protect the brain and spinal cord, typically caused by a bacterial or viral infection. Sometimes fatal. (23)

metastasis A process in which cancer cells break away from the original tumor and travel to other areas of the body, where they form new tumors. (26)

mitochondrion An important cellular organelle. The mitochondria (plural) are often referred to as the power plants of a cell because many of the reactions that produce energy take place in mitochondria. (19)

mitosis Nuclear division plus cytokinesis (the actual cellular division) that produces two identical daughter cells during prophase, prometaphase, metaphase, anaphase, and telophase. (19)

molecule The smallest part of a substance called a compound that still is that substance; for example, a molecule of water is the smallest bit of water that still is water. Molecules are composed of atoms joined together chemically. (19)

multiple sclerosis (MS) A chronic autoimmune disease in which the body directs the antibodies and white cells to attack the myelin sheath surrounding nerves in the brain and spinal cord, which causes inflammation and injury and, eventually, scarring, which results in difficulty with movement, vision, or sensation. (23)

muscle cramps Pain in the absence of electrolyte or pH disturbance, commonly indicating a peripheral nerve disorder and less commonly an abnormality in muscle fibers. (22)

muscular dystrophy (MD) One of a group of genetic diseases characterized by progressive weakness and muscle degeneration. There are a number of major forms of the disease, some involving the skeletal, or voluntary, muscles that control movement and others involving the heart and other involuntary muscles and other organs as well. (22)

myasthenia gravis A chronic neuromuscular disease characterized by varying degrees of weakness of the skeletal, or voluntary, muscles of the body. (22)

myocardial infarction (MI) Also called heart attack. Condition that occurs when the blood supply to a part of the myocardium is severely reduced or stopped, usually due to atherosclerosis, potentially resulting in disability or death. (25)

myocardium The middle muscular layer of the heart wall. (25)

myomectomy Surgery used to treat uterine fibroids, involving removal of the fibroids without removing the healthy tissue. (31)

myxedema A rare, life-threatening condition that can result from long-term, untreated hypothyroidism. (30)

nephrons The functional units of the kidney that remove the waste products of metabolism from the blood plasma. (29)

neuralgia An intense burning or stabbing pain caused by irritation of or damage to a nerve from a variety of sources. (23)

neutrophils White blood cells, the most common type of phagocyte, that primarily attack bacteria. (26)

non–insulin-dependent diabetes mellitus (NIDDM) Also known as type 2 diabetes, adult-onset diabetes. A condition in which the body is unable to properly control its blood sugar level, resulting from insulin resistance combined with a relative insulin deficiency, often diagnosed later in life and having a very strong correlation with obesity. (30)

nucleus The center part of a cell containing the cell's DNA. (19)

oncogenes The genes controlling cell growth and multiplication that are transformed into cancer cells by cancer-causing agents. (26)

oral cancer Cancer of the mouth, usually starting in the flat squamous cells that line it. (28)

organelles Small structures that help carry out the day-to-day operations of a cell. (19)

organs Groups of tissues that serve a common purpose or function. (19)

origin In locations at which skeletal muscles attach, the attachment point on the bone that is more fixed or still. (22)

osteoarthritis The most common type of arthritis, resulting from years of wear and tear on joints and occurring most frequently in the hips, knees, and finger joints. (21)

osteoporosis The loss of bone density and the thinning of bone tissue, a condition seen most commonly in older adults, especially postmenopausal women, and in individuals who do not consume enough calcium. (21)

otitis media Inflammation of the middle ear caused by viral or bacterial infections. (24)

otosclerosis A condition in which the tissue surrounding the bone of the stapes grows abnormally around it, preventing it from transmitting sound vibrations to the inner ear and resulting in profound hearing loss. (24)

ovarian cancer The three main types are epithelial cell cancer, the most common, which starts in the outer covering of the ovary, germ cell tumors, which start in the egg cells within the ovary and generally occur in younger women and even children, and stromal tumors, which start in the cells that form the structural framework of the ovary. (31)

ovarian cyst Sac filled with a fluid or semisolid material that develops on or within the ovary, typically not disease related and disappearing on its own, when the grown follicle fails to rupture and release an egg and instead of being reabsorbed forms a cyst. (31)

ovulation The process of producing an ovum and releasing it into the pelvic cavity and the fallopian tube. (31)

oxygen debt The inability of the body to absorb enough oxygen to supply the energy required to sustain a high level of activity, resulting in its utilizing the anaerobic energy system and in the buildup of lactic acid in the muscles. (22)

pancreatic cancer The two types are adenocarcinoma, the more common, which arises from the exocrine glands, and neuroendocrine carcinoma, or islet cell tumor, which is rare. (28)

paraplegia Paralysis from approximately the waist down. (23)

Parkinson's disease A progressive disorder caused by degeneration of the nerve cells in the parts of the brain that control movement, resulting in a shortage of the neurotransmitter dopamine, which impairs movement. (23)

passive transport Process in cells that does not require energy to transport materials to, from, and within the cell. Passive transport mechanisms include diffusion, osmosis, and filtration. (19)

pathophysiology The study of diseases or disorders caused by a malfunction or by aging. (19)

pediculosis An infestation of the hairy parts of the body or clothing with the eggs, larvae, or adults of lice. (20)

pelvic inflammatory disease (PID) An infection of the upper genital area that occurs when disease-carrying organisms migrate upward from the urethra and cervix, potentially affecting the uterus, ovaries, and fallopian tubes and potentially leading to scarring and infertility or to tubal pregnancy. (31)

peptic ulcer disease (PUD) A condition in which a disruption occurs in the lining of the esophagus, stomach, or duodenum. (28)

pericardium The outer lining of the heart wall. (25)

perimysium Connective tissue responsible for dividing a muscle into sections. (22)

perineum The external region between the vulva and the anus, composed of muscle covered with skin. (31)

periosteum The membrane that forms the covering of long bones, except at their articular surfaces. (21)

phagocytes Several types of white blood cells that attack invading organisms, the most common being neutrophils, which primarily attack bacteria. (26)

physiology The study of the function of an organism. (19)

platelets Fragments of cells (thrombocytes) found in the bloodstream. (25)

pleurisy Also called pleuritis. An inflammation of the pleura, the membrane surrounding the lungs, generally stemming from an existing respiratory infection, disease, or injury. (27)

pneumonia An inflammation of the lungs, caused by bacteria, viruses, fungi, or chemical irritants, often following influenza in the elderly and debilitated and with the most common bacterial cause in the United States being *Streptococcus pneumoniae* (pneumococcus pneumonia). (27)

polycystic kidney disease (PKD) A disorder in which clusters of cysts, noncancerous sacs of water-like fluid, develop, primarily within the kidneys. (29)

premenstrual syndrome (PMS) A condition affecting women who menstruate that may include such symptoms as constipation, diarrhea, nausea, anorexia, appetite cravings, headache, backache, muscular aches, edema, insomnia, clumsiness, malaise, irritability, indecisiveness, mental confusion, and depression. (31)

presbycusis Hearing loss from the gradual deterioration of the sensory receptors located in the cochlea, seen most frequently in older adults and caused by such factors as long exposures to loud noises, infection, injury, and in some cases side effects caused by certain medications. (24)

presbyopia A disorder that causes the loss of elasticity in the eye's lens as a result of aging. (24)

prime mover A muscle that is the primary actor in a given movement, that is, the muscle that produces the movement in muscle contraction. (22)

pronation The process of lying prone, or face downward; the process of turning the hand so that the palm points downward. (21)

prostate cancer A malignant tumor that grows in the prostate gland. (31)

protraction The process of moving a body part forward. (21)

psoriasis A common skin condition characterized by frequent episodes of redness, itching, and thick, dry scales that result from the accelerated movement of new skin from the lower layers of the skin to the top, causing a buildup of dead skin cells. (20)

pulmonary edema A condition in which fluid accumulates in the lungs, usually caused by failure of the heart's left ventricle but also caused by lung problems such as pneumonia, an excess of intravenous fluids, some types of kidney disease, bad burns, liver disease, nutritional problems, and Hodgkin's disease. (27)

pulmonary embolism (PE) A blood clot in the lung, usually originating in smaller vessels in the leg, pelvis, arms, or heart and traveling to the lung, where it ultimately becomes wedged in a vessel too small to allow it to pass, causing that portion of the lung to die due to lack of oxygen. (27)

Purkinje fibers Specialized conductive fibers located within the walls of the ventricles, responsible for relaying cardiac impulses to the cells of the ventricles, which allow the ventricles to contract. The Purkinje system includes the bundle of His and the peripheral fibers. (25)

pyelonephritis An infection of the kidney and renal pelvis caused by bacteria, usually *E. coli*, entering the kidneys from the bladder. (29)

pyloric stenosis A condition in which a baby's pylorus (the connection between the stomach and the duodenum) gradually swells and thickens, which interferes with food entering the intestine. (28)

quadriplegia Paralysis from approximately the shoulders down. (23)

radiation therapy Cancer treatment using high-energy waves, such as X rays, to damage and destroy cancer cells. (26)

renal calculi Also called kidney stones. Deposits of mineral salts in the kidney, usually benign there, that can pass into the ureter, slowing down or blocking urine flow and irritating the ureter, causing bleeding. (29)

renal pelvis A sac-like area of the kidney for collecting urine. (29)

retinal detachment Separation of the retina from the underlying choroids layer. (24)

retraction The process of moving a body part backward. (21)

rheumatoid arthritis An immune system disorder in which the body's defenses attack the tissue in the joints, leading to inflammation, degeneration of the articular cartilage, and deformation of the joints. (21, 26)

RhoGAM Drug administered to a pregnant woman to inhibit the production of antibodies against the Rh antigen. (25)

ribosome An important cellular organelle that participates in protein synthesis. (19)

RNA (ribonucleic acid) A single chain of chemical bases important for protein synthesis. The two types of RNA molecules are mRNA and tRNA. (19)

rosacea A chronic and potentially life-disruptive disorder, primarily of the facial skin and often characterized by flare-ups and remissions. (20)

rotation The process of moving a body part around a central axis. (21)

scabies A contagious disorder of the skin caused by very small, wingless insects or mites called the human itch mite or scabies itch mite. (20)

sciatica Pain along the large sciatic nerve that runs from the lower back down the back of each leg, usually caused by pressure on the sciatic nerve from a herniated disc. (23)

sebaceous glands Glands in the skin that produce sebum, an oil that acts to protect the body from dehydration and the possible absorption of harmful substances. (20)

seizure A temporary interference with muscle control, movement, speech, vision, or awareness. (23)

selective permeability The attribute of a cell membrane that allows certain substances to enter the cell while preventing other substances from doing so. (19)

severe acute respiratory syndrome (SARS) A newly identified respiratory illness caused by a previously unknown virus, denoted SARS-CoV, of the coronavirus family, whose members often cause mild to moderate upper respiratory illness, such as the common cold. (27)

sexually transmitted infection (STI) Also called venereal disease. An infection transmitted through exchange of semen, blood, and other body fluids or by direct contact with the affected area of another person, caused by such organisms as chlamydia, human papillomavirus (HPV), genital herpes, gonorrhea, syphilis, and human immunovirus (HIV) and potentially resulting in birth defects, blindness, bone deformities, brain damage, cancer, heart disease, infertility and other abnormalities of the reproductive system, mental retardation, or death. (31)

sinoatrial node Also called SA node, "pacemaker." One of the three areas of specialized neuromuscular tissue that initiate the heartbeat, it is located in the upper wall of the right atrium, just below the opening of the superior vena cava, and discharges the electrical impulses that cause contractions of the atria, thus initiating the heartbeat. (25)

sinusitis An infection or inflammation of the mucous membranes that line the inside of the nose and sinuses, causing them to swell and thus block the drainage of fluid from the sinuses into the nose and throat. (27)

skeletal muscle Type of voluntary muscle found in the locomotive system that controls movement by being attached to bones in the body, made up of cylindrical fibers of striated cells with the nucleus of each cell tending to be toward the edge of the cell. (22)

smooth muscle Type of involuntary muscle found throughout the body, composed of elongated, spindle-shaped cells with the nucleus centrally located and without striations. (22)

spina bifida The most frequently occurring, permanently disabling birth defect, resulting from the failure of the spine to close properly during the first month of pregnancy. (23)

sprain A stretching or tearing injury to a ligament. (22)

squamous cell carcinoma A malignant tumor that affects the middle layer of the skin. (20)

stomach ulcers Also called peptic ulcers, gastric ulcers. A condition in which the lining of the stomach or upper part of the small intestine (duodenum) is damaged and the sensitive tissue underneath is exposed to stomach acid. (28)

strabismus Also called crossed eyes. A disorder in which the eyes are not able to focus on the same image. (24)

strain A stretching or tearing injury to a muscle or a tendon. (22)

stroke Also called cerebrovascular accident (CVA). Result of a clot or hemorrhage in the brain blocking the blood supply and causing brain cells to die from a lack of oxygen. (23)

sudoriferous glands Also called sweat glands. Glands that occur in nearly all regions of the skin but are most numerous in the palms and soles. The two types of sweat glands are the apocrine glands and eccrine glands. (20)

supination The process of lying supine, or face upward; the process of turning the palm or foot upward. (21)

sweat glands Also called sudoriferous glands. Glands that occur in nearly all regions of the skin but are most numerous in the palms and soles. The two types of sweat glands are the apocrine glands and eccrine glands. (20)

synarthrotic joint An articulation, or joint, that produces no movement. (21)

synergist A muscle that acts with another muscle to produce movement. (22)

system A group of organs that work together to perform a specific function. (19)

systemic lupus erythematosus (SLE) System-wide immune system disorder in which the body produces abnormal antibodies that attack its own tissues rather than foreign organisms. Lupus refers to a type of skin rash and erythematosus means red. (26)

systolic blood pressure Pressure recorded in an artery when the left ventricle contracts. In standard notation it is recorded above the diastolic pressure. (25)

T lymphocytes White blood cells created in the bone marrow and matured in the thymus gland that destroy invading organisms identified by the B lymphocytes. (26)

tachycardia An abnormally fast heartbeat of more than 100 beats per minute. The rhythm may be regular or irregular and may not allow the ventricle of the heart to fill properly, causing a lack of oxygen to the brain and body. (25)

tendonitis Inflammation and irritation of the tendon, caused by microscopic tearing. (22)

tendons The connective tissue that attaches muscles to bones. (22)

tetanus Also called lockjaw. Disease that results from the bacteria *Clostridium tetani* releasing a toxin that affects the motor nerves, characterized by painful spasms of muscles. Often fatal. (22)

thrombophlebitis Condition that occurs when a blood clot causes inflammation in one or more veins, typically those in the lower extremities. The two types are superficial, in which the affected vein is near the surface of the skin, and deep vein, in which the affected vein lies deep within a muscle. (25)

tinnitus A symptom associated with many forms of hearing loss, caused by loud noises, medicines, and health problems, such as allergies, tumors, and problems arising from the cardiovascular system, with severe cases

causing the individual difficulty hearing, working, or even sleeping. (24)

tissue A grouping of cells that performs a specialized function. There are four types of tissues in the body: epithelial, connective, muscle, and nerve. (19)

trabeculae Inward-pointing structures that subdivide lymph nodes into different compartments. (26)

tricuspid valve The heart valve from the right atrium to the right ventricle. (25)

tuberculosis (TB) A contagious disease caused by the bacillus *Mycobacterium tuberculosis*, which can grow anywhere in the body but are most commonly found in the lungs, producing granular tumors in the infected tissues. (27)

ureters Tubes that carry newly formed urine from each kidney down to the bladder, made up of an inner coat of mucous membrane, a middle coat of smooth muscle, and an outer layer of fibrous tissue. (29)

urethra The musculomembranous tube extending from the bladder to the urinary meatus, the external opening of the urinary system. (29)

urethritis Inflammation of the urethra. (31)

urinary bladder The muscular sac, located in the pelvic cavity, that serves as a reservoir for urine and whose wall consists of an inner layer of epithelium, a layer of smooth muscle, an outer layer of longitudinal muscle, and a fibrous layer. (29)

urinary meatus The external opening of the urinary system. (29)

uterine cancer Also called endometrial cancer, adenocarcinoma. Cancer that starts in the cells of the lining of the uterus and usually develops in the glandular tissue of the endometrium. (31)

uterine fibroids Benign tumors made up of muscle cells and other tissues that grow within the wall of the uterus, manifesting as a single growth or a cluster. (31)

vaginitis An inflammation of the vagina usually caused by a change in the normal balance of vaginal bacteria or by an infection, with the most common types being bacterial, yeast infections, trichomoniasis, and atrophic vaginitis. (31)

ventricles The two lower pumping chambers of the heart. (25)

wart A type of infection caused by viruses in the human papillomavirus (HPV) family that can grow on all parts of the body, including on the skin, inside the mouth, on the genitals, and in the rectal area. (20)

Index

Cancer, 467
  breast, 544, 546–547
  causes and treatment of, 467
  cervical, 547
  colon, 498
  endometrial, 552–553
  and immune system, 467
  lung, 483
  oral, 502–503
  ovarian, 549
  pancreatic, 503–504
  prostate, 556
  skin, 364–365
  uterine, 552–553
Canthus, 424
Capillaries, 440, 444f, 476
  alveoli with, 477f
Carbon dioxide
  exhalation of, 474
  removal of, 474
  transfer, 477f
Carcinogens, 467
Cardiac cycle, 439
  phases of, 439
Cardiac muscles, 396, 438
Cardiomegaly, 533
Cardiopulmonary resuscitation (CPR), 452
Cardiovascular system. See also Circulatory
    system
  disorders of, 456t–457t
Carditis, 453
Carpal tunnel syndrome, 386–387
Cataracts, 426
Cauda equine, 411
Cavities, 351, 353, 353f
Cecum, 494
Cell membrane, 345
Cells, 344–347
  cancer, 467. See also Cancer
  cell membrane, 345
  chemistry and, 354–355
  cytoplasm, 345–346
  of islets of Langerhans, 525
  in lungs, 477
  major parts of, and structures inside, 345f
  muscle fibers, 394. See also Muscles;
    Muscular system
  nucleus, 345, 346
  phagocytic, 463. See also Macrophages
  types of blood, 442
Cellulitis, 368, 368f
Centers for Disease Control and Prevention
    (CDC), 550–551
Central lymphoid tissue, 462
Central nervous system (CNS),
    408–411, 409f
  nerves in, 407
Centrioles, 346
Cerebellum, 411
Cerebral aqueduct, 410
Cerebral hemispheres, 409
Cerebrospinal fluid, 411
Cerebrovascular accident (CVA), 419, 455
Cerebrum, 409
  lobes of, 409
Cerumen, 430
Cervical cancer, 547
Cervicitis, 547–54
Cervix, 538
Chemotherapy, 467, 483, 547, 556
Children
  bones in, 379
  circulatory system development in, 438
  dehydration in, 513
  digestive system and, 495
  drinking bottles, proper angle for, 429
  endocrine system in, 526
  immune response in, 462
  muscular development in, 395

  nervous system in, 408
  otitis media in, 429
  prescriptions to be kept at school for, 480
  reproductive system in, 540
  respiratory system in, 477
  skin conditions in, 365
Chime, 493
Cholelithiasis, 494
Cholesterol, 450
Choroid plexus, 411
Choroids, 424
Chromosomes, 346
Chronic fatigue syndrome (CFS), 468
Chronic obstructive pulmonary disease
    (COPD), 479
Chronic renal failure, 517
Cilia
  in bronchial tubes, 477
  in cells, 346
  in lungs, 477
  in nose, 474
Circulatory system, 435–458. See also
    Lymphatic system
  blood, 442–446
  blood vessels, 439–440
  common disorders associated with,
    450–458. See also specific disorders
  lymphatic system, 449–450
  overview of, 436
  pulmonary and systemic circulation,
    442, 444f
Circumcision, 543
Circumduction, 381
Cirrhosis, 497–498
Cleft palate, 356
Clitoris, 541
Closed fracture, 387
Clots, 444
Cluster headaches, 417
Coagulation, 444, 445
  defined, 446
Cochlea, 428, 429f
Colitis, 498
Colles's fracture, 388
Colon, 494f
  with diverticulosis, 500f
Colon cancer, 498
Color deficiency, 356
Colorectal cancers, 498
Comminuted fracture, 388
Common cold, 481
Compact bone, 380
Complement, 464
Complete decongestive therapy
    (CDT), 469
Compound fracture, 387
Compression fracture, 388
Conductive hearing loss, 430
Congenital disorders, 356
Congestive heart failure (CHF), 452
Conjunctiva, 425
Conjunctivitis, 426
Connective tissue, 347
Constipation, 495, 498–499
Contact dermatitis, 368
Convolutions, in brain, 409
COPD. See Chronic obstructive pulmonary
    disease (COPD)
Cornea, 424
  lesions or abrasions to, 427
Corneal abrasion, 427
Coronal plane (frontal plane), 350
Coronary artery bypass graft (CABG), 452
Coronary artery disease (CAD), 450
Coronary heart disease (CHD), 450–451
Coronary occlusion, 451
Coronary thrombosis, 451
Coronavirus, 484
Corpus callosum, 408, 409

Cortex
  adrenal, 525–526
  of brain, 409–410
  of kidney, 511
  of lymph node, 463
Corticosterone, 525
Corticotropin-releasing factor (CRF), 522
Cortisol, 523, 525
Cowper's glands, 544
Crab lice, 371
Cranial cavity, 353
Cranial nerves, 411–414
  12 pairs of, 413t
Cretinism, 524
Crohn's disease, 499
Cultural considerations
  addressing issues of diabetes, 530
  assumptions regarding curative
    measures, 547
  attitudes toward tobacco smoking, 481
  dietary habits, 449
  modesty requirements, 516
  patient's rights and need for modesty, 369
  psychological implications of some immune
    system diseases and, 465
  risk factors for osteoporosis, 389
  role of diet and disorders of digestive
    system, 503
  role of, regarding exercise and holistic
    health, 399
  stereotypes about neurological diseases, 418
  use of interpreters, 354
Cushing's disease, 530, 531f
Cyanosis, 483
Cystic fibrosis (CF), 356, 481–482
Cystitis, 513–514
Cysts, 516
Cytokinesis, 346, 347
Cytoplasm, 345–346
Cytoplasmic streaming, 345–346
Cytosol. See Cytoplasm

D

Deafness, 430
Deciduous teeth, 491, 492f
  eruption of, 493
Decubitus ulcers, 368–369
  four stages of, 369
Defibrillation, 452
Dendrites, 407
Dermis, 363
  touch originating in, 431
Diabetes, 517
Diabetes mellitus, 526, 530–531
Dialysis, 517–518
Diaphragm, 351, 474
Diaphysis, 380
Diarrhea, 499
Diarthrotic joints, 380
Diastolic blood pressure, 442, 526
Diencephalon, 409, 410–411
Diffusion, 355
Digestion, 490
  accessory organs of, 494–495
  elimination of waste products of, 494
  organs of, 490f
  in small intestine, 493
Digestive system, 489–505, 490f
  common disorders associated with,
    495–505. See also specific disorders
  disorders and pathology of, 496t–497t
  main functions of, 490
  organs of, 491–494
Diseases
  autoimmune. See Autoimmune diseases
  genetic, 399–400. See also Genetic
    disorders
  genetics, heredity, and, 356–358

Dislocations, 388–389
Diverticulitis, 500
Diverticulosis, 500
DNA (deoxyribonucleic acid), 345, 346
    fingerprinting, 355–356
Documentation, legal importance of, 346
Dopamine, 526
Dorsal cavity, 351
Dorsiflexion, 381
Down syndrome (trisomy 21), 356
Ductus deferens, 544
Dura mater, 409
Dwarfism, 526, 531–532
Dysmenorrhea, 548
Dysplasia, 364
Dysplastic nevi, 364
Dyspnea, 453
Dysuria, 514

E

Ear
    anatomy of, 428
    external ear, 428
    inner ear, 428, 429
    middle ear, 428
    and sense of hearing, 428
    wax in, 430
Eardrum, 428
Eczema, 369
Edema, 450, 452
Efferent neurons, 407
Electroencephalogram (EEG), 416
Electrolytes, 355, 511
Electrons, 342
Elimination, 490. See also Urinary system
Embolism, 455
Emphysema, 480–481
Encephalitis, 415–416
Endocarditis, 453
Endocardium, 436
Endocrine system, 521–534
    common disorders associated with,
        527–533. See also specific disorders
    disorders of, 529t–530t
    function of, 522
    homeostasis and, 522
    primary glands of, 522, 522f. See also
        specific glands
Endometrial cancer, 552–553
Endometriosis, 548
Endomysium, 396
Endoplasmic reticulum, 346
Endosteum, 380
Epidermis, 362–363
Epididymitis, 555
Epididymus, 542, 544
Epiglottis, 476
Epilepsy, 416
Epimysium, 396
Epinephrine, 523, 526
Epiphyseal fracture, 388
Epiphysis, 380
Episiotomy, 541
Epithelial tissue, 347
Epstein-Barr virus (EBV), 468
Erectile dysfunction, 555
Erythrocytes, 444. See also Red blood cells
Esophagus, 493
Estrogen, 526, 527, 540, 541
Eustachian tube, 429
Eversion, 381
Exhalation, 478
Exophthalmos, 532, 532f
Expiration, 478f. See also Inhalation
Extension, 381
External ear, 428, 428f

Externship
    asking questions, 388
    being respectful and polite, 368
    defining problem and remedy, 401
    evaluating strengths, 482
    focusing on patients, 516
    in gynecology, obstetrical, or urological
        practice, 553
    importance of clear writing, 356
    patient communication, 498
    patient presentations in neurological
        practices, 418
    professional attire, 454
    relating to teammates, 469
    thinking ahead, 426
    treating patients with equal respect, 528
Eye
    anatomy of, 424–425
    common disorders associated with,
        425–427. See also specific disorders
    eyeball and anatomical structures, 424f
    and sense of vision, 424

F

Fallopian tubes, 538–539
False ribs, 383
Falx cerebri, 409
Farsightedness, 426
Fascia, 394, 396
Fascicles, 396
Female-pattern hair loss, 368
Female reproductive system, 538–542, 538f
    common disorders associated with,
        544–554. See also specific disorders
    disorders and pathology of, 545t–546t
    function of, 538
Fibrinogen, 445
Fibrocystic breast disease, 548–549, 549f
Fibroids, 553
Fibromyalgia, 399
Fibrosis, 497
"Fight or flight" syndrome, 526
Filtration, 355, 512
Fissures, 409
Flexion, 381
Flu, 482
Follicle-stimulating hormone, 523, 540–541
Folliculitis, 369
Foreskin, 543
Fractures, 387–388
    various types of, 388f
Fragile X syndrome, 357
FRAXA syndrome, 357
Frontal lobe, 409, 410

G

Gallbladder, 494
Gallstones, 494
Gastrin, 527
Gastroesophageal reflux disease (GERD),
    500–501
Gastrointestinal mucosa, 527
Genes, 346
Genetic disorders, 356–358, 481
Genetic engineering, 355
Genetic fingerprinting, 355–356
Genetics, 355
    hair color and, 363
    heredity, and disease, 356–358
Genital herpes, 370
Germinal centers, 463
Gestational diabetes, 531
Gigantism, 526, 532. See also Acromegaly
Glands
    of endocrine system, 522–527. See also
        specific glands
    primary, of endocrine system, 522f

Glasgow seven-point scale, 366–367
Glaucoma, 426
Glomerular disease, 514–515
Glomerular excretion, 512
Glomerulonephritis, 514–515
Glomerulus, 511
Goiter, 533, 533f
Golgi apparatus, 346
Gonadotropin, 524
Gonadotropin-releasing hormone (GTRH),
    522
Gout, 389
Graafian follicle, 540, 542
    rupture of, 541
    stages of development, 539f
Granulocytes, 444
Graves' disease, 532
Gray matter, 408, 411
Greenstick fracture, 388
Growth hormone (GH), 523, 526
    excess production of, 527–528
Growth hormone-releasing factor (GHRF),
    522
Gyri, 409

H

Hair follicles, 363
    inflammation or infection of, 369
Hashimoto's thyroiditis, 533
Hay fever, 482
HDL cholesterol, 450
Headaches, 416–417
Head lice, 371
Health Insurance Portability and
    Accountability Act (HIPAA), 444
Hearing loss, 430
Heart, 436–439
    blood flow through, 436–437, 437f
    cardiac cycle, 439
    chambers, interior view of, 437f
    circulation in, 439f
    conduction system of, 438–439, 440f
    linings of, 437f
    location of, 436f
    physiology of, 437–438
    sounds, 439
    valves of, 438f
    vascular system of, 438
Heart attack, 438, 450
    symptoms of, 451–452
Heart murmur, 437, 439
Hematocrit, 443
Hematopoiesis, 443, 462
Hemochromatosis, 357
Hemodialysis, 517–518
Hemoglobin, 444, 454
Hemoglobin S disease, 455. See also Sickle
    cell anemia
Hemolytic anemias, 454
Hemophilia, 357
Hemoptysis, 485
Hemorrhage, 455
Hemorrhoids, 501
Hemostasis, 446
Heredity
    defined, 356
    genetics, disease, and, 356–358
Hernia, 501–502
Herpes simplex, 370
    symptoms of, 370
Herpes zoster, 370
Herpetic whitlow, 370
Hiatal hernia, 501
High blood pressure, 455, 516
Hilum, 511
Homeostasis, 342
    contribution of white blood cells to, 444
    maintenance of, 522

Hordeolums, 427
Hormones, 522–523
  adrenal cortex, 525–526
  adrenal medulla, 526
  defined, 522
  gastrointestinal mucosal, 527
  gonadotropic, production of, 540
  pancreatic, 525
  parathyroid gland, 524
  pineal gland, 524
  pituitary gland, 523–524
  placental, 527
  produced by ovaries, 527
  release of, 540
  of testes, 527
  thymus gland, 527
  thyroid gland, 524
Hormone therapy, 556
HSV-1 (herpes simplex virus type 1), 370
HSV-2 (herpes simplex virus type 2), 370
Human body
  anatomical locations and positions, 350–354
  anatomical planes of, 350, 352f
  basic building blocks of, 344f. See also Cells
  cavities and abdominal regions, 351, 353
  defense of. See Immune system
  directional anatomical terms, 350, 351f
  landmarks, 354t
  levels of organization in, 342–347, 343f
  organs and systems, 347
  organ systems of, with major functions, 349f
  primary pulse points of, 442f
  types of movements in, 381f
  types of tissue in, 348f
Human immunodeficiency virus (HIV), 547
Human papillomavirus (HPV), 373, 547
Hydrocele, 556
Hydrocephalus, 419
Hyperopia, 426
Hypertension, 455, 458
  chronic renal failure and, 517
Hyperthyroidism, 524, 532
Hypotension, 458
Hypothalamus, 410–411
  hormones of, 522–523
Hypothyroidism, 524, 532–533, 533f
Hysterectomy, 548, 553

I

Ileum, 493
Immune response, 462, 464
  cancer and, 467
  inappropriate, excessive, or lacking, 465
Immune system, 449, 461–470. See also Tonsils
  anatomy of, 462–464
  and body's defense, 464–465
  cancer and, 467
  common disorders associated with, 465–469, 466t
  structures central to, 462–464
Immunity, 464–465
  types of, 464
Immunizations, 464
Immunoglobulins, 464–465
Impacted cerumen, 430
Impetigo, 370–371, 371f
Incontinence, 513, 515
Incus (anvil), 428
Infectious mononucleosis, 468
Inflammatory bowel disease (IBD), 499
Influenza, 482
Infundibulum, 411
Inguinal hernia, 501–502, 502f
Inhalation, 478
Innate immunity, 465

Inner ear, 428
  common disorders associated with, 429–430
Insertion, 397
Inspiration, 478, 478f. See also Inhalation
Insula, 409
Insulin, 525, 531, 534, 541
Insulin-dependent diabetes mellitus (IDDM), 531
Integumentary system, 361–374. See also Skin
  accessory structures in, 362
  common disorders associated with, 364–374. See also specific disorders
  functions of, 362
  overview of, 362
International Headache Society (IHS), 417
Interneurons, 407
Interstitial cystitis (IC), 514
Interventricular foramina, 410
Intrapleural pressure, 478
Intrapulmonic pressure, 478
Inversion, 381
Iris, 424
Iron deficiency anemia, 454
Irritable bowel syndrome (IBS), 502
Ischemia, 455
Islets of Langerhans, 525

J

Jejunum, 493, 527
Joints, 380
  movement and, 380–381
  typical, 380f
Juvenile diabetes, 531

K

Keratin, 362, 363
Kidneys, 511
  external structure of, 511
  internal structure of, 511
  nephrons of, 511
  transplants of, 518
  waste products of, 511
Kidney stones, 515–516
  types of, 515f
Klinefelter's syndrome, 357
Korotkoff sounds, 441
Kyphosis, 384, 385f

L

Labia majora, 541
Labia minora, 541
Lacrimal apparatus, 425
Lactic acid, buildup of, 396
Lactogenic hormone, 524
Landmark terms, human body, 354f
Large intestine, 494, 494f
Larynx, 476
Laser surgery, 426, 427
Lasik procedure, 426
LDL cholesterol, 450
Legal and ethical issues
  checking patient's past medical history, 387
  confidentiality standards, 444
  dealing with reproductive issues, 547
  digestive disorders and lifestyle, 500
  documentation and, 346
  driving and neurological disorders, 416
  immunodeficiency disorders, emotional lifestyle and, 467
  laws regarding diabetes and driving public transportation vehicles, 530
  patient privacy, 512
  prescriptions to be kept at school, 480

  removal of clothing and, 372
  visual difficulties and driving, 427
Legionellosis, 482
Legionnaire's disease, 482
Lens, 424
Lesions
  corneal, 427
  tumors of skin, 364
Leukemia, 455
Leukocytes, 442, 444, 445f, 464
  defenses performed by, 445
Lifespan considerations
  bones and, 379
  circulatory system, 438
  digestive system, 495
  effect of aging on senses, 425
  endocrine system, 526
  immune system, 462
  kidneys, 513
  movement and exercise, 395
  nervous system, 408
  reproductive system, 540
  skin and, 365
Lipoatrophy, 399
Lipodystrophy, 399
Lipolysis, 523
Lipoproteins, 450
Lithotripsy, 516
Liver, 494–495
  substances manufactured by, 495
Lobes, 409
Long bones, 380
  features found in, 380f
Longitudinal fissure, 409
Loop of Henle, 511
Lordosis, 384, 385f
Lou Gehrig's disease, 415
Low blood pressure, 458
Lower respiratory system, 474
Lumpectomy, 547
Lung cancer, 483
Lungs, 477
  cells in, 477
  roles of, 477
Luteinizing hormone, 524, 541
Lymph, 449–450
Lymphatic system, 449–450, 449f. See also Circulatory system
  central lymphoid tissue, 462
  components of, 449, 463f
  function of, 449
  peripheral, 462–464
  primary responsibility of, 462
  spleen, 450
  thymus gland, 450
  tissue fluid, lymph, and lymph nodes, 449–450
Lymphedema, 468
Lymph nodes, 449, 463
  functions of, 463
  structure of, 450f
Lymphocytes, 450, 464
Lysosomes, 345, 346

M

Macrophages, 463
Macular degeneration, 426–427
Male-pattern baldness, 368
Male reproductive system, 542–544, 542f
  common disorders associated with, 554–556. See also specific disorders
  disorders of, 554t
  external organs, 542–543
  internal organs, 543–544
Malignant melanoma, 364, 366–367
Malleus (hammer), 428
Mammary glands, 541
Manual decongestive therapy (MDT), 469